W9-BFQ-288

Workbook for

Insurance Handbook for the Medical Office

Workbook for Insurance Handbook for the Medical Office

Thirteenth Edition

MARILYN TAKAHASHI FORDNEY
CMA-AC (AAMA)
Formerly Instructor of Medical Insurance, Medical Terminology,
Medical Machine Transcription, and Medical Office Procedures
Ventura College
Ventura, California

ELSEVIER

ELSEVIER
SAUNDERS

3251 Riverport Lane
St. Louis, Missouri 63043

Workbook For
INSURANCE HANDBOOK FOR THE MEDICAL OFFICE

ISBN: 978-1-4557-4811-2

Executive Content Strategist: Jennifer B. Janson
Senior Content Development Specialist: Jennifer L. Bertucci
Publishing Services Manager: Hemamalini Rajendrababu
Project Manager: Saravanan Thavamani
Design Direction: Paula Catalano
Associate Marketing Manager: Kristin Winfrey

Printed in the United States

Last digit is the print number: 9 8 7 6 5 4 3

Acknowledgments

This edition of the *Workbook* for *Insurance Handbook for the Medical Office* has had considerable input from many medical professionals. Expert consultation has been necessary because of the impact of the health care reform, complexities of the managed care environment, intricacies of procedural coding, adoption of a newer diagnostic coding system, impact of technology on electronic medical record keeping and insurance claims processing, and the more sophisticated role the insurance billing specialist has in today's workforce.

I owe an immense debt of gratitude to the reviewers of the *Workbook* assignments and to Karen Levein, instructor at Monrovia Adult School, who helped me update the coding data. Also a debt of gratitude is extended to Linda Smith, CPC, CPC-1, CEMC, PCS, CMBS; Karen Levein, CPC, CPC-I; Payel Bhattacharya Madero, RHIT, MBA; and Norma Jean Scott, who acted as contributors and technical collaborators and helped update the assignments in the *Workbook* exercises and tests.

Most important, I express overwhelming gratitude to the professional consultants who provided vital information to make this *Workbook* better than previous editions. They are listed in the following section.

Contributors

Karen Levein, CPC, CPC-I
Medical Professions Instructor
Burbank Adult School
Burbank, California

Payel Bhattacharya Madero, RHIT, MBA
AHIMA-Approved ICD-10 Trainer
COO, PPJ Enterprises
Upland, California

Linda Smith, CPC, CPC-I, CEMC, PCS, CMBS
Consultant/Educator
MedOffice Resources
Greene, New York

EDITORIAL REVIEW BOARD

Pamela Audette, MBA, MT(ASCP), RMA
Assistant Professor and Program Director
Finlandia University
Hancock, Michigan

Megan Baez, CPC, CMA (AAMA)
Medical Coding and Billing Instructor
Everest University
Lakeland, Florida

Kelly Berge, MSHA, CPC, CBCS
Assistant Dean, Online
Berkeley College
Clifton, New Jersey

Ruth Berger, MS, RHIA
Instructor, Health Information Technology
Chippewa Valley Technical College
Eau Claire, Wisconsin

Peggy Black, RN, CCS
AHIMA-Approved ICD-10-CM/PCS Trainer
Medical Coding and Billing Instructor
Winter Park Tech
Winter Park, Florida

Carrie Cosson, CMA (NCCT), RMA (AMT)
Medical Assisting Instructor
Everest University
Lakeland, Florida

Gerard Cronin, DC, CCA
Assistant Professor
Salem Community College
Carneys Point, New Jersey

Brian Edward Dickens, MBA, RMA, CHI
Program Director, Medical Assisting
Southeastern College
Greenacres, Florida

Jennifer Flippin, CPC
Medical Billing and Coding Program Coordinator
Pinnacle Career Institute
Kansas City, Missouri

Carol Hendrickson, MSEd, CCS-P
Medical Coding and Health Information Management Instructor
Pasco-Hernando Community College
New Port Richey, Florida

Mary A. Johnson, BA, CPC
Program Manager, Medical Record Coding
Central Carolina Technical College
Sumter, South Carolina

Geri Kale-Smith, MS, CMA
Coordinator, Medical Office Programs, Associate Professor
Harper College
Palatine, Illinois

Colleen O. Kim, BS
Certified SHIP Counselor, Adjunct Professor
Manchester Community College
Manchester, Connecticut

Judith Leonhart, MBA
Instructor, Adult Education
OCM BOCES
Liverpool, New York

Angela MacLeod, MS, RHIA
Medical Coding and Billing Instructor
Certified Medical Assistant Program Director
Gogebic Community College
Ironwood, Michigan

Cassondra Major, MBA
Academic Program Director, Medical
Everest College
Henderson, Nevada

JanMarie C. Malik, MBA, RHIA, CCS-P
Coding, Billing, Reimbursement and Office Procedures Instructor
Shasta Community College; National University
Redding, California

Michelle C. Maus, MBA
Facilitator/Professor Health Care Administration
Ivy Bridge College of Tiffin University
Tiffin, Ohio

Laura Melendez, BS, RMA, RT BMO
Allied Health Instructor, Medical Assisting
Southeastern College
Greenacres, Florida

Deborah Newton, MA, PhD
Program Director, Medical Billing/Coding
Great Falls College Montana State University
Great Falls, Montana

Bhamini Patel BSHIM, CPC, CPC-H
Medical Coding and Billing Instructor
Everest University
Lakeland, Florida

Jeanice Porta, BSEd, CPC, CPC-I
Medical Coding/Billing Instructor
Lee County High Tech Center North
Cape Coral, Florida

Susan Shear, MHA, CPC
Assistant Professor, Medical Information Technology
Bluegrass Community and Technical College
Danville, Kentucky

Tara Shepherd, CMA (AAMA)
Allied Health Director
Apollo Career Center
Lima, Ohio

Phaedra Spartan, RMA, CMAS, BS, MSHA
Healthcare Programs
Director, Medical
Vatterott College
Springfield, Missouri

Mia K. Thompson
MIBC, MAA Program Director
Everest Institute
Marietta, Georgia

Deanne Ulrich, CPC-A
Instructor, Business
Hawkeye Community College
Waterloo, Iowa

Chris Welch, MBA, CPC, CMC, CEC, CMPE
Medical Insurance Billing and Coding, Program Director
Everest University
Orange Park, Florida

Nancy C. Withee, CPC, CPMA
Program Coordinator
Medical Office Administration and Health Information Technology
Great Bay Community College
Portsmouth, New Hampshire

Contents

Instruction Guide to the *Workbook*

LEARNING OBJECTIVES

The student will be able to:

- Define and spell key terms and key abbreviations for each chapter.
- Answer review questions for each chapter of the *Handbook*.
- Complete assignments to enhance and develop better critical thinking skills.
- Define abbreviations as they appear on a patient record.
- Abstract subjective and objective data from patient records.
- Review documentation on patient records.
- Code professional services properly, using the *Current Procedural Terminology* (CPT) Code Book or Appendixes A and B.
- Select diagnostic code numbers, using the *International Classification of Diseases, Tenth Revision, Clinical Modification (ICD-10-CM) or International Classification of Diseases, Ninth Revision, Clinical Modification* (ICD-9-CM).
- Locate errors on insurance claims before submission to insurance companies.
- Locate errors on returned insurance claims.
- Complete an insurance claim tracer form.
- Carry out collection procedures on delinquent accounts.
- Execute financial management procedures for tracing managed care plans.
- Abstract information necessary to complete insurance claim forms from patient records and billing statement/ledger cards.
- Post payments, adjustments, and balances to patients' statement/ledger cards when submitting insurance claims.
- Compute mathematic calculations for Medicare and TRICARE cases.
- Analyze insurance claims in both hospital inpatient and outpatient settings.
- Prepare a cover letter, résumé, job application, and follow-up letter when searching for employment.
- Access the Internet and visit websites to research and/or obtain data.

INSTRUCTIONS TO THE STUDENT

The thirteenth edition of *Workbook* for *Insurance Handbook for the Medical Office* has been prepared for those who use the textbook, *Insurance Handbook for the Medical Office* (hereafter referred to as the *Handbook*). It is designed to assist the learner in a practical approach to doing insurance billing and coding. It will also help the learner develop a better understanding of the differences among the insurance programs when completing and electronically transmitting the 837 P (Professional) or the paper claim CMS-1500 (02-12).

The key terms and key abbreviations are repeated for quick reference when studying. Each chapter's outline serves as a lecture guide to use for note taking. The review questions in the form of short answer, true/false, multiple choice, and matching are presented to reinforce learning of key concepts for each topic.

Some assignments give students hands-on experience in completing claim forms using National Uniform Claim Committee (NUCC) guidelines. Insurance claim forms and other sample documents that are easily removable are included for practice.

Current procedural and diagnostic code exercises are used throughout to facilitate and enhance coding skills for submitting a claim or making up an itemized billing statement.

Icons appearing throughout the *Workbook* are used to indicate assignment types. An illustration of each icon, along with its description, is outlined below.

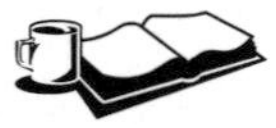

Self-study assignments encompass important points from each chapter and allow you to study at your own pace.

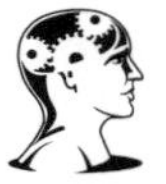

Critical thinking assignments require skills that help prepare you for real-world scenarios encountered in insurance billing.

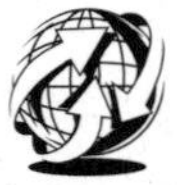

The **Student Software Challenge** located on the **Evolve** website is required for completing selected assignments for several chapters. **Internet** assignments point you to the World Wide Web for resources.

KEY TERMS AND KEY ABBREVIATIONS

Key terms and key abbreviations are presented for each chapter, and definitions may be located in the glossary at the end of the *Handbook*. It is suggested that you make up 3- by 5-inch index cards for each term or abbreviation and write in the definitions as you encounter them while reading each chapter in the *Handbook*. Doing this will reinforce your knowledge and help you learn the words and abbreviations. Your instructor may wish to select certain words for you to study for pop quizzes. In addition, on the Evolve website, crossword puzzles are provided for each chapter to reinforce learning key words and their definitions.

NOTE TAKING

Taking notes is an important key to success in studying and learning. Note taking helps an individual pay attention during class and retain information. Each chapter has a study outline for organizational purposes, and the outline may be used as a guide for writing down key points during lectures or when studying or reviewing from the *Handbook* for tests. Use file cards, notepads, notebook, computer, or tablet for taking notes. Underline or highlight important words or phrases. To improve the usefulness of notes, try the following format:

1. Using a tablet note-taking app, notepad sheet, or file card, draw a margin 3 inches from the left.
2. Use the left side for topic headings and the right side for notes.
3. Skip a few lines when the topic changes.
4. Write numbers or letters to indicate sub-ideas under a heading.
5. Be brief; do not write down every word except when emphasizing a quotation, rule, or law. Write notes in your own words because that is what you will understand.
6. Use abbreviations that you know how to translate.
7. Listen carefully to the lecture.
8. After the lecture, reread your notes. Highlight the word(s) on the left side of the page to identify the topic of the notes on the right.
9. For study purposes, cover the right side and see if you can explain to yourself or someone else the topic or word.
10. Remember: Learning is by doing, and doing is up to you. So take notes for better understanding.

REVIEW QUESTION ASSIGNMENTS

Review questions have been designed to encompass important points for each chapter to assist you in studying insurance billing and coding theory. Additional quizzes are available on the Evolve website.

SIMULATION ASSIGNMENTS

Assume that you have been hired as an insurance billing specialist and that you are working in a clinic setting for an incorporated group of medical doctors, other allied health specialists, and a podiatrist. You will be asked to complete various assignments. These doctors will be on the staff of a nearby hospital. Appendix A details this clinic's policies and procedures, which you must read completely before beginning the competency-based assignments.

Within each chapter, the simulation assignments progress from easy to more complex. Some assignments are given with critical thinking problems, which the instructor may use for class discussion.

Always read the assignment entirely before beginning it. There are *Workbook* assignments. Table I.1 is a reference guide that lists chapter numbers and titles, along with the corresponding assignment numbers.

MEDICAL TERMINOLOGY AND ABBREVIATIONS

A list of abbreviations is provided in Appendix A to help you learn how to abstract and read physicians' notes. Decode any abbreviations that you do not understand or that are unfamiliar to you. To reinforce learning these abbreviations, write their meanings on the assignment pages. If you do not have a background in medical terminology, it may be wise to use a good medical dictionary as a reference or, better yet, enroll in a terminology course to master that skill.

PATIENT RECORDS

Patient records, financial accounting records (ledgers), and encounter forms are presented as they might appear in a physician's office, so the learner may have the tools needed to extract information to complete claim forms. Patient records have been abbreviated because of space and page constraints. The records contain pertinent data for each type of case, but it was necessary to omit a lengthy physical examination. Because detailed documentation is encouraged in medical practices, the records all appear typewritten rather than in handwritten notes. The physician's signature appears after each dated entry on the record.

All the materials included in the assignments have been altered to prevent identification of the cases or parties involved. The names and addresses are fictitious, and no reference to any person living or dead is intended. No evaluation of medical practice or medical advice is to be inferred from the patient records, nor is any recommendation made toward alternative treatment methods or prescribed medications.

FINANCIAL RECORDS

Financial accounting record statements (ledgers) are included for practice in posting, totaling fees, and properly recording appropriate information when an insurance claim is submitted. Refer to Appendix A to obtain information about the Mock Fee Schedule and the physicians' fees for posting to the statements.

CMS-1500 (02-12) CLAIM FORM

If you have access to a computer, use the practice management software that accompanies the *Workbook* to complete each assignment and print it out for evaluation. To complete the CMS-1500 (02-12) claim form properly for each type of program, refer to the section in Chapter 7 of the *Handbook* that describes in detail the correct information to be put in each block. Also view

TABLE I-1

***Workbook* Assignments**

Handbook Chapter	Corresponding *Workbook* Chapter	Assignments
1	Role of an Insurance Billing Specialist	1–1 through 1–3
2	Compliance, Privacy, Fraud, and Abuse in Insurance Billing	2–1 through 2–5
3	Basics of Health Insurance	3–1 through 3–7
4	Medical Documentation and the Electronic Health Record	4–1 through 4–7
5	Diagnostic Coding	5–1 through 5–12
6	Procedural Coding	6–1 through 6–10
7	The Paper Claim CMS-1500 (02-12)	7–1 through 7–7
8	The Electronic Claim	8–1 through 8–9
9	Receiving Payments and Insurance Problem Solving	9–1 through 9–9
10	Office and Insurance Collection Strategies	10–1 through 10–7
11	The Blue Plans, Private Insurance, and Managed Care Plans	11–1 through 11–6
12	Medicare	12–1 through 12–11
13	Medicaid and Other State Programs	13–1 through 13–5
14	TRICARE and Veteran's Health Care	14–1 through 14–7
15	Workers' Compensation	15–1 through 15–6
16	Disability Income Insurance and Disability Benefits Programs	16–1 through 16–6
17	Hospital Billing	17–1 through 17–11
18	Seeking a Job and Attaining Professional Advancement	18–1 through 18–8

the templates found at the end of Chapter 7 for each insurance type.

Do's and don'ts for claim completion and National Uniform Claim Committee (NUCC) guidelines are mentioned in Chapter 7. If you do not have access to a computer, type or neatly write in the information on the insurance form as you abstract it from the patient record.

PERFORMANCE EVALUATION CHECKLIST

The thirteenth edition features a competency-based format for each assignment indicating performance objectives to let you know what is to be accomplished. The task (job assignment), conditions (elements needed to perform and complete the task), and standards (time management), as well as directions for the specific task, are included. Use of a checklist with points projected and points earned is available on the Evolve website; the checklist assists in scoring the assignments and helps you develop the skill of speed in completing tasks.

A two-part performance evaluation checklist used when completing a CMS-1500 (02-12) claim form is depicted in Figures I–1 and I–2. Reproduce these sheets only for the assignments that involve completing the CMS-1500 (02-12) claim form. Your instructor will give you the number of points to be assigned for each step.

APPENDIXES

Refer to Table I.2, which shows what is included in each of the appendixes.

STUDENT REFERENCE NOTEBOOK

A student reference notebook is recommended so that you can access information quickly to help you complete the *Workbook* assignments. Before beginning the assignments, tear out Appendix A and place it in a three-ring binder with chapter indexes. Appendix A includes the clinic policies and guidelines, data about the clinic staff, medical and laboratory abbreviations, and Mock Fee Schedule used while working as an insurance billing specialist for the College Clinic.

Besides these suggestions, you may wish either to tear out or to make photocopies of other sections of the *Handbook* for your personal use. In addition, your instructor may give you handouts from time to time, pertaining to regional insurance program policies and procedures, to place in your notebook.

Content Suggestions From the *Workbook*

- ✓ Appendix A: College Clinic policies, data about staff physicians, medical and laboratory abbreviations, and Mock Fee Schedule
- ✓ Appendix B: HCPCS Level II codes
- ✓ Appendix C: ICD-10-PCS Section 0 Medical and Surgical, Character 3, Operation Definitions
- ✓ Appendix D: ICD-10-PCS Section 0 Medical and Surgical, Character 5, Approach Definitions
- ✓ CMS-1500 (02-12) claim form (photocopy if extra copies are needed for making rough drafts or retyping an assignment)

Content Suggestions From the *Handbook*

- ✓ Evaluation and Management CPT codes: Tables 6-3 and 6-4
- ✓ Insurance form templates from Chapter 7: Figures 7–3 through 7–11
- ✓ Terminology used in coding procedures: Table 4-1
- ✓ CMS-1500 (02-12) block-by-block claim form instructions from Chapter 7
- ✓ Glossary (key terms and key abbreviations)

TESTS

Tests appear at the end of the *Workbook* to provide a complete, competency-based educational program.

REFERENCE MATERIAL

To do the assignments in this *Workbook* and gain expertise in coding and insurance claims completion, an individual must have access to the books listed here. Addresses for obtaining these materials are given in parentheses. Additional books and booklets on these topics, as well as on Medicaid, Medicare, TRICARE, and more, can be found at bookstores or online retailers.

Dictionary

Dorland's Illustrated Medical Dictionary, 32nd edition, Elsevier, 2012 (6277 Sea Harbor Drive, Orlando, FL 32821-9989; 1-800-545-2522).

Code Books

Current Procedural Terminology, American Medical Association, published annually (515 North State Street, Chicago, IL 60610; 1-800-621-8335).

International Classification of Diseases, Tenth Revision, Clinical Modification, Elsevier, published annually (6277 Sea Harbor Drive, Orlando, FL 32821-9989; 1-800-545-2522).

Word Book

Sloane's Medical Word Book, 5th edition, by Ellen Drake, CMT, FAAMT, Elsevier (6277 Sea Harbor Drive, Orlando, FL 32821-9989; 1-800-545-2522).

Pharmaceutical Book

Optional publications for drug names and descriptions might be either drug books used by nurses (e.g., *Mosby's Gen RX*, Elsevier, published annually [3251 Riverport Lane, St. Louis, MO 63043; 1-800-325-4177; www.elsevier.com]) or ones used by physicians (e.g., *Physician's*

PERFORMANCE EVALUATION CHECKLIST

Assignment No. ____________

Name: ____ Date: ____________________________

Performance Objective

Task: Given access to all necessary equipment and information, the student will complete a CMS-1500 health insurance claim form.

Standards: Claim Productivity Management
Time ____________ minutes
Note: Time element may be given by instructor.

Directions: See assignment.

NOTE TIME BEGAN ____________ **NOTE TIME COMPLETED** ____________

PROCEDURE STEPS	ASSIGNED POINTS	STEP PERFORMED SATISFACTORY	COMMENTS
1. Assembled CMS-1500 claim form, patient record, E/M code slip, ledger card, computer, pen or pencil, and code books.	____________	____________	____________
2. Posed ledger card correctly.	____________	____________	____________
3. Proofread form for spelling and typographical errors while form remained in on computer screen.	____________	____________	____________
4. Points earned for correct completion of CMS-1500 block-by-block data.	____________	____________	____________

Figure I-1

PERFORMANCE EVALUATION CHECKLIST

BLOCK	INCORRECT	MISSING	NOT NEEDED	REMARKS	BLOCK	INCORRECT	MISSING	NOT NEEDED	REMARKS
					18				
1A					19				
2					20				
3					21				
4									
5					22				
6					23				
7					24A				
8					24B				
					24C				
9					24D				
9A									
9B									
9C					24E				
9D									
					24F				
10A					24G				
10B					24H, 24I				
10C					24J				
10D									
11					25, 26				
11A					27				
11B					28				
11C					29				
11D									
12					30				
13									
14					31				
15									
16					32				
17									
17A					33				
					Reference Initials				

TOTAL POINTS EARNED: __________ TOTAL POINTS POSSIBLE: __________

Evaluator's signature ______________________________ NEED TO REPEAT: ______________

Figure I-2

TABLE I-2

Appendix	Contents
A	College Clinic College Clinic Staff Abbreviations and Symbols Laboratory Abbreviations Mock Fee Schedule
B	Medicare Level II Healthcare Common Procedure Coding System (HCPCS) Codes
C	ICD-10-PCS Section 0 Medical and Surgical, Character 3, Operation Definitions
D	ICD-10-PCS Section 0 Medical and Surgical, Character 5, Approach Definitions

Desk Reference [PDR], Medical Economics Company, published annually [5 Paragon Drive, Montvale, NJ, 07645; 1-800-432-4570]).

EMPLOYEE INSURANCE PROCEDURAL MANUAL

If you currently work in a medical office, you may custom design an insurance manual for your physician's practice as you complete insurance claims in this *Workbook*. Obtain a three-ring binder with indexes and label them "Group Plans," "Private Plans," "Medicaid," "Medicare," "Managed Care Plans," "State Disability," "TRICARE," and "Workers' Compensation." If many of your patients have group plans, complete an insurance data or fact sheet for each plan and organize them alphabetically by group plan (Figure I–3). For managed care plans, type a form as shown in Figure 11-6 of the *Handbook*.

An insurance manual with fact sheets listing benefits can keep you up to date on policy changes and ensure maximum reimbursement. Fact sheets can be prepared from information obtained when patients bring in their benefit booklets. Obtain and insert a list of the procedures that must be performed as an outpatient and those that must have second opinions for each of the insurance plans.

As you complete the assignments in this *Workbook*, place them in the insurance manual as examples of completed claims for each particular program.

STUDENT SOFTWARE CHALLENGE (LOCATED ON EVOLVE)

The Student Software Challenge is another user-friendly software program located on the Evolve website. The software simulates a realistic experience by having students gather necessary documents and extract specific information to complete the CMS-1500 (02-12) insurance claim form. All source documents appear on screen and may be viewed simultaneously or printed for 10 patient cases that escalate in difficulty.

Student Software Challenge exercises are located in Chapters 7, 12, and 14. Some added features on the Evolve site are blank forms that students can fill out and print or save for additional practice or for use in the classroom. Documents available for printing include letterheads, authorization request forms, financial accounting statements (ledgers), and the CMS-1500 (02-12) form.

INSURANCE DATA

1. Employer's name ______________________________
2. Address ______________________ Telephone Number ______________________
3. Insurance Company Contact Person ______________________________
4. Insurance Carrier ______________________________
5. Address ______________________ Telephone Number to Call for Benefits ______________________
6. Group Policy Number ______________________________
7. Group Account Manager ______________________ Telephone Number ______________________
8. **Insurance Coverage:**
   Annual Deductible ______________________ Patient Copayment Percentage ______________________
   Noncovered Procedures ______________________________
   Maximum Benefits ______________________________
9. **Diagnostic Coverage:**
   Limited Benefits ______________________________
   Maximum Benefits ______________________________
   Noncovered Procedures ______________________________
10. **Major Medical:**
   Annual Deductible ______________________ Patient Copayment Percentage ______________________
   Limited Benefits ______________________________
   Maximum Benefits ______________________________
   Noncovered Procedures ______________________________

Mandatory Outpatient Surgeries ______________________________

Second Surgical Opinions ______________________________

Preadmission Certification Yes ______ No ______ Authorized Labs ______________________

Payment Plan:

UCR ______________ Schedule of Benefits ______________ CPT ______________ RVS ______________

Send claims to: ______________________________

____

Date Entered ______________________ Date Updated ______________________

Figure I-3

1 Role of an Insurance Billing Specialist

Marilyn T. Fordney

KEY TERMS

Your instructor may wish to select some specific words pertinent to this chapter for a test. For definitions of the terms, further study, and/or reference, the words, phrases, and abbreviations may be found in the glossary at the end of the Handbook. *Key terms for this chapter follow.*

American Health Information Management Association
American Medical Association
cash flow
claims assistance professional
ethics
etiquette
insurance billing specialist
list service
medical billing representative
multiskilled health practitioner
reimbursement specialist
respondeat superior
senior billing representative

KEY ABBREVIATIONS

See how many abbreviations and acronyms you can translate and then use this as a handy reference list. Definitions for the key abbreviations are located near the back of the Handbook *in the glossary.*

AAMA ____________________

ACA ____________________

AHIMA ____________________

AMA ____________________

ASHD ____________________

CAP ____________________

e-mail ____________________

GED ____________________

HIPAA ____________________

listserv ____________________

MSHP ____________________

MSO ____________________

NPP ____________________

PERFORMANCE OBJECTIVES

The student will be able to:

- Define and spell the key terms and key abbreviations for this chapter, given the information from the *Handbook* glossary, within a reasonable time period and with enough accuracy to obtain a satisfactory evaluation.
- Answer the fill-in-the-blank, multiple choice, and true/false review questions after reading the chapter, with enough accuracy to obtain a satisfactory evaluation.
- Use critical thinking to write one or two grammatically correct paragraphs with sufficient information to obtain a satisfactory evaluation.
- Visit websites and site-search information via the Evolve website, with sufficient information to obtain a satisfactory evaluation.

STUDY OUTLINE

Background of Insurance Claims, Coding, and Billing
Role of the Insurance Billing Specialist
- Job Responsibilities
- Educational and Training Requirements
- Career Advantages
- Self-Employment or Independent Contracting
- Flexible Hours
- Disabled Workers
- Qualifications
- Skills
- Personal Image
- Behavior

Medical Etiquette
Medical Ethics
Employer Liability
Employee Liability
Scope of Practice
Future Challenges

ASSIGNMENT 1-1 REVIEW QUESTIONS

Part I Fill in the Blank

Review the objectives, key terms, and chapter information before completing the following review questions.

1. Read the job descriptions in Chapter 1 in the *Handbook*. The ability to input data and transmit insurance claims accurately either directly or through a clearinghouse, as well as update and maintain software applications to requirements of third-party payers, is a technical skill required in the job of a/an

   ______________________________.

2. Name some of the facilities where facility billing is used.

   a. ______________________________
   b. ______________________________
   c. ______________________________
   d. ______________________________
   e. ______________________________

3. Name examples of non-physician practitioners (NPPs).

   a. ______________________________
   b. ______________________________
   c. ______________________________
   d. ______________________________
   e. ______________________________
   f. ______________________________
   g. ______________________________
   h. ______________________________

4. Identify three career opportunities (job titles) available after training in diagnostic and procedural coding and insurance claims completion.

   a. ______________________________
   b. ______________________________
   c. ______________________________

5. List some of the responsibilities and duties an insurance billing specialist might perform generally, as well as when acting as a collection manager. Refer to the section on "Job Responsibilities" on p. 5 in the text.

   a. ______________________________

   b. ______________________________

   c. ______________________________

   d. ______________________________

   e. ______________________________

   f. ______________________________

   g. ______________________________

6. List the duties of a claims assistance professional.

   a. ______________________________

   b. ______________________________

   c. ______________________________

7. Insurance claims must be promptly submitted within ____________ business days to ensure continuous cash flow.

8. Define cash flow.

   ____

9. Reasons for a medical practice's large accounts receivable are

   a. ______________________________

   b. ______________________________

   c. ______________________________

   d. ______________________________

10. Skills required for an insurance billing specialist are

    a. ______________________________

    b. ______________________________

    c. ______________________________

    d. ______________________________

    e. ______________________________

    f. ______________________________

    g. ______________________________

    h. ______________________________

    i. ______________________________

    j. ______________________________

11. Standards of conduct by which an insurance billing specialist determines the propriety of his or her behavior in a relationship are known as ____________.

12. Complete these statements with either the word *illegal* or *unethical*.
   a. To report incorrect information to the Aetna Casualty Company is ______________________________.
   b. To report incorrect information to a Medicare fiscal intermediary is ______________________________.
   d. In certain circumstances, it may be ______________ for two physicians to treat the same patient for the same condition.

13. When a physician is legally responsible for an employee's conduct performed during employment, this is known as ______________________________.

14. A claims assistance professional neglects to submit an insurance claim to a Medicare supplemental insurance carrier within the proper time limit. What type of insurance is needed for protection against this loss for the client?

   ____

Part II Multiple Choice

Choose the best answer.

15. Two billing components are facility billing and professional billing. Professional billing is done for
   a. hospitals.
   b. skilled nursing facilities.
   c. ambulatory surgical centers.
   d. physicians.

16. *Physician extenders* are health care personnel trained to provide medical care under the direct or indirect supervision of a physician, such as
   a. multiskilled health practitioners (MSHPs).
   b. claims assistance professionals (CAPs).
   c. non-physician practitioners (NPPs).
   d. insurance billing specialists.

17. The individual responsible for documenting the patient's clinical notes and assigning a diagnosis code and a procedure code for medical services rendered is a/an
   a. physician.
   b. insurance biller.
   c. office manager.
   d. financial accounting clerk.

18. An individual cross-trained to function in more than one job is known as a/an
   a. administrative medical assistant.
   b. receptionist.
   c. claims assistance professional.
   d. multiskilled health practitioner.

19. Third-party payers that require the provider to submit insurance claims for the patient are
   a. federal and state programs.
   b. private insurance plans.
   c. managed care programs.
   d. health care insurance plans.

Part III True/False

Write "T" or "F" in the blank to indicate whether you think the statement is true or false.

________ 20. Physicians are paid according to relative value units that are based on cost of delivering care, malpractice insurance, and the physician's work.

________ 21. It is not necessary to refer to coding books because medical practices use a fee schedule.

________ 22. It is the coder's responsibility to inform administration or his or her immediate supervisor if unethical or illegal coding practices are occurring.

_______ 23. When one code is available that includes all of the services, it is permissible to bill using separate codes for the services.

_______ 24. Depending on the circumstances of the case, an insurance billing specialist can be held personally responsible under the law for billing errors.

CRITICAL THINKING

To enhance your critical thinking skills, problems will be interspersed throughout the *Workbook*. Thinking is the goal of instruction and a student's responsibility. When trying to solve a problem by critical thinking, it is desirable to have more than one solution and to take time to think out answers. Remember that an answer may be changed when additional information is provided in a classroom setting.

ASSIGNMENT 1-2 CRITICAL THINKING

Performance Objective

Task: Describe why you are training to become an insurance billing specialist.

Conditions: Use one or two sheets of white typing paper and pen or pencil.

Standards: Time: ______________ minutes

Accuracy: ______________

(Note: The time element and accuracy criteria may be given by your instructor.)

Directions: Write one or two paragraphs describing why you are training to become an insurance billing specialist. Or, if enrolled in a class that is part of a medical assisting course, explain why you are motivated to seek a career as a medical assistant. Make sure grammar, punctuation, and spelling are correct.

ASSIGNMENT 1-3 VISIT WEBSITES

Performance Objective

Task: Access the Internet and visit several websites of the World Wide Web.

Conditions: Use a computer with printer and/or pen or pencil to make notes.

Standards: Time: _______________ minutes

Accuracy: _______________

(Note: The time element and accuracy criteria may be given by your instructor.)

Directions: For active web links to the following resources, visit the Evolve website at http://evolve.elsevier.com/Fordney/handbook and do the following site searches:

1. Access the Internet and find one of the web search engines (Yahoo, Excite, Google, Bing). Begin a web search (e.g., key in "insurance billers") to search for information about insurance billers or go to the career path website listed on Evolve. List three to five websites found. Go to one or more of those resources and list the benefits that those sites might have for a student in locating job opportunities or networking with others for professional growth and knowledge. Bring the website addresses to share with the class.

2. Site-search information on standards of ethical coding by visiting the website of the American Health Information Management Association (AHIMA). Download and print a hard copy of this code of ethics developed by AHIMA. Next, obtain information on the eHealth code of ethics, and respond to the following:

   A. Write a brief definition for each of the following terms: health information, health products, and health services.
   B. State the eight guiding principles of organizations and individuals who provide health information over the Internet.

2 Compliance, Privacy, Fraud, and Abuse in Insurance Billing

Linda Smith

KEY TERMS

Your instructor may wish to select some specific words pertinent to this chapter for a test. For definitions of the terms, further study, and/or reference, the words, phrases, and abbreviations may be found in the glossary at the end of the Handbook. *Key terms for this chapter follow.*

abuse
American Recovery and Reinvestment Act
authorization
authorization form
breach
breach of confidential communication
business associate
civil monetary penalty
clearinghouse
compliance
compliance plan
Comprehensive Error Rate Testing
confidential communication
confidentiality
consent
consent form
covered entity
disclosure
electronic media
embezzlement
fraud
Health Care Fraud Prevention and Enforcement Action Team
health care provider
individually identifiable health information
nonprivileged information
Notice of Privacy Practices
phantom billing
privacy
privacy officer, privacy official
privileged information
protected health information
qui tam
Recovery Audit Contractor
security officer
Security Rule
Self-Disclosure Protocol
state preemption
transaction
use
Zone Program Integrity Contractor

KEY ABBREVIATIONS

See how many abbreviations and acronyms you can translate and then use this as a handy reference list. Definitions for the key abbreviations are located near the back of the Handbook *in the glossary.*

ARRA ______________________

CD ______________________

CERT ______________________

CLIA ______________________

CMP ______________________

CMS ______________________

DHHS ______________________

DOJ ______________________

FBI ______________________

FCA ______________________

FDIC ______________________

FTP ______________________

HCFAP ______________________

HEAT ______________________

HIPAA ______________________

HITECH ______________________

IIHI ______________________

MIP ______________________

NPP ______________________

OCR ______________________

OIG ______________________

ORT ______________________

OSHA ______________________

P&P ______________________

PHI ______________________

PO ______________________

RAC ______________________

SDP ______________________

TPO ______________________

ZPIC ______________________

PERFORMANCE OBJECTIVES

The student will be able to:

- Define and spell the key terms and key abbreviations for this chapter, given the information from the *Handbook* glossary, within a reasonable time period and with enough accuracy to obtain a satisfactory evaluation.
- Answer the fill-in-the-blank, multiple choice, and true/false review questions after reading the chapter, with enough accuracy to obtain a satisfactory evaluation.
- Make decisions after reading scenarios whether the situations are considered fraud, abuse, or neither, with sufficient information to obtain a satisfactory evaluation.
- Decide when a situation is an incidental disclosure, HIPAA violation, or neither, with sufficient information to obtain a satisfactory evaluation.
- Make a choice after reading scenarios whether to ask for consent or authorization, or perform other office procedures, with sufficient information to obtain a satisfactory evaluation.
- Visit websites and site-search information via the Evolve website, with sufficient information to obtain a satisfactory evaluation.

STUDY OUTLINE

Compliance Defined
Health Information Portability and Accountability Act
- Title I: Health Insurance Reform
- Title II: Administrative Simplification
- Defining HIPAA Roles, Relationships, and Key Terms
- HIPAA in the Practice Setting

The Privacy Rule: Confidentiality and Protected Health Information
- Confidential Information
- Patients' Rights
- Obligations of the Health Care Provider

The Security Rule: Administrative, Physical, and Technical Safeguards
Health Information Technology for Economic and Clinical Health Act (HITECH Act)
- Business Associates
- Notification of Breach
- HIPAA Compliance Audits
- Increased Civil Penalties for Noncompliance With the Provisions of HIPAA
- Consequences of Noncompliance With the Provisions of HIPAA

Application to Practice Setting
- Organization and Staff Responsibilities in Protecting Patient Rights

Fraud and Abuse Laws
- Defining Fraud and Abuse Roles, Responsibilities, and Key Terms
- Criminal False Claims Act (18 US Code §287)
- False Claims Act (31 US Code §3729-3733)
- Qui Tam Provision (42 US Code §1320a-7a)
- Exclusion Statute
- Civil Monetary Penalties Law (41 US Code §1320a-7)
- Stark I and II Laws (42 US Code §1395nn)
- Anti-Kickback Statute (42 US Code §1320a-7b[b])
- Safe Harbors
- Operation Restore Trust
- Additional Laws and Compliance
- Increased Compliance Audits and Oversight
- Special Alerts, Bulletins, and Guidance Documents

Compliance Program Guidance for Individual and Small Group Physician Practices
- Increased Productivity and Decreased Penalties with Compliance Plan
- Seven Basic Components of a Compliance Plan
- Conducting Internal Monitoring and Auditing
- Implementing Compliance and Practice Standards
- Designating a Compliance Officer or Contact
- Conducting Appropriate Training and Education
- Responding Appropriately to Detected Offenses and Developing Corrective Action
- Developing Open Lines of Communication
- Enforcing Disciplinary Standards through Well-Publicized Guidelines

What to Expect from Your Health Care Practice

ASSIGNMENT 2-1 REVIEW QUESTIONS

Part I Fill in the Blank

Review the objectives, key terms, and chapter information before completing the following review questions.

1. Compliance is the process of ____.

2. What is the first step health insurance specialists should take toward achieving compliance so they do not violate laws, which may result in penalties or fines? ______________________________

3. What is the primary purpose of HIPAA Title I: Insurance Reform? ______________________________

4. The focus on the health care practice setting and reduction of administrative costs and burdens are the goals of which part of HIPAA? ______________________________

5. An independent organization that receives insurance claims from the physician's office, performs edits, and transmits claims to insurance carriers is known as a/an ______________________________.

6. Under HIPAA guidelines, a health care coverage carrier, such as Blue Cross/Blue Shield, that transmits health information in electronic form in connection with a transaction is called a/an ______________________________.

7. Dr. John Doe contracts with an outside billing company to manage claims and accounts receivable. Under HIPAA guidelines, the billing company is considered a/an ____________ of the provider.

8. An individual designated to assist the provider by putting compliance policies and procedures in place and training office staff is known as a/an ______________________________ under HIPAA guidelines.

9. If you give, release, or transfer information to another entity, this is known as ______________________________.

10. Define protected health information (PHI).

____

11. Unauthorized release of a patient's health information is called ______________________________.

12. A confidential communication related to the patient's treatment and progress that may be disclosed only with the patient's permission is known as ______________________________.

13. Under HIPAA, exceptions to the right of privacy are those records involving

    a. ______________________________
    b. ______________________________
    c. ______________________________
    d. ______________________________
    e. ______________________________
    f. ______________________________
    g. ______________________________
    h. ______________________________
    i. ______________________________

14. At a patient's first visit under HIPAA guidelines, the document that must be given so the patient acknowledges the provider's confidentiality of his or her protected health information is the ______________________________.

15. If a breach of privacy is discovered, the health care provider is required to take affirmative action to respond to the breach and alleviate the severity of it. This is known as ______________________________.

16. Name the three main sections of the HIPAA Security Rule for protecting electronic health information.

    a. ______________________________
    b. ______________________________
    c. ______________________________

17. Name the three specific areas of significant change that resulted from the HITECH Act.

    a. ______________________________
    b. ______________________________
    c. ______________________________

18. Indicate whether each of the following situations is one of fraud or abuse.

    a. Under the False Claims Act, billing a claim for services not medically necessary ______________
    b. Changing a figure on an insurance claim form to get increased payment ______________
    c. Dismissing the copayment owed by a Medicare patient ______________
    d. Neglecting to refund an overpayment to the patient ______________
    e. Billing for a complex fracture when the patient suffered a simple break ______________

Part II Multiple Choice

Choose the best answer.

19. One of the agencies charged with enforcing laws that regulate the health care industry is:
    a. Drug Enforcement Agency (DEA).
    b. Office of Inspector General (OIG).
    c. National Committee on Vital and Health Statistics (NCVHS).
    d. Department of Internal Affairs (DIA).

20. HIPAA transaction standards apply to the following, which are called covered entities. They are
    a. health care third-party payers.
    b. health care providers.
    c. health care clearinghouses.
    d. all of the above.

21. Enforcement of the privacy standards of HIPAA is the responsibility of
    a. Health Care Fraud and Abuse Control Program (HCFAP).
    b. National Committee on Vital and Health Statistics (NCVHS).
    c. Office for Civil Rights (OCR).
    d. Federal Bureau of Investigation (FBI).

22. Verbal or written agreement that gives approval to some action, situation, or statement is called
    a. authorization.
    b. consent.
    c. disclosure.
    d. release.

23. An individual's formal written permission to use or disclose his or her personally identifiable health information for purposes other than treatment, payment, or health care operations is called
    a. authorization.
    b. disclosure.
    c. release.
    d. consent.

24. The Notice of Privacy Practices (NPP) document is given to patients
    a. at the first visit to the practice.
    b. at every visit to the practice.
    c. on an annual basis.
    d. only on request of the patient.

25. Privacy regulations allow patients the right to obtain a copy of PHI
    a. under all circumstances.
    b. if they have a court order.
    c. only if the health care provider has determined that it would be appropriate and would not endanger the patient or any other person.
    d. only if the patient can pay the associated fee for the copies.

26. Under HIPAA, patient sign-in sheets
    a. are never permissible.
    b. are permissible.
    c. are permissible but limit the information that is requested.
    d. are permissible but require the practice to give the patient a number to be used when calling the patient.

27. Under HITECH, if a breach occurs, the covered entity
    a. does not have to notify the affected party.
    b. only has to notify the affected party if they feel it is reasonable.
    c. must notify the affected party no later than 30 calendar days after the discovery of the breach.
    d. must notify the affected party no later than 60 calendar days after the discovery of the breach.

28. Measurable solutions that have been taken, based on accepted standards and are periodically monitored to demonstrate that an office is in compliance with HIPAA Privacy rules is referred to as
    a. reasonable safeguards.
    b. privacy safeguards.
    c. security safeguards.
    d. standards.

29. Stealing money that has been entrusted in one's care is referred to as
    a. fraud.
    b. abuse.
    c. embezzlement.
    d. obstruction.

30. Under the Criminal False Claims Act, fines and imprisonment penalties for making a false claim in connection with payment for health care benefits can be imposed on
    a. the physician who provided the services.
    b. the health care billing specialist who prepared the claim.
    c. the health care administrator who oversees the practice or organization.
    d. anyone who knowingly and willfully participated in the scheme.

31. The FCA provision that allows a private citizen to bring civil action for a violation on behalf of the federal government and share in any money recovered is referred to as
    a. minimum necessary.
    b. qui tam.
    c. privileged information.
    d. exclusion statute.

32. The initiative that established hotlines for the public to report issues that might indicate fraud, abuse, or waste is
    a. ORT.
    b. CMP.
    c. HEAT.
    d. RAC.

33. Health care providers who determine that they have submitted false claims, should resolve the issue by seeking the HHS and OIG guidance established in 2006 and referred to as
    a. Operation Restore Trust.
    b. Stark I and II.
    c. Self-Disclosure Protocol.
    d. Safe Harbor.

34. The OIG recommends that health care staff should attend trainings in "general" compliance
    a. as part of their initial orientation.
    b. at least annually.
    c. every 6 months.
    d. every 6 years.

35. When faced with the discovery of an offense or an error, the health insurance specialist should immediately report concerns
    a. using the established chain of command outlined in your compliance plan.
    b. to the OIG through their telephone hotline.
    c. to the OIG through their e-mail address.
    d. directly to the Department of Health and Human Services.

Part III True/False

Write "T" or "F" in the blank to indicate whether you think the statement is true or false.

________ 36. Individually identifiable health information (IIHI) is any part of a person's health data (e.g., demographic information, address, date of birth) obtained from the patient that is created or received by a covered entity.

________ 37. HIPAA requirements protect disclosure of protected health information outside of the organization but does not protect against internal use of health information.

________ 38. Under HIPAA, patients may request confidential communications and may restrict certain disclosures of protected health information.

________ 39. It is not necessary to turn documents over or lock them in a secure drawer if you are only leaving your desk for a few moments.

________ 40. Under HIPAA Privacy regulations, patients do not have the right to access psychotherapy notes.

________ 41. The HITECH Act requires that business associates comply with the HIPAA Security Rule in the same manner that a covered entity would.

________ 42. Under HITECH, civil penalties for HIPAA violations are $100 for each violation with a maximum penalty of $25,000 for all violations of the same provision in a calendar year.

________ 43. To submit an insurance claim for medical services that were not medically necessary is a violation of the False Claims Act (FCA).

________ 44. Organizations who hire or contract with individuals who have been convicted of a misdemeanor or criminal offense and are on the OIG's list of excluded individuals may be subject to civil monetary penalties.

________ 45. In the federal health care program, accepting discounts, rebates, or other types of reductions in price is encouraged.

________ 46. Recovery audit contractors are highly motivated to find claim errors as they are paid a percentage of the money they recover.

________ 47. If fraud and abuse are detected, ZPIC contractors report to the DOJ for further investigation.

________ 48. In the event of an OIG audit, the presence of an OIG compliance program will prevent penalties and fines from being imposed.

ASSIGNMENT 2-2 CRITICAL THINKING: INCIDENTAL DISCLOSURE VERSUS HIPAA VIOLATION

Performance Objective

Task: Make a decision using your best judgment after reading each case study, whether it should be considered an incidental disclosure, a HIPAA violation, or neither.

Conditions: Use pen or pencil.

Standards: Time: ______________ minutes

Accuracy: ______________

(Note: The time element and accuracy criteria may be given by your instructor.)

Directions: Read through each case study. Use your best judgment and circle whether you think it is an incidental disclosure issue (ID), a HIPAA violation (V), or neither (N). Briefly explain the answer that you selected.

Scenarios

1. Dr. Practon's office sign-in sheets ask patients to fill in their names, appointment times, and physicians' names.

   ID V N

   Explain: ______________________________

2. It is Monday morning and you are inundated with work that needs to be done. You receive a telephone call and give patient information without confirming who is on the line.

   ID V N

   Explain ______________________________

3. You send a fax, but accidentally you switch the last two digits of the fax number and the patient's billing information is received in the wrong location.

   ID V N

   Explain: ______________________________

4. You are in a high-traffic area where patients might overhear protected health information, and you are careful to keep your voice down.

   ID V N

   Explain: ______________________________

5. It is 10:30 AM, and you go on a coffee break leaving two patients' charts on the checkout counter.

   ID V N

   Explain: ______________________________

6. In the reception room, a patient, Martha Havasi, overhears your telephone conversation even though you spoke quietly and shut the glass window.

ID V N

Explain: ___

7. You telephone a patient, Alex Massey, to remind him of tomorrow's appointment and leave a voicemail message on his answering machine.

ID V N

Explain: ___

8. Three patients near the reception area of the office overhear you telling another staff member that Daisy Dotson is scheduled for a Pap smear tomorrow at 4:00 PM.

ID V N

Explain: ___

9. You telephone a patient, Janet Hudson. She is not home so you leave a message on her answering machine that her breast cancer biopsy results came back negative.

ID V N

Explain: ___

10. You call out Fran O'Donnell's complete name in the waiting room where other patients are sitting.

ID V N

Explain: ___

11. You do not close the glass window to the reception room when talking on the telephone with your sister.

ID V N

Explain: ___

12. The office nurse tells a patient, Hugo Wells, his test results in front of his relatives in a treatment area.

ID V N

Explain: ___

13. You leave Katy Zontag's medical chart open at the receptionist's counter.

ID V N

Explain: ___

14. You telephone a patient, José Ramirez, and leave your name, the physician's name, and telephone number on his answering machine.

ID V N

Explain: ____

15. A patient, Kim Lee, is in the examination room and overhears a conversation concerning blood test results of another patient in an adjoining room.

ID V N

Explain: ____

16. While waiting in the reception room, a patient, Xavier Gomez, overhears a receptionist talking with another patient on the telephone about a colonoscopy appointment.

ID V N

Explain: ____

17. Betty Burton, a patient who is being weighed on the office scale by the medical assistant, overhears a conversation between an insurance billing specialist and an insurance company representative in which the billing specialist is trying to obtain preauthorization for another patient's medical procedure.

ID V N

Explain: ____

18. In a restaurant, a waitress overhears an insurance biller talking to a friend and telling her about a famous actress who visited her physician's office yesterday.

ID V N

Explain: ____

ASSIGNMENT 2-3 CRITICAL THINKING: FRAUD VERSUS ABUSE

Performance Objective

Task: Make a decision after reading each case study, whether it is considered fraud, abuse, or neither.

Conditions: Use pen or pencil.

Standards: Time: ______________ minutes

Accuracy: ______________

(Note: The time element and accuracy criteria may be given by your instructor.)

Directions: Read through each scenario and circle whether it is a fraud (F) issue, practice of abuse (A), or neither (N). To distinguish the difference between fraud and abuse situations, remember that under the Medicare program, abuse relates to incidents or practices that are inconsistent with accepted sound business practices, whereas fraud is intentional deception that an individual knows, or should know, to be false, and the individual knows the deception could result in some unauthorized benefit to himself or herself or to some other person(s). Briefly explain the answer you selected.

Scenarios

1. Dr. Pedro Atrics has a friend whose child needs elective surgery. He agrees to perform the surgery and bill as an "insurance only" case.

   F A N

   Explain: ______________________________

2. A patient, Carl Skinner, calls the office repeatedly about his prescriptions. When seen in the office the next time, Dr. Input bills a higher level of evaluation and management service to allow for the additional time.

   F A N

   Explain: ______________________________

3. Dr. Skeleton sets a simple fracture and puts a cast on Mr. Davis. He bills for a complex fracture.

   F A N

   Explain: ______________________________

4. A patient, Maria Gomez, asks a friendly staff member to change the dates on the insurance claim form. The medical assistant complies with the request.

   F A N

   Explain: ______________________________

5. A patient, Roberto Loren, asks the physician to restate a diagnosis so the insurance company will pay because payment would be denied based on the present statement. The physician complies with the request.

   F A N

   Explain: ______________________________

6. Dr. Rumsey sees a patient twice on the same day but bills as though the patient was seen on two different dates.

   F A N

   Explain: ______________________________

7. A Medicare patient, Joan O'Connor, is seen by Dr. Practon, and the insurance claim shows a charge to the Medicare fiscal intermediary at a fee schedule rate higher than and different from that of non-Medicare patients.

   F A N

   Explain: ______________________________

8. A patient, Hazel Plunkett, receives a service that is not medically necessary to the extent rendered, and an insurance claim is submitted.

   F A N

   Explain: ______________________________

9. A patient, Sun Cho, paid for services that were subsequently declared not medically necessary, and Dr. Cardi failed to refund the payment to the patient.

   F A N

   Explain: ______________________________

10. Dr. Ulibarri tells the insurance biller not to collect the deductible and copayments from Mrs. Gerry Coleman.

   F A N

   Explain: ______________________________

ASSIGNMENT 2-4 CRITICAL THINKING: CONSENT VERSUS AUTHORIZATION

Performance Objective

Task: Make a decision using your best judgment after reading each scenario and determine whether you should ask for consent or authorization, or do other procedures.

Conditions: Use pen or pencil.

Standards: Time: ______________ minutes

Accuracy: ______________

(Note: The time element and accuracy criteria may be given by your instructor. Class discussion may offer other possible ways of handling the given situations.)

Directions: Read through each case study and determine whether you should ask for consent or authorization, or perform other office procedures.

Scenarios

1. Dr. Practon's patient, Mary Ann Bailey, goes to the College Hospital's emergency department complaining of severe stomach cramps. Subsequently, she is admitted to the hospital for pancreatitis. The floor nurse at the hospital telephones Dr. Practon's office asking for the patient's medical records to be brought over immediately. What should you do?

   Response: ____

   ____

   ____

2. Robert Fellow, a patient, telephones the College Clinic and states that he has hired a lawyer and is filing a lawsuit against another driver for an automobile accident that happened about a month ago. The attorney for the other driver needs your patient's medical records to find out what injuries your patient suffered as a result of the accident. The attorney also wants to know if there are any preexisting injuries. Mr. Fellow requests that you send a copy of his medical records to the other attorney. What should you do?

   Response: ____

   ____

   ____

3. Consuelo Lopez, the mother of a minor patient, Johnnie Lopez, telephones your office stating that Johnnie is having difficulty staying focused and loses his concentration during classroom activities at school. Mrs. Lopez has made an appointment for him to be seen by a psychologist and has requested that you send his medical records to the psychologist before the date of the appointment. What should you do?

   Response: ____

   ____

   ____

4. Eric Jacobs, a patient, receives psychiatric counseling (not psychotherapy) and treatment for diabetes at the College Clinic. The patient requests a copy of his medical record. (A) Is it necessary to remove the documentation pertaining to the psychiatric counseling sessions before giving the patient a copy of his medical record? (B) Can you disclose to the patient his medical records? Explain.

   Response: (A) ____

   ____

   ____

   Response: (B) ____

   ____

   ____

ASSIGNMENT 2-5 VISIT WEBSITES

Performance Objective

Task: Access the Internet and visit several websites of the World Wide Web.

Conditions: Use a computer with printer and/or pen or pencil to make notes.

Standards: Time: ______________ minutes

Accuracy: ______________

(Note: The time element and accuracy criteria may be given by your instructor.)

Directions: For active web links to the following resources, visit the Evolve website at http://evolve.elsevier.com/Fordney/handbook and do the following three site searches.

1. Site-search information on patient confidentiality by visiting the website of the American Medical Association (www.ama-assn.org). Click on Physician Resources/Legal Issues/Patient Physician Relationship Topics/Patient Confidentiality.

2. Site-search information on patient confidentiality in health care by visiting the Google search engine. Key in patient confidentiality in health care. Locate an article and print a hard copy to share and discuss with the class.

3. Site-search for information on fraud and abuse by visiting one or more of the federal websites. See what you can discover and either print out or take notes and bring back information to share with the class for discussion. Try one or more of the CMS websites listed on Evolve.

3 Basics of Health Insurance

Linda Smith

KEY TERMS

Your instructor may wish to select some words pertinent to this chapter for a test. For definitions of the terms, further study, and/or reference, the words, phrases, and abbreviations may be found in the glossary at the end of the Handbook. *Key terms for this chapter follow.*

accounts receivable management
applicant
assignment
blanket contract
cancelable
Civilian Health and Medical Program of the Department of Veterans Affairs
claim
coinsurance
competitive medical plan
conditionally renewable
Consumer Directed Health Plan
contract
coordination of benefits
copayment
daysheet
deductible
disability income insurance
electronic signature
eligibility
emancipated minor
encounter form
exclusions
exclusive provider organization
expressed contract
extended
financial accounting record
foundation for medical care
guaranteed renewable
guarantor
Health Care and Education Reconciliation Act
healthcare flexible spending account
health insurance
health maintenance organization
high risk
implied contract
indemnity
indemnity health insurance
independent or individual practice association
insured
major medical
Maternal and Child Health Program
Medicaid
Medicare
Medicare/Medicaid
member
noncancelable policy
nonparticipating physician or provider
optionally renewable
participating physician or provider
Patient Protection and Affordable Care Act
patient registration form
personal insurance
point-of-service (POS) plan
posted
preauthorization
precertification
predetermination
preexisting conditions
preferred provider organization
premium
running balance
Small Business Health Option Program
State Children's Health Insurance Program
State Disability Insurance
subscriber
TRICARE
unemployment compensation disability insurance
Veterans Affairs outpatient clinic
workers' compensation insurance

KEY ABBREVIATIONS

See how many abbreviations and acronyms you can translate and then use this as a handy reference list. Definitions for the key abbreviations are located near the back of the Handbook *in the glossary.*

AAMB ____________________

AAPC ____________________

ADSM ____________________

A/R ____________________

CDHP ____________________

CHAMPVA ____________________

CMP ____________________

COB ____________________

COBRA ____________________

DoD ____________________

DOS ____________________

EPO ____________________

FMC ____________________

HBMA ____________________

HCERA ____________________

HDHP ____________________

HFMA ____________________

HFSA ____________________

HMO ____________________

HRA ____________________

HSA ____________________

IPA ____________________

MAB ____________________

MCHP ____________________

Medi-Medi ____________________

MGMA ____________________

MSA ____________________

nonpar ____________________

NPP ____________________

PAHCOM ____________________

par ____________________

PMS ____________________

POS plan ____________________

PPACA ____________________

PPO ____________________

ROA ____________________

SCHIP ____________________

SDHP ____________________

SDI ____________________

SHOP ____________________

SOF ____________________

UCD ____________________

VA ____________________

PERFORMANCE OBJECTIVES

The student will be able to:

- Define and spell the key terms and key abbreviations for this chapter, given the information from the *Handbook* glossary, within a reasonable time period and with enough accuracy to obtain a satisfactory evaluation.
- Answer the fill-in-the-blank, multiple choice, and true/false review questions after reading the chapter, with enough accuracy to obtain a satisfactory evaluation.
- Arrange 18 administrative processing steps of an insurance claim in proper sequence, given data from the textbook, within a reasonable time period and with enough accuracy to obtain a satisfactory evaluation.
- Use critical thinking to explain some of the differences in insurance key terms, given data from the textbook, within a reasonable time period and with enough accuracy to obtain a satisfactory evaluation.
- Prepare a financial accounting record, given data from the textbook, within a reasonable time period and with enough accuracy to obtain a satisfactory evaluation.
- Abstract data from some insurance identification cards, given data from the textbook, within a reasonable time period and with enough accuracy to obtain a satisfactory evaluation.

STUDY OUTLINE

History
Insurance in the United States
Health Care Reform
- Health Benefit Exchanges

Legal Principles of Insurance
- Insurance Contracts

Physician–Patient Contracts and Financial Obligation
- Implied or Expressed Contracts

The Insurance Policy
- Policy Application
- Policy Renewal Provisions
- Policy Terms
- Coordination of Benefits
- General Policy Limitations
- Case Management Requirements

Choice of Health Insurance
- Group Contract
- Individual Contract

Types of Health Insurance Coverage
- CHAMPVA
- Competitive Medical Plan
- Consumer-Directed Health Plans
- Disability Income Insurance
- Exclusive Provider Organization
- Foundation for Medical Care
- Health Maintenance Organization
- Indemnity Health Insurance
- Independent or Individual Practice Association
- Maternal and Child Health Program
- Medicaid
- Medicare
- Medicare/Medicaid
- Point-of-Service Plan
- Preferred Provider Organization
- State Children's Health Insurance Program
- TRICARE
- Unemployment Compensation Disability Insurance
- Veterans Affairs Outpatient Clinic
- Workers' Compensation Insurance

Examples of Insurance Billing
Handling and Processing Insurance Claims
- Life Cycle of an Insurance Claim

Keeping Up to Date
Procedure 3-1: Prepare and Post to a Patient's Financial Accounting Record

ASSIGNMENT 3-1 REVIEW QUESTIONS

Part I Fill in the Blank

Review the objectives, key terms, glossary definitions to key terms, chapter information, and figures before completing the following review questions.

1. A/an ______________________________ is a legally enforceable agreement or contract.

2. An individual promising to pay for medical services rendered is known as a/an

   ______________________________.

3. List five health insurance policy renewal provisions.

   a. ______________________________

   b. ______________________________

   c. ______________________________

   d. ______________________________

   e. ______________________________

4. Insurance reimbursement or payment is also called ______________________.

5. Name two general health insurance policy limitations.

   a. ______________________________

   b. ______________________________

6. Under the health care reform legislation of 2010, health plans must allow employees to keep their children on their plans until the children are __________ years old.

7. The act of determining whether treatment is covered under an individual's health insurance policy is called ______________________________.

8. The procedure to obtain permission for a procedure before it is done, to determine whether the insurance program agrees it is medically necessary, is termed

   ______________________________.

9. Determining the maximum dollar amount the insurance company will pay for a procedure before it is done is known as ______________________________.

10. Name two ways an individual may obtain health insurance.

    a. ______________________________

    b. ______________________________

11. List four methods a physician's practice may use to submit insurance claims to insurance companies.

    a. ______________________________

    b. ______________________________

    c. ______________________________

    d. ______________________________

12. A document signed by the insured directing the insurance company to pay benefits directly to the physician is known as a/an ________________________________.

13. A patient service slip personalized to the practice of the physician and used as a communications/billing tool during routing of the patient is also known as a/an

a. ____.

b. ____.

c. ____.

d. ____.

14. For electronic access to computer data, computerized signatures may consist of the following verification or access methods:

a. ____

b. ____

c. ____

d. ____

e. ____

f. ____

g. ____

15. A method of making an automatic deposit of funds from the payer into the provider's bank account and used in place of a mailed paper check is referred to as

____.

Part II Mix and Match

16. Match the following insurance terms in the right column with their descriptions, and fill in the blank with the appropriate letter.

_______	An insurance company taking into account benefits payable by another carrier in determining its own liability	a. Adjuster
_______	Benefits paid by an insurance company to an insured person	b. Assignment
_______	Transfer of one's right to collect an amount payable under an insurance contract	c. Carrier
_______	Time that must elapse before an indemnity is paid	d. Coordination of benefits (COB)
_______	Acts for insurance company or insured in settlement of claims	e. Deductible
_______	Periodic payment to keep insurance policy in force	f. Exclusions
_______	Amount insured person must pay before policy will pay	g. Indemnity
_______	Time period in which a claim must be filed	h. Premium
_______	Certain illnesses or injuries listed in a policy that the insurance company will not cover	i. Subscriber
_______	Insurance company that carries the insurance	j. Time limit
_______	One who belongs to an insurance plan	k. Waiting period

Part III Multiple Choice

Choose the best answer.

17. When a patient goes to a physician's office seeking medical services, the physician accepts the patient and agrees to render treatment, and both parties agree, this contract is known as a/an
    a. expressed contract.
    b. agreed contract.
    c. implied contract.
    d. written contract.

18. The process of checking and confirming that a patient is covered under an insurance plan is known as
    a. precertification.
    b. eligibility verification.
    c. coordination of benefits (COB).
    d. predetermination.

19. A provision that allows the policyholder the right to refuse to renew the insurance policy on a premium due date is called
    a. conditionally renewable.
    b. guaranteed renewable.
    c. optionally renewable.
    d. noncancelable.

20. A provision in a health insurance policy in which two insurance carriers work together for payment so that there is no duplication of benefits paid between the primary insurance carrier and the secondary insurance carrier is called
    a. copayment.
    b. coinsurance.
    c. coordination of benefits (COB).
    d. cost-share rider.

21. A type of tax-free savings account that allows individuals and their employers to set aside money to pay for health care expenses is known as
    a. a health savings account.
    b. a medical savings account.
    c. a flexible spending account.
    d. all of the above.

22. Time limits for filing insurance claims to a commercial carrier may have a range of
    a. 10 days from the date medical service is received to 1 year.
    b. 30 days from the date of service to 1½ years.
    c. 60 days from the date of service.
    d. no time limit.

Part IV True/False

Write "T" or "F" in the blank to indicate whether you think the statement is true or false.

________ 23. If a physician belongs to a preferred provider organization (PPO) and does not follow his or her contract with the PPO, the patient is liable for the bill.

________ 24. The birthday law is a change in the order of determination of coordination of benefits (COB) regarding primary and secondary insurance carriers for dependent children.

________ 25. The Consolidated Omnibus Budget Reconciliation Act of 1985 (COBRA) mandates that when an employee is laid off from a company, the group health insurance coverage must continue at group rates for up to 18 months.

________ 26. A group policy usually provides better benefits; however, the premiums are generally higher than an individual contract would be.

________ 27. A signature stamp is acceptable by all insurances as proof of the provider's signature on a CMS-1500 claim form.

ASSIGNMENT 3-2 CRITICAL THINKING: ADMINISTRATIVE SEQUENCE OF PROCESSING AN INSURANCE CLAIM

Performance Objective

Task: Number from 1 to 18 the proper sequence of processing an insurance claim.

Conditions: Use given data and pen or pencil.

Standards: Time: __________ minutes

Accuracy: __________

(Note: The time element and accuracy criteria may be given by your instructor.)

Directions: Arrange the listed steps 1 through 18 in proper sequence by placing the correct number to the left of the statement. (Note: Each medical practice has its own order of the way office procedures are carried out; thus, these steps may vary slightly from practice to practice.)

_______ Bank deposit made and unpaid claims followed up

_______ Patient's financial account

_______ Insurance information (obtained and verified)

_______ Payer processing/payment received with explanation of benefits document

_______ Patient's financial data posted and patient checkout

_______ Patient appointment and preregistration

_______ CMS-1500 (02-12) paper claim forms submitted

_______ Provider's signature

_______ Electronic (HIPAA X12 837) claims transmitted

_______ Insurance claims preparation

_______ HIPAA Notice of Privacy

_______ Balance due statement mailed to patient

_______ Track pending insurance claims

_______ Patient's signature requirements

_______ Assignment of benefits

_______ Medical services performed and encounter form completed

_______ Insurance identification card photocopied

_______ Full payment received and financial records retained

ASSIGNMENT 3-3 CRITICAL THINKING: DIFFERENCES IN INSURANCE KEY TERMS

Performance Objective

Task: Describe and/or explain your response to five questions.

Conditions: Use one or two sheets of white typing paper and pen or pencil.

Standards: Time: ______________ minutes

Accuracy: ______________

(Note: The time element and accuracy criteria may be given by your instructor.)

Directions: Respond verbally or in writing to these questions or statements.

1. Explain the difference between the following:

Blanket contract ____

Individual contract ____

2. Explain the difference between a participating provider and a nonparticipating provider for the following:

Commercial insurance company or managed care plan participating provider:

____

Commercial insurance company or managed care plan nonparticipating provider:

____

Medicare participating provider:

____

Medicare nonparticipating provider:

____

3. State the difference between the following:

Implied contract: ____

Expressed contract: ____

4. Explain the birthday law (rule) and when it is used.

____

ASSIGNMENT 3-4 PREPARE A FINANCIAL ACCOUNTING RECORD

Performance Objective

Task: Prepare, insert descriptions, and post fees, payments, credit adjustments, and balances due to a patient's ledger card. If you have access to copy equipment, make a photocopy.

Conditions: Use one patient account form or ledger form (Figure 3-1), pen or pencil, and calculator.

Standards: Time: ______________ minutes

Accuracy: ______________

(Note: The time element and accuracy criteria may be given by your instructor.)

Directions:

1. Locate a financial accounting record (ledger) (see Figure 3-1) form. Refer to the step-by-step procedure at the end of Chapter 3 in the *Handbook*. In addition, see Figures 3-14 and 10-3 in the *Handbook* for graphic examples of financial accounting records (ledgers).
2. Insert the patient's name and address, including ZIP code, in the box.
3. Enter the patient's personal data.
4. Ledger lines: Insert date of service (DOS), reference (CPT code number, check number, or dates of service for posting adjustments or when insurance was billed), description of the transaction, charge amounts, payments, adjustments, and running current balance. The posting date is the actual date the transaction is recorded. If the DOS differs from the posting date, list the DOS in the reference or description column.

(Note: A good bookkeeping practice is to use a red pen to draw a line across the financial accounting record [ledger] from left to right to indicate the last entry billed to the insurance company.)

Scenario:

A new patient, Miss Carolyn Wachsman, of 4590 Ashton Street, Woodland Hills, XY 12345, was seen by Dr. Practon; her account number is 3-3. Her home telephone number is (555) 340-8876, and her work telephone number is (555) 509-7091. She was born on 5-8-75. She is insured by Blue Cross, and her subscriber number is 540-xx-3209.

Miss Wachsman was seen on March 24 of the current year for a level III evaluation and management office visit ($). She also received an ECG ($). Locate these fees in the Mock Fee Schedule in Appendix A of this *Workbook*.

An insurance claim form was sent to Blue Cross on March 25. On May 15, Blue Cross sent an explanation of benefits stating the patient had previously met her deductible. Check number 433 for $76 was attached to the EOB and $19 was indicated as the adjustment to be made by the provider. On May 25, the patient was billed for the balance.

After the instructor has returned your work to you, either make the necessary corrections and place it in a three-ring notebook for future reference, or, if you received a high score, place it in your portfolio for reference when applying for a job.

Acct No. 3-3

Financial Statement

COLLEGE CLINIC
4567 Broad Avenue
Woodland Hills, XY 12345-0001
Tel. 555-486-9002
Fax No. 555-487-8976

Phone No. (H) ____________________ (W) ____________________ Birthdate ____________________

Primary Insurance Co. ____________________ Policy/Group No. ____________________

Secondary Insurance Co. ____________________ Policy/Group No. ____________________

DATE	REFERENCE	DESCRIPTION	CHARGES	CREDITS PYMNTS.	CREDITS ADJ.	BALANCE
				BALANCE FORWARD →		

PLEASE PAY LAST AMOUNT IN BALANCE COLUMN

THIS IS A COPY OF YOUR FINANCIAL ACCOUNT AS IT APPEARS ON OUR RECORDS

Figure 3-1

ASSIGNMENT 3-5 ABSTRACT DATA FROM AN INSURANCE IDENTIFICATION CARD

Performance Objective

Task: Answer questions in reference to an insurance identification card for Case A.

Conditions: Use an insurance identification card (Figure 3-2), the questions presented, and pen or pencil.

Standards: Time: ______________ minutes

Accuracy: ______________

(Note: The time element and accuracy criteria may be given by your instructor.)

Directions: An identification card provides much of the information needed to establish a patient's insurance coverage. You have photocopied the front and back sides of three patients' cards and placed copies in their patient records, returning the originals to the patients. Answer the questions by abstracting or obtaining the data from the cards.

CASE A

1. Name of patient covered by the policy. ______________________________
2. Provide the insurance policy's effective date. ______________________________
3. List the telephone number for preauthorization. ______________________________
4. State name and address of insurance company. ______________________________
5. List the telephone number to call for provider access. ______________________________
6. Name the type of insurance plan. ______________________________
7. List the insurance identification number (a.k.a. subscriber, certificate, or member numbers). ______________________________

   ____
8. Furnish the group number. ______________ Plan or coverage code. ______________
9. State the copay requirements. ______________________________
10. Does the card indicate the patient has hospital coverage? ______________________________

    ____

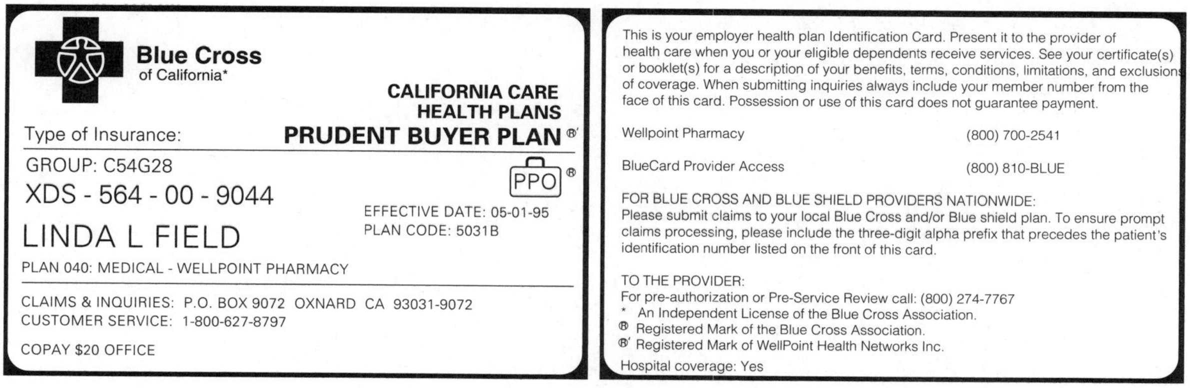

Figure 3-2

ASSIGNMENT 3-6 ABSTRACT DATA FROM AN INSURANCE IDENTIFICATION CARD

Performance Objective

Task: Answer questions in reference to the insurance identification card for Case B.

Conditions: Use an insurance identification card (Figure 3-3), the questions presented, and pen or pencil.

Standards: Time: ______________ minutes

Accuracy: ______________

(Note: The time element and accuracy criteria may be given by your instructor.)

CASE B

1. Name of patient covered by the policy. ______________________________
2. Provide the insurance policy's effective date. ______________________________
3. List the telephone number for preauthorization. ______________________________
4. State name of insurance company. ______________________________
5. List the telephone number to call for patient benefits and eligibility. ______________________________
6. Name the type of insurance plan. ______________________________
7. List the insurance identification number (a.k.a. subscriber, certificate, or member numbers). ______________________________

   ____
8. Furnish the group number. ______________ Plan or coverage code. ______________
9. State the copay requirements, if any. ______________________________
10. List the Blue Shield website. ______________________________

Blue Shield of California
An Independent Member of the Blue Shield Association

Preferred Plan

PPO

SUBSCRIBER NAME: M T FORDHAM

EFFECTIVE DATE: 010120XX

SUBSCRIBER ID NUMBER: AJC557469969

GROUP NUMBER: 00P1901

PLAN CODE: 542

CUSTOMER SERVICE: (800) 331-2001

07/16/20XX

Use Blue Shield of California Preferred Physicians and Hospitals to receive maximum benefits.

Carry the Blue Shield Identification Card with you at all times and present it whenever you or one of your covered dependents receives medical services. Read your employee booklet/Health Services Agreement which summarizes the benefits, provisions, limitations and exclusions of your plan. Your health plan may require prior notification of any hospitalization and notification, within one business day, of an emergency admission. Review of selected procedures may be required before some services are performed. To receive hospital pre-admission and pre-service reviews, call 1-800-343-1691. Your failure to call may result in a reduction of benefits.

For questions, including those related to benefits, and eligibility, call the customer service number listed on the front of this card.

The PPO logo on the front of this ID Card identifies you to preferred providers outside the state of California as a member of the Blue Card PPO Program.

When you are outside of California call 1-800-810-2583 to locate the nearest PPO Provider. Remember, any services you receive are subject to the policies and provisions of your group plan.

ID-23200-PPO REVERSE www.blueshieldca.com

Figure 3-3

ASSIGNMENT 3-7 ABSTRACT DATA FROM AN INSURANCE IDENTIFICATION CARD

Performance Objective

Task: Answer questions in reference to the insurance identification card for Case C.

Conditions: Use an insurance identification card (Figure 3-4), the questions presented, and pen or pencil.

Standards: Time: ______________ minutes

Accuracy: ______________

(Note: The time element and accuracy criteria may be given by your instructor.)

CASE C

1. Name of patient covered by the policy. ______________
2. Provide the insurance policy's effective date, if there is one. ______________
3. List the number to call for out-of-network preauthorization. ______________
4. State name and address of insurance company. ______________
5. List the telephone number to call for member inquiries. ______________
6. Name the type of insurance plan. ______________
7. List the insurance identification number (a.k.a. subscriber, certificate, or member numbers). ______________
8. Furnish the group number. ______________
9. State the copay requirements, if any. ______________
10. Who is the patient's primary care physician? ______________

UNITEDhealthcare

LINDA L. FLORES
Member # 52170-5172

CALMAT

Group # 176422
COPAY: Office Visit $10 ER $50
Urgent $35

Electronic Claims Payor ID 87726

POS PCP Plan
WITH RX D - UHC
and MH/CD
PCP: G. LOMAN
805-643-9973

MTH

Call 800-842-5751 for Member Inquiries

This identification card is not proof of membership nor does it guarantee coverage. Persons with coverage that remains in force are entitled to benefits under the terms and conditions of this group health benefit plan as detailed in your benefit description.

IMPORTANT MEMBER INFORMATION
In non-emergencies, call your Primary Care Physician to receive the highest level of benefits. If you have an emergency and are admitted to a hospital, you are required to call your Primary Care Physician within two working days.
For out of network services that require authorization, call the Member Inquiries 800 number on the front of this card.

Claim Address: P.O. Box 30990, Salt Lake City, UT 84130-0990

Figure 3-4

4 Medical Documentation and the Electronic Health Record

Linda Smith

KEY TERMS

Your instructor may wish to select some words pertinent to this chapter for a test. For definitions of the terms, further study, and/or reference, the words, phrases, and abbreviations may be found in the glossary at the end of the Handbook. *Key terms for this chapter follow.*

acute
attending physician
chief complaint
chronic
cloned note
comorbidity
comprehensive
concurrent care
consultation
consulting physician
continuity of care
counseling
critical care
degaussing
detailed
documentation
electronic health record
emergency care
eponym
established patient
expanded problem focused
external audit
facsimile
family history
health record/medical record
high complexity
history of present illness
internal review
legible
low complexity
meaningful use
medical decision making
medical necessity
medical report
moderate complexity
new patient
non-physician practitioner
ordering physician
past history
physical examination
primary care physician
problem focused
prospective review
referral
referring physician
resident physician
retrospective review
review of systems
social history
straightforward
subpoena
subpoena duces tecum
teaching physician
treating or performing physician
zeroization

KEY ABBREVIATIONS

See how many abbreviations and acronyms you can translate and then use this as a handy reference list. Definitions for the key abbreviations are located near the back of the Handbook *in the glossary.*

ARRA ______________________

C level of history or examination ______________________

CC ______________________

CCU ______________________

D level of history or examination ______________________

dx or Dx ______________________

ED or ER ______________________

EHR ______________________

E/M service ______________________

EMR ______________________

EPF level of history or examination ______________________

ESI ______________________

fax ____________________

FH ____________________

HC medical decision making ____________________

HIM ____________________

HIV ____________________

HPI ____________________

ICU ____________________

LC medical decision making ____________________

LLQ ____________________

LUQ ____________________

MC medical decision making ____________________

MU ____________________

MDM ____________________

NLP ____________________

NP ____________________

NPP ____________________

PCP ____________________

PE or PX ____________________

PF level of history or examination ____________________

PFSH ____________________

PH ____________________

PO ____________________

POR system ____________________

RCU ____________________

RLQ ____________________

R/O ____________________

ROS ____________________

RUQ ____________________

SF medical decision making ____________________

SH ____________________

SNOMED-CT ____________________

SOAP style ____________________

SOR system ____________________

WNL ____________________

PERFORMANCE OBJECTIVES

The student will be able to:

- Define and spell the key terms and key abbreviations for this chapter, given the information from the *Handbook* glossary, within a reasonable time period and with enough accuracy to obtain a satisfactory evaluation.
- Answer the fill-in-the-blank, mix and match, multiple choice, and true/false review questions after reading the chapter, with enough accuracy to obtain a satisfactory evaluation.
- Use critical thinking to solve an office problem about patients' medical records.
- Abstract subjective and objective data from patient records, within a reasonable time period and with enough accuracy to obtain a satisfactory evaluation.
- Review a patient record and obtain answers to questions about the documentation presented, within a reasonable time period and with enough accuracy to obtain a satisfactory evaluation.
- Select the correct medicolegal form, create a letter with appropriate content, prepare an envelope, and properly complete U.S. Postal Service documents for the physician's signature, given the patients' chart notes and ledger cards, within a reasonable time period and with enough accuracy to obtain a satisfactory evaluation.

STUDY OUTLINE

The Documentation Process
- Health Record
- Electronic Health Records

Incentive Programs for Adoption of Electronic Health Records
- Physician Quality Reporting System Incentive Program
- E-Prescribing Incentive Program
- Electronic Health Record Incentive Program
- Meaningful Use

General Principles of Health Record Documentation
- Documenters
- Legible Documentation
- Medical Necessity
- Legalities of Health Record Billing Patterns

Documentation Guidelines for Medical Services
- Evaluation and Management Services
- Audit Point System
- Documentation of History
- Documentation of Examination
- Documentation of Medical Decision Making

Documentation Terminology
- Terminology for Evaluation and Management Services
- Diagnostic Terminology and Abbreviations
- Directional Terms
- Surgical Terminology

Abstracting From Medical Records
- Life or Health Insurance Applications

Review and Audit of Health Records
- Internal Reviews
- Software Edit Checks

Release and Retention of Health Records
- Faxing Documents
- Sensitive Information
- Subpoena
- Retention of Records
- Termination of a Case
- Prevention of Legal Problems

Procedure 4-1: Abstract Data From a Health Record

Procedure 4-2: Compose, Format, Key, Proofread, and Print a Letter

ASSIGNMENT 4-1 REVIEW QUESTIONS

Part I Fill in the Blank

Review the objectives, key terms, glossary definitions to key terms, chapter information, and figures before completing the following review questions.

1. Written or graphic information about patient care is termed a/an ______________.

2. List three of the various types of health record systems that can be used in a medical practice.

   ____

   ____

   ____

3. The difference between an EMR and an EHR is that the ______________ is an individual physician's record of the patient's care, whereas the ______________ is all of the patient's records, from many different information systems and providers.

4. The greatest advantage of an EHR system is the improvement of quality of care and patient safety through the ______________ of medical records between providers and other health care organizations.

5. Providers who are not participating in the E-Prescribing Incentive Program in 2014 will have Medicare claims processed with a ______________ percent adjustment/reduction in their payments.

6. Stage 2 of the Meaningful Use Incentive Program will focus on ______________, which will expand the criteria in areas of disease management, clinical decision support, medication management, transitions in care, quality measurement, and research.

7. What is the CMS definition of *legible documentation?*

   ____

8. Performance of services or procedures consistent with the diagnosis, done with standards of good medical practice and a proper level of care given in the appropriate setting is known as ______________________________.

9. Medicare administrative contractors have ______________ to access a medical practice without an appointment or search warrant to conduct a review of documentation, audits, and evaluations.

10. A list of all staff members' names, job titles, signatures, and their initials is known as a/an ______________________________.

11. For electronic health records, how should an insurance billing specialist correct an error on a patient's record? ______________________________.

12. For paper-based records, how should an error be corrected on a patient's record?

    ______________________________.

13. If a medical practice is audited by Medicare officials and intentional miscoding is discovered, ______________ may be levied and providers may be ______________.

14. Name the six documentation components of a patient's history.

a. ______________________________

b. ______________________________

c. ______________________________

d. ______________________________

e. ______________________________

f. ______________________________

15. List the eight descriptive elements that can be documented in the HPI.

____

____

____

16. List the body systems that are recognized for reporting of the ROS.

____

____

____

17. A problem-focused examination is a ______________ examination of the affected body area or organ system.

18. MDM is the process performed after taking the patient's history and performing the examination, which results in a ______________________________.

19. Define the following terms in relationship to billing.

a. New patient ______________________________

b. Established patient ______________________________

20. Explain the difference between a consultation and the referral of a patient.

a. Consultation ______________________________

b. Referral ______________________________

21. Medical care for a patient who has received treatment for an illness and is referred to a second physician for treatment of the same condition is a situation called

______________________________.

22. An emergency medical condition, as defined by Medicare, is a medical condition manifesting itself by ______________ of ______________ such that the absence of immediate medical attention could reasonably be expected to result in placing the patient's health in serious jeopardy, serious impairment to body functions, or serious dysfunction of any body organ or part.

23. Whenever the words "rule out" are used to describe a patient's condition, do not code these conditions as if they existed; instead code the ______________ or

______________________________.

24. Any charts that are amended with additional notes must be labeled "________________" or "late entry" and dated on the day of the amendment, and signed by the physician.

25. If a fax is misdirected, either ______________________ or ______________________.

Part II Mix and Match

26. Match the following terms in the right column with their descriptions, and fill in the blank with the appropriate letter.

________	Renders a service to a patient	a. Attending physician
________	Directs selection, preparation, and administration of tests, medication, or treatment	b. Consulting physician
________	Legally responsible for the care and treatment given to a patient	c. Non-physician practitioner
________	Gives an opinion regarding a specific problem that is requested by another doctor	d. Ordering physician
________	Sends the patient for tests or treatment or to another doctor for consultation	e. Primary care physician
________	Oversees care of patients in managed care plans and refers patients to see specialists when needed	f. Referring physician
________	Responsible for training and supervising medical students	g. Resident physician
________	Clinical nurse specialist or licensed social worker who treats a patient for a specific medical problem and uses the results of a diagnostic test in managing a patient's medical problem	h. Teaching physician
________	Performs one or more years of training in a specialty area while working at a hospital (medical center)	i. Treating or performing physician

Part III Multiple Choice

Choose the best answer.

27. Chart chasing is eliminated when using which type of record system?
    a. Paper-based system
    b. Electronic health record system
    c. Problem-oriented system
    d. Integrated record system

28. Which of the following is NOT an incentive program for the adoption of EHR?
    a. PQRS
    b. MPFS
    c. ERx
    d. MU

29. Which MU stage focuses on electronically capturing health information into coded format to track conditions, communicate information for care coordination, and report on clinical quality measures and public health information?
    a. Stage 1
    b. Stage 2
    c. Stage 3
    d. Stage 4

30. Regarding the SOAP style of documentation that a physician uses to chart a patient's progress in the health record, SOAP stands for
    a. signature, observations, assessment, and progress.
    b. subjective, objective, assessment, and plan.
    c. symptoms, objective findings, and professional services.
    d. subjective, opinions, assistance, and present illness.

31. A physical examination of a patient performed by a physician is
    a. descriptive.
    b. comprehensive.
    c. subjective.
    d. objective.

32. During the performance of an external audit to review a medical practice's health records, the system used to show deficiencies in documentation is called a/an
    a. SOAP system.
    b. electronic recording system.
    c. information record system.
    d. point system.

33. Which of these elements is a requirement for all levels of history?
   a. CC
   b. HPI
   c. ROS
   d. PFSH

34. When there is an underlying disease or other conditions are present at the time of the patient's office visit, this is termed
   a. mortality.
   b. continuity.
   c. comorbidity.
   d. complexity.

35. Critical care is rendered in
   a. the coronary care unit.
   b. the intensive care unit.
   c. the emergency room.
   d. all of the above.

Part IV True/False

Write "T" or "F" in the blank line to indicate whether you think the statement is true or false.

________ 36. A patient's hospital discharge summary contains the discharge diagnosis but not the admitting diagnosis.

________ 37. An eponym should not be used when a comparable anatomic term can be used in its place.

________ 38. If the phrase "rule out" appears in a patient's health record in connection with a disease, then code the condition as if it existed.

________ 39. During a prospective review or prebilling audit, all procedures or services and diagnoses listed on the encounter form must match the data on the insurance claim form.

________ 40. Both civil and criminal subpoenas can be served via a fax machine.

________ 41. Willful disregard of a subpoena is punishable as contempt of court.

________ 42. Based on Medicare Conditions of Participation, hospitals must retain medical records for a period of at least 4 years.

________ 43. Assigned insurance claims for Medicaid and Medicare cases must be kept for a period of 7 years.

________ 44. If a patient fails to make payment on an overdue account, the physician has the right to formally withdraw from providing care to the patient.

________ 45. There are very few circumstances that insurance billers may be faced with when executing their job duties that may lead a case of lawsuit.

ASSIGNMENT 4-2 REVIEW DIAGNOSTIC TERMINOLOGY AND ABBREVIATIONS

In the *Handbook,* review Table 4-1 and anatomic figures, as well as Appendix A in the *Workbook,* which has a list of abbreviations and symbols.

Mix and Match

1. Match the following terms in the right column with the descriptions, and fill in the blank with the appropriate letter.

______	Taking or letting out fluids from a body part	a. Alteration
______	Act of cutting out	b. Bypass
______	Modifying a body part without affecting function	c. Control
______	Taking out or off a device from a body part	d. Drainage
______	Stop or attempt to stop bleeding	e. Excision
______	Altering the route of passage with anastomoses	f. Removal

Fill in the Blank

2. Write in the meaning for these abbreviations and/or symbols commonly encountered in a patient's medical record.

RLQ ________________________________

DC ________________________________

WNL ________________________________

R/O ________________________________

URI ________________________________

c̄ ________________________________

3. When documenting incisions, the unit of measure length should be listed in ________________________________.

Multiple Choice

Circle the letter that gives the best answer to each question.

4. If a physician called and asked for a patient's medical record STAT, what would he or she mean?
   a. The physician wants a statistic from a patient's record.
   b. The physician wants the record delivered on Tuesday.
   c. The physician wants the record delivered immediately.

5. If a physician asks you to locate the results of the last UA, what would you be searching for?
   a. A urinalysis report
   b. An x-ray report of the ulna
   c. Uric acid test results

6. If a physician telephoned and asked for a copy of the last H&P to be faxed, what is being requested?
   a. Heart and pulmonary findings
   b. H2 antagonist test results
   c. History and physical

7. If a hospital nurse telephoned and asked you to read the results of the patient's last CBC, what would you be searching for?
   a. Carcinoma basal cell report
   b. Complete blood count
   c. Congenital blindness, complete report

8. If you were asked to make a photocopy of the patient's last CT, what would you be searching for?
   a. Chemotherapy record
   b. Connective tissue report
   c. Computed tomography scan

ASSIGNMENT 4-3 CRITICAL THINKING: SOLVE AN OFFICE PROBLEM

Performance Objective

Task: Answer questions after reviewing the case study using critical thinking skills.

Conditions: Use a case study and a pen or pencil.

Standards: Time: ____________ minutes

Accuracy: ____________

Directions: Answer questions after reviewing the case study using your critical thinking skills. Record your answer on the blank lines.

1. A patient comes into the office for treatment. He does not return, because he is dissatisfied with Dr. Practon's treatment. Is it necessary to keep his records when he obviously will not return? ______________________________.

   Why? ____

   ____

ASSIGNMENT 4-4 ABSTRACT SUBJECTIVE OBSERVATIONS AND OBJECTIVE FINDINGS FROM PATIENT RECORDS

Performance Objective

Task: List subjective observations and objective findings after reading each of the case studies.

Conditions: Use a pencil and four case studies.

Standards: Time: ______________ minutes

Accuracy: ______________

(Note: The time element and accuracy criteria may be given by your instructor.)

Case Study 1 Mrs. Smith is 25 years old and was brought into the emergency department of College Hospital with complaints of difficulty breathing and chest pain. Her vital signs show an elevated temperature of 101° F and pulse rate of 90. Respirations are labored at 30/min. BP is 140/80. Her skin is warm and diaphoretic (perspiring). She states, "This condition has been going on for the past 3 days."

Subjective observations: ____

Objective findings: ____

Case Study 2 Mr. Jones is 56 years old and was admitted to the hospital with chest pain and elevated pulse and blood pressure. His skin is cold and clammy.

Subjective observations: ____

Objective findings: ____

Case Study 3 You are assisting the radiology technician with Sally Salazar, a 6-year-old Hispanic girl who was brought into the pediatrician's office with a suspected fracture of the right arm. Sally states she was "running at school, tripped on my shoelace, and fell." She tells you her "arm hurts," points out how "funny my arm looks," and starts to cry. You notice her arm looks disfigured and is covered with dirt. Sally is cradling her arm against her body and is unwilling to let go because "it's going to fall off."

Subjective observations: ____

Objective findings: ____

Case Study 4 You are working in the business office of College Hospital. A former patient in your hospital comes in complaining of his billing. He states he was never catheterized, never had any of the medications listed on his itemized bill, and has "never been in this hospital for that length of time." His face is red, his voice is gradually getting louder, and you notice he is standing with the aid of crutches because his left leg is in a full cast.

Subjective observations: ____

Objective findings: ____

ASSIGNMENT 4-5 REVIEW OF A PATIENT RECORD

Performance Objective

Task: Answer questions after reviewing a patient's record.

Conditions: Use a pencil, internal record review sheet, medical dictionary, abbreviation reference list, drug reference book (e.g., *Mosby's MD Consult*), and laboratory reference book.

Standards: Time: ______________ minutes

Accuracy: ______________

(Note: The time element and accuracy criteria may be given by your instructor.)

Directions: In many instances, when developing the skill of reviewing a patient record, you may need critical thinking in addition to efficient use of reference books. Answer only those questions you think can be justified by the documentation presented in the patient's record. Because the content of each record is variable, you may or may not have answers to all eight questions.

Answer the questions by recording on the blank lines the documentation found identifying the components from the patient's record.

If your answers vary, perhaps you have a reason for them that may or may not be valid. List your reasons in the response section. Differences may be reviewed with your instructor privately or via class discussion.

Patient Record

10-21-20xx
HPI
This new pt is an 80-year-old white male who has had problems with voiding since 9-5-20xx.

During the night, the pt had only 50 mL output and was catheterized this morning because of his poor urinary output (200 mL). He was thought to have a distended bladder; he complains of pressure in the suprapubic region. He has not had any gross hematuria. He has difficulty voiding, especially lying down. His voiding pattern is improved while standing and sitting.

Gene Ulibarri, MD

mtf

1. Location: In what body system is the sign or symptom occurring?

   Response: ____

2. Quality: Is the symptom or pain burning, gnawing, stabbing, pressure-like, squeezing, fullness?

   Response: ____

3. Severity: In this case, how would you rank the symptom (how was distress relieved) or pain (slight, mild, severe, persistent)?

   Response: ____

4. Duration: How long has the symptom been present, or how long does it last?

   Response: ____

5. Timing: When does(do) a sign(s) or symptom(s) occur (AM, PM, after or before meals)?

   Response: ____

6. Context: Is the pain/symptom associated with big meals, dairy products, etc.?

   Response: ____

7. Modifying factors: What actions make symptoms worse or better?

   Response: ____

8. Associated signs and symptoms: What other system or body area produces complaints when the presenting problem occurs? (Example: Chest pain leads to shortness of breath.)

   Response: ____

ASSIGNMENT 4-6 KEY A LETTER OF WITHDRAWAL

Performance Objective

Task: Key letter for physician's signature with envelope, prepare U.S. Postal Service forms, and complete an authorization form.

Conditions: Use one sheet of letterhead (print from Evolve website), U.S. Postal Service forms for certified mail with return receipt requested (Figure 4-1), Authorization for Release of Information form (Figure 4-2), a number 10 envelope, thesaurus, English dictionary, medical dictionary, computer, printer, and pen or pencil.

Standards: Time: ______________ minutes

Accuracy: ______________

(Note: The time element and accuracy criteria may be given by your instructor.)

Directions: Mrs. McLean is negligent about following Dr. Ulibarri's advice after she received surgery. Refer to *Workbook* Assignment 7-2 for information from the patient record of Mrs. Merry M. McLean. Use a letterhead and type in modified block style to write an appropriate letter to Mrs. McLean advising her of the doctor's withdrawal from the case (see *Handbook* Figure 4-21). Date the letter June 30 of the current year. Dr. Ulibarri will be available to this patient for 30 days after receipt of this letter.

This letter must be prepared for Dr. Ulibarri's signature because it is a legal document. Type Mrs. McLean's address on a number 10 envelope, referring to *Workbook* Figure 4-3. Send the letter by certified mail with return receipt requested, referring to *Handbook* Figure 4-22, and enclose a completed Authorization for Release of Information form (see Figure 4-2).

After the instructor has returned your work to you, either make the necessary corrections and place it in a three-ring notebook for future reference, or, if you receive a high score, place it in your portfolio for reference when applying for a job.

UNITED STATES POSTAL SERVICE

First-Class Mail
Postage & Fees Paid
USPS
Permit No. G-10

• Sender: Please print your name, address, and ZIP+4 in this box •

SENDER: *COMPLETE THIS SECTION*

- Complete items 1, 2, and 3. Also complete item 4 if Restricted Delivery is desired.
- Print your name and address on the reverse so that we can return the card to you.
- Attach this card to the back of the mailpiece, or on the front if space permits.

1. Article Addressed to:

COMPLETE THIS SECTION ON DELIVERY

A. Signature

x ☐ Agent ☐ Addressee

B. Received by (*Printed Name*) | C. Date of Delivery

D. Is delivery address different from item 1? ☐ Yes
If YES, enter delivery address below: ☐ No

3. Service Type
☐ Certified Mail ☐ Express Mail
☐ Registered ☐ Return Receipt for Merchandise
☐ Insured Mail ☐ C.O.D.

4. Restricted Delivery? *(Extra Fee)* ☐ Yes

2. Article Number
(Transfer from service label)

PS Form 3811, February 2004 Domestic Return Receipt 102595-02-M-1540

7006 0810 0001 6207 8857

PLACE STICKER AT TOP OF ENVELOPE TO THE RIGHT
OF THE RETURN ADDRESS, FOLD AT DOTTED LINE

CERTIFIED MAIL™

7006 0810 0001 6207 8857
7006 0810 0001 6207 8857

U.S. Postal Service™
CERTIFIED MAIL™ RECEIPT
(Domestic Mail Only; No Insurance Coverage Provided)

For delivery information visit our website at www.usps.com®

OFFICIAL USE

Postage	$
Certified Fee	
Return Receipt Fee (Endorsement Required)	
Restricted Delivery Fee (Endorsement Required)	
Total Postage & Fees	**$**

Postmark Here

Sent To

Street, Apt. No.; or PO Box No.

City, State, ZIP+4

PS Form 3800, June 2002 See Reverse for Instructions

Figure 4-1

AUTHORIZATION FOR RELEASE OF INFORMATION

Section A: Must be completed for all authorizations.

I hereby authorize the use or disclosure of my individually identifiable health information as described below.
I understand that this authorization is voluntary. I understand that if the organization to receive the information is not a health plan or health care provider, the released information may no longer be protected by federal privacy regulations.

Patient name: ______________________ **ID Number:** ______________

Persons/organizations providing information: ______________________

Persons/organizations receiving information: ______________________

Specific description of information [including date(s)]: ______________________

Section B: Must be completed only if a health plan or a health care provider has requested the authorization.

1. The health plan or health care provider must complete the following:
   a. What is the purpose of the use or disclosure? ______________________
   b. Will the health plan or health care provider requesting the authorization receive financial or in-kind compensation in exchange for using or disclosing the health information described above? Yes____ No ____
2. The patient or the patient's representative must read and initial the following statements:
   a. I understand that my health care and the payment of my health care will not be affected if I do not sign this form.
   Initials: __________
   b. I understand that I may see and copy the information described on this form if I ask for it, and that I get a copy of this form after I sign it.
   Initials: __________

Section C: Must be completed for all authorizations.

The patient or the patient's representative must read and initial the following statements:

1. I understand that this authorization will expire on ____/____ /____ (DD/MM/YR).
   Initials: __________
2. I understand that I may revoke this authorization at any time by notifying the providing organization in writing, but if I do not it will not have any effect on actions they took before they received the revocation.
   Initials: __________

______________________ ______________
Signature of patient or patient's representative **Date**
(Form MUST be completed before signing)

Printed name of patient's representative: ______________________

Relationship to patient: ______________________

***YOU MAY REFUSE TO SIGN THIS AUTHORIZATION**
You may not use this form to release information for treatment or payment except when the information to be released is psychotherapy notes or certain research information.

Figure 4-2

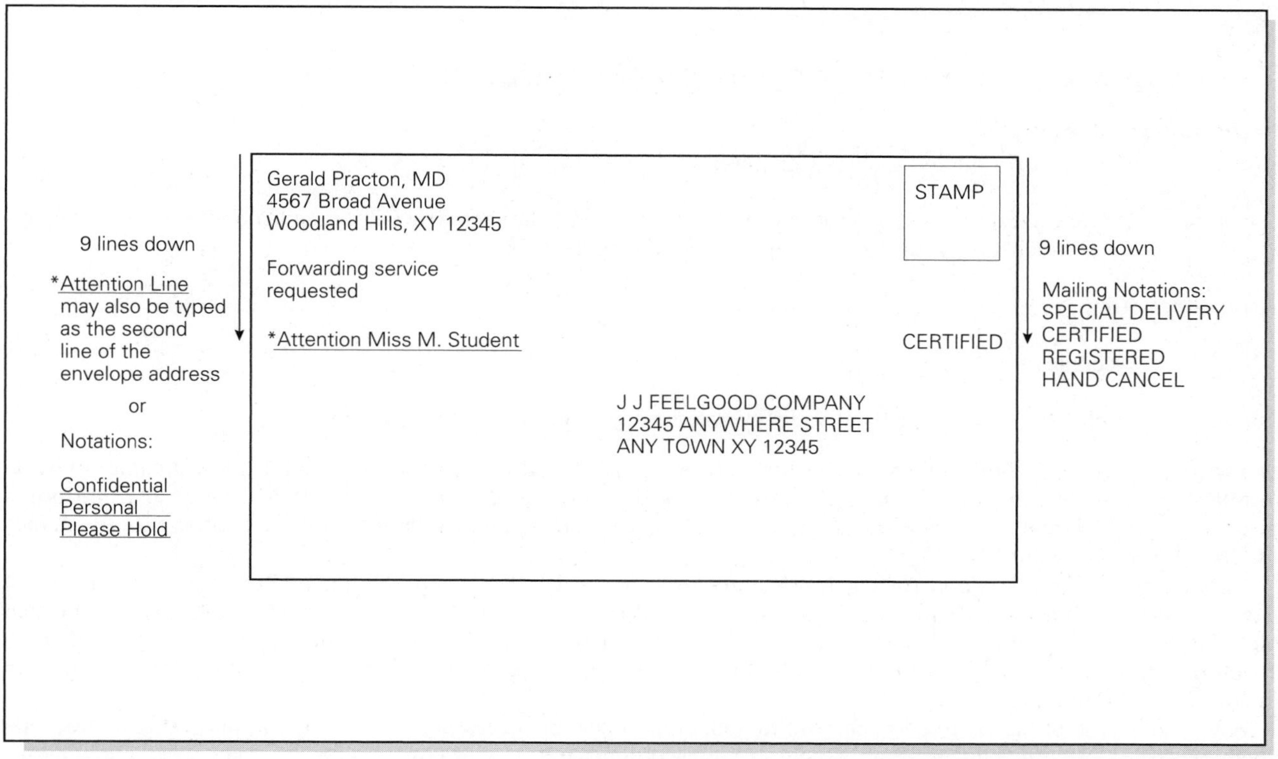

9 lines down
*Attention Line may also be typed as the second line of the envelope address
or
Notations:
Confidential
Personal
Please Hold
Gerald Practon, MD
4567 Broad Avenue
Woodland Hills, XY 12345
Forwarding service requested
*Attention Miss M. Student
STAMP
CERTIFIED
J J FEELGOOD COMPANY
12345 ANYWHERE STREET
ANY TOWN XY 12345
9 lines down
Mailing Notations:
SPECIAL DELIVERY
CERTIFIED
REGISTERED
HAND CANCEL

Figure 4-3

ASSIGNMENT 4-7 KEY A LETTER TO CONFIRM DISCHARGE BY THE PATIENT

Performance Objective

Task: Key letter for the physician's signature.

Conditions: Use one sheet of letterhead (print from Evolve website), number 10 envelope, and U.S. Postal Service forms for certified mail with return receipt requested (Figure 4-4).

Standards: Time: ______________ minutes

Accuracy: ______________

(Note: The time element and accuracy criteria may be given by your instructor.)

Directions: Mr. Walter J. Stone telephones on June 3, sounding extremely upset and irrational. He says that he is unable to return to work on June 22 and that he does not want to be seen by Dr. Input again. Type a letter to confirm this discharge by the patient (see *Handbook* Figure 4-23). Suggest that he contact the local medical society for the names of three internists for further care.

This letter must be prepared for Dr. Input's signature because it is a legal document. Refer to Assignment 7-4 for information from the patient record. Use a letterhead (printed from the Evolve website) and key in modified block style as shown in *Handbook* Figure 4-21. Use the current date. Key Mr. Stone's address on a number 10 envelope, referring to *Workbook* Figure 4-3. Send the letter by certified mail with return receipt requested, referring to *Handbook* Figure 4-22.

After the instructor has returned your work to you, either make the necessary corrections and place it in a three-ring notebook for future reference, or, if you receive a high score, place it in your portfolio for reference when applying for a job.

UNITED STATES POSTAL SERVICE

First-Class Mail
Postage & Fees Paid
USPS
Permit No. G-10

• Sender: Please print your name, address, and ZIP+4 in this box •

SENDER: *COMPLETE THIS SECTION*

- Complete items 1, 2, and 3. Also complete item 4 if Restricted Delivery is desired.
- Print your name and address on the reverse so that we can return the card to you.
- Attach this card to the back of the mailpiece, or on the front if space permits.

1. Article Addressed to:

COMPLETE THIS SECTION ON DELIVERY

A. Signature

X

☐ Agent
☐ Addressee

B. Received by (*Printed Name*) | C. Date of Delivery

D. Is delivery address different from item 1? ☐ Yes
If YES, enter delivery address below: ☐ No

3. Service Type
☐ Certified Mail ☐ Express Mail
☐ Registered ☐ Return Receipt for Merchandise
☐ Insured Mail ☐ C.O.D.

4. Restricted Delivery? (*Extra Fee*) ☐ Yes

2. Article Number
(*Transfer from service label*)

PS Form 3811, February 2004 Domestic Return Receipt 102595-02-M-1540

7006 0810 0001 6207 8857

PLACE STICKER AT TOP OF ENVELOPE TO THE RIGHT OF THE RETURN ADDRESS, FOLD AT DOTTED LINE

CERTIFIED MAIL™

7006 0810 0001 6207 8857

7006 0810 0001 6207 8857

U.S. Postal Service™
CERTIFIED MAIL™ RECEIPT
(Domestic Mail Only; No Insurance Coverage Provided)

For delivery information visit our website at www.usps.com®

OFFICIAL USE

Postage	$	Postmark Here
Certified Fee		
Return Receipt Fee (Endorsement Required)		
Restricted Delivery Fee (Endorsement Required)		
Total Postage & Fees	**$**	

Sent To

Street, Apt. No.; or PO Box No.

City, State, ZIP+4

PS Form 3800, June 2002 **See Reverse for Instructions**

Figure 4-4

5 Diagnostic Coding

Linda Smith

KEY TERMS

Your instructor may wish to select some words pertinent to this chapter for a test. For definitions of the terms, further study, and/or reference, the words, phrases, and abbreviations may be found in the glossary at the end of the Handbook. *Key terms for this chapter follow.*

adverse effect
benign tumor
chief complaint
combination code
computer-assisted coding
conventions
eponym
essential modifiers
etiology
Excludes 1
Excludes 2
external causes of morbidity
in situ
International Classification of Diseases, Ninth Revision, Clinical Modification
International Classification of Diseases, Tenth Revision, Clinical Modification
International Classification of Diseases, Tenth Revision, Procedure Coding System
intoxication
late effect
malignant tumor
metastasis
neoplasm
nonessential modifiers
not elsewhere classifiable
not otherwise specified
Official ICD-9-CM Guidelines for Coding and Reporting
physician's fee profile
placeholder
poisoning
primary diagnosis
principal diagnosis
secondary diagnosis
sequela
syndrome
Z codes

KEY ABBREVIATIONS

AHA ____________________

AHIMA ____________________

CAC ____________________

CC ____________________

CM ____________________

CPT ____________________

DM ____________________

DRG ____________________

ICD-9-CM ____________________

ICD-10-CM ____________________

ICD-10-PCS ____________________

MRI ____________________

NCHS ____________________

NEC ____________________

NOS ____________________

Z codes ____________________

PERFORMANCE OBJECTIVES

The student will be able to:

- Define and spell the key terms and key abbreviations for this chapter, given the information from the *Handbook* glossary, within a reasonable time period and with enough accuracy to obtain a satisfactory evaluation.
- Answer the fill-in-the-blank, multiple choice, and true/false review questions after reading the chapter, with enough accuracy to obtain a satisfactory evaluation.
- Assignment 5-2: Indicate main terms, subterms, subterms to subterms, and carryover lines, given a section of a page from the ICD-10-CM code book, with enough accuracy to obtain a satisfactory evaluation.
- Assignment 5-3: Answer questions given a section of a page from the ICD-10-CM code book, with enough accuracy to obtain a satisfactory evaluation.
- Assignment 5-4: Select the correct diagnostic code numbers, given diagnoses, and locate the conditions using Volumes 1 and 2 of the ICD-10-CM code book, with enough accuracy to obtain a satisfactory evaluation.
- Assignments 5-5 through 5-12: Select the correct diagnostic code numbers, given a series of scenarios and diagnoses using Volumes 1 and 2 of the ICD-10-CM code book, with enough accuracy to obtain a satisfactory evaluation.

STUDY OUTLINE

The Diagnosis Coding for Outpatient Professional Services
- Physician's Fee Profile
- Assigning a Diagnosis Code
- Sequencing of Diagnostic Codes
- Admitting Diagnoses
- Medical Necessity

International Classification of Diseases
- History
- Transition From ICD-9-CM to ICD-10-CM

ICD-10 Diagnosis and Procedure Codes
- ICD-10-CM
- ICD-10-PCS

Organization and Format of ICD-10-CM
- Standard Transaction Code Sets
- Alphabetic Index to Diseases and Injuries
- Tabular List of Diseases and Injuries

Official Coding Guidelines for ICD-10-CM
- Diagnostic Code Book Conventions
- General Coding Guidelines
- Chapter-Specific Coding Guidelines
- Diagnostic Coding and Reporting Guidelines for Outpatient Services
- Handy Hints for Diagnostic Coding
- Computer-Assisted Coding

Procedure 5-1: Basic Steps in Selecting Diagnostic Codes From ICD-9-CM

Procedure 5-2: Basic Steps in Selecting Diagnostic Codes From ICD-10-CM

ASSIGNMENT 5-1 REVIEW QUESTIONS

Part I Fill in the Blank on ICD-10-CM

Review the objectives, key terms, and chapter information before completing the following review questions.

1. Insurance carriers keep ______________, which are a compilation of statistics regarding services and payments made to the physician over a period of time.

2. When submitting insurance claims for patients seen in a physician's office or in an outpatient hospital setting, the ______________ diagnosis is listed first, but in the inpatient hospital setting, the ______________ diagnosis is used.

3. Claims to insurance carriers often are denied because of lack of ______________, which indicates that the procedure provided was not payable for the diagnosis submitted.

4. Diagnosis coding for services provided by a physician are reported using ICD-10-CM effective with dates of service ______________________________.

5. The abbreviation ICD-10-CM means ______________________________
____.

6. The official version of the International Classification of Disease was developed by the ____.

7. ICD-10-CM requires ______________ documentation in the medical record than the previous coding system, ICD-9-CM.

8. ICD-10-CM is the coding system for reporting inpatient services by hospitals and replaces ______________ of the ICD-9-CM coding system.

9. ICD-10-CM is the standard code set required under ______________ legislation and must be used by covered entities when assigning diagnostic codes.

10. Volume 2, Diseases, is a/an ______________ index or listing of code numbers.

11. Volume 1, Diseases, is a/an ______________ listing of code numbers.

12. When using the ICD-10-CM coding system, the ______________ is used as a placeholder to save space for future code expansion.

13. Conventions are ______________ used in the diagnostic code books to assist in the selection of correct codes for the diagnosis encountered.

14. The abbreviation NEC appearing in the ICD-10-CM code book means ______________.

15. ______________ are used to enclose synonyms in the Tabular List.

16. If a condition is documented in the medical record, but it is not specified as to whether the condition is acute or chronic, then the ______________ code should be assigned.

17. When selecting a code that corresponds with the condition stated in the medical record, the coder should first locate the term in the ______________ and then confirm the code in the ____.

18. The instructional note ______________ listed in the Tabular List assists the coder as to when it is appropriate to report a secondary code.

19. A condition that is produced after the acute phase of an illness is listed as the main term ______________ in the Alphabetic Index.

20. When reporting a condition that affects the left side of the patient, the character ______________ is reported to indicate laterality.

21. The neoplasm table has column headings for ______________, ______________, ______________, and ______________.

22. In juvenile diabetes, the patient's ______________ does not function and produce enough insulin.

23. When coding for diabetes in pregnancy, a code from category ______________ is assigned as the primary diagnosis.

24. ______________ hypertension is indicative of a life-threatening condition.

25. Full-term uncomplicated ______________ deliveries are always reported with the code O80.

26. When reporting accidents and injuries, a seventh character of "A" identifies that the encounter is ____.

27. Additional external cause codes are ______________ when reporting poisonings using combination codes from T36 through T65.

28. If documentation states that the incident related to a poisoning was a suspected suicide attempt, the code would be reported from the column titled ______________.

29. If a patient falls and fractures his or her wrist, the fracture code is the primary code, followed by a/an ______________ code to explain how the accident occurred.

30. When a person encounters health services to receive a vaccination, the diagnosis is reported with a ____.

Part II Multiple Choice on ICD-10-CM

Directions: Choose the best answer.

31. The consequences of inaccurate assignment of diagnostic codes include
    a. delay in payment of claim.
    b. denial of claim.
    c. change in level of reimbursement.
    d. all of the above.

32. Diagnosis codes should be reported to the highest level of
    a. specificity.
    b. medical necessity.
    c. etiology.
    d. sequel.

33. When a provider makes a hospital visit, the encounter should be reported with a diagnosis code that represents
    a. the reason the patient was admitted to the hospital.
    b. the condition the provider evaluated and treated during the encounter.
    c. the condition that was requested by the admitting physician.
    d. the final discharge diagnosis.

34. To determine the diagnosis codes that would support medical necessity of a specific procedure such as an MRI under Medicare guidelines, the coder should consult
    a. CPT guidelines.
    b. LCDs and NCDs.
    c. all of the above.
    d. none of the above.

35. Passage of which legislation, in 1988, placed requirements on physicians to report appropriate diagnosis codes on all claims to Medicare?
    a. Affordable Care Act
    b. HIPAA
    c. American Recovery and Reinvestment Act
    d. Medicare Catastrophic Coverage Act

36. GEMS is a common translation tool used to
    a. convert ICD-9-CM codes to ICD-10-CM codes.
    b. convert ICD-10-CM codes to ICD-10-PCS codes.
    c. convert ICD-10-CM codes to ICD-9-CM codes.
    d. a and c.
    e. All of the above.

37. ICD-10-PCS (Procedure Coding System) was developed by 3M Health Information Systems under contract with the
    a. National Center for Health Statistics.
    b. World Health Organization.
    c. Centers for Disease Control.
    d. Centers for Medicare and Medicaid Services.

38. Annual updates to ICD-10-CM are published
    a. by the AMA and AHA.
    b. by the AHA and AHIMA.
    c. by the AHA, AHIMA, and U.S. Printing Office.
    d. by the AMA, AHA, AHIMA, and U.S. Printing Office.

39. The Alphabetic Index to Diseases and Injuries is placed
    a. after Volume 1, the Tabular Index.
    b. first in the coding manual.
    c. after the Table of Drugs and Chemicals.
    d. after the Index to External Causes.

40. How many chapters does the Tabular List contain?
    a. 17
    b. 17 with two supplementary classifications
    c. 19
    d. 21

41. When two diagnoses are classified with a single code, it is referred to as
    a. a combination code.
    b. a manifestation.
    c. an external cause code.
    d. a Z code.

42. An essential modifier is also referred to as a
    a. main term.
    b. nonessential modifier.
    c. subterm.
    d. convention.

43. The equivalent of unspecified is
    a. NEC.
    b. NOS.
    c. nonessential.
    d. secondary.

44. Signs and symptoms are acceptable for reporting purposes
    a. in all situations.
    b. in addition to the definitive diagnosis.
    c. when a definitive diagnosis has not been determined.
    d. under no circumstances.

45. When conditions documented as "threatened" are referenced in the Alphabetic Index and there is no entry for the threatened condition, report
    a. with signs and symptoms.
    b. as if the patient has the condition.
    c. the existing underlying condition.
    d. all of the above.

46. When reporting laterality, the final character "3" is reported to indicate
   a. right side.
   b. left side.
   c. bilateral.
   d. unspecified.

47. When reporting an encounter for testing of HIV, the code should be assigned as
   a. B20.
   b. R75.
   c. Z11.4.
   d. Z21.

48. When fractures are documented, but there is no indication of whether the fracture is open or closed,
   a. report as closed.
   b. report as open.
   c. it does not matter if it is reported as open or closed.
   d. report as unspecified.

49. When identifying the total body surface area of a burn, the front torso is considered as
   a. 1%.
   b. 9%.
   c. 18%.
   d. 36%.

50. External cause codes are used to
   a. generate additional revenue.
   b. establish injury prevention programs.
   c. a and b.
   d. none of the above.

Part III True/False

Write "T" or "F" in the blank to indicate whether you think the statement is true or false.

________ 51. Diagnoses that relate to the patient's previous medical problem must always be reported.

________ 52. The concept of "principal diagnosis" is applicable to outpatient and inpatient cases.

________ 53. The diagnosis coding system is designed to provide statistical mortality rate data that include information about causes of diseases.

________ 54. The process for looking up a diagnosis code in the ICD-9-CM coding system is the same as in the ICD-10-CM coding system.

________ 55. ICD-10 was published by the WHO and clinically modified by CMS.

________ 56. The Alphabetic Index contains the Table of Drugs and Chemicals.

________ 57. ICD-10-CM codes can contain up to seven characters.

________ 58. Signs and symptoms that are not typically associated with a disease process should be reported when documented.

________ 59. When a person who is not currently sick encounters health services for some specific purpose, such as to receive a vaccination, then a Z code is used.

________ 60. Code conventions are rules or principles for determining a diagnostic code when using a diagnostic code book.

________ 61. Because there are annual ICD-10-CM code revisions, there is a 3-month grace period to implement these changes and revisions.

________ 62. An external cause code may never be sequenced as the primary diagnosis in the first position.

ASSIGNMENT 5-2 LOCATING INFORMATION IN ICD-9-CM, VOLUME 2

Performance Objective

Task: Answer questions pertaining to categories 320 and 321 of ICD-9-CM, Volume 2.

Conditions: Use the abstracted section from ICD-9-CM, Volume 2 and pen or pencil.

Standards: Time: ______________ minutes

Accuracy: ______________

(Note: The time element and accuracy criteria may be given by your instructor.)

Directions: Refer to a section from a page of ICD-9-CM, Volume 2 (Figure 5-1), and answer questions pertaining to categories 320 and 321.

1. Locate the section title. ____

2. Refer to the INCLUSION TERMS listed under category code 320, titled "Bacterial meningitis." Place an "X" in front of each of the following diagnostic statements that are included in category 320.

______________ purulent meningitis

______________ bacterial meningomyelitis

______________ meningitis

______________ meningoencephalitis

______________ pyogenic meningitis

______________ meningococcal

3. Refer to the EXCLUSION TERMS located under code 320.7, titled "Meningitis in other bacterial diseases classified elsewhere." Place an "X" in front of the following code number(s) that are excluded.

______________ secondary syphilis 091.81

______________ acquired syphilis 097.9

______________ gonococcal meningitis 098.82

______________ congenital syphilis 090.42

______________ primary syphilis 091.2

______________ gram-negative anaerobes 320.81

6. NERVOUS SYSTEM AND SENSE ORGANS (320-389)

INFLAMMATORY DISEASES OF THE CENTRAL NERVOUS SYSTEM (320-326)

320 Bacterial meningitis

Includes: arachnoiditis, leptomeningitis, meningitis, meningoencephalitis, meningomyelitis, pachymeningitis } bacterial

320.0 *Haemophilus* meningitis

Meningitis due to *Haemophilus influenzae* [*H. Influenzae*]

320.1 Pneumococcal meningitis

320.2 Streptococcal meningitis

320.3 Staphylococcal meningitis

320.7 Meningitis in other bacterial diseases classified elsewhere

Code first underlying diseases as:
actinomycosis (039.8)
listeriosis (027.0)
typhoid fever (002.0)
whooping cough (033.0-033.9)

Excludes: *meningitis (in):*
epidemic (036.0)
gonococcal (098.82)
meningococcal (036.0)
salmonellosis (003.21)
syphilis:
NOS (094.2)
congenital (090.42)
meningovascular (094.2)
secondary (091.81)
tuberculous (013.0)

320.8 Meningitis due to other specified bacteria

320.81 Anaerobic meningitis

Bacteroides (fragilis)
Gram-negative anaerobes

320.82 Meningitis due to gram-negative bacteria, not elsewhere classified

Aerobacter aerogenes
Escherichia coli [E. coli]
Friedländer bacillus
Klebsiella pneumoniae
Proteus morganii
Pseudomonas

Excludes: *gram-negative anaerobes (320.81)*

320.89 Meningitis due to other specified bacteria

Bacillus pyocyaneus

320.9 Meningitis due to unspecified bacterium

Meningitis:
bacterial NOS
purulent NOS
pyogenic NOS
suppurative NOS

321 Meningitis due to other organisms

Includes: arachnoiditis, leptomeningitis, meningitis, pachymeningitis } due to organisms other than bacteria

321.0 Cryptococcal meningitis

Code first underlying disease (117.5)

Figure 5-1

4. Place an "X" in front of each of the following diagnostic statements included in category code 320 and its subcategories.

_______________ leptomeningitis

_______________ meningitis resulting from *E. coli*

_______________ pyogenic meningitis

_______________ epidemic meningitis

_______________ tuberculous meningitis

5. Write the code numbers for category 320 that require fifth digits.

____

ASSIGNMENT 5-3 LOCATING INFORMATION IN ICD-10-CM, VOLUME 2

Performance Objective

Task: Answer questions pertaining to categories G00-G09 of ICD-10-CM, Volume 2.

Conditions: Use the abstracted section from ICD-10-CM, Volume 2 and pen or pencil.

Standards: Time: ______________ minutes

Accuracy: ______________

(Note: The time element and accuracy criteria may be given by your instructor.)

Directions: Refer to a section from a page of ICD-10-CM, Volume 2 (Figure 5-2), and answer questions pertaining to categories G00 through G09.

1. Locate the section title. ____

2. Place an "X" in front of each of the following diagnostic statements included in category code G00 and its subcategories.

______________ bacterial leptomeningitis

______________ bacterial meningitis

______________ bacterial meningomyelitis

______________ leptospirosis

______________ tuberculous meningitis

______________ meningoencephalitis

______________ bacterial arachnoiditis

3. Refer to the EXCLUSION 1 note located under category code G01, titled "Meningitis in bacterial diseases classified elsewhere." Place an "X" in front of the following code number(s) that are excluded.

______________ gonococcal meningitis A54.81

______________ Meningitis due to measles (B05.1)

______________ Meningitis in Neurosyphilis (A52.13)

______________ Hemophilus meningitis (G00.0)

______________ Meningitis due to candidal (B37.5)

______________ Lyme disease (A69.21)

INFLAMMATORY DISEASES OF THE CENTRAL NERVOUS SYSTEM (G00-G09)

● **G00 Bacterial meningitis, not elsewhere classified**

An infection of the cerebrospinal fluid surrounding the spinal cord and brain.

Includes bacterial arachnoiditis
bacterial leptomeningitis
bacterial meningitis
bacterial pachymeningitis

Excludes1 bacterial:
meningoencephalitis (G04.2)
meningomyelitis (G04.2)

G00.0 Hemophilus meningitis
Meningitis due to Hemophilus influenzae

G00.1 Pneumococcal meningitis

G00.2 Streptococcal meningitis
Use additional code to further identify organism (B95.0-B95.5)

G00.3 Staphylococcal meningitis
Use additional code to further identify organism (B95.61-B95.8)

G00.8 Other bacterial meningitis
Meningitis due to Escherichia coli
Meningitis due to Friedländer bacillus
Meningitis due to Klebsiella
Use additional code to further identify organism (B96.-)

■ **G00.9 Bacterial meningitis, unspecified**
Meningitis due to gram-negative bacteria, unspecified
Purulent meningitis NOS
Pyogenic meningitis NOS
Suppurative meningitis NOS

●◗ ***G01 Meningitis in bacterial diseases classified elsewhere***

Code first underlying disease

Excludes1 meningitis (in):
gonococcal (A54.81)
leptospirosis (A27.81)
listeriosis (A32.11)
Lyme disease (A69.21)
meningococcal (A39.0)
neurosyphilis (A52.13)
tuberculosis (A17.0)
meningoencephalitis and meningomyelitis in bacterial diseases classified elsewhere (G05)

Figure 5-2

Continued

G02 ***Meningitis in other infectious and parasitic diseases classified elsewhere***

Code first underlying disease, such as:

African trypanosomiasis (B56.-)

poliovirus infection (A80.-)

Excludes1 candidal meningitis (B37.5)

coccidioidomycosis meningitis (B38.4)

cryptococcal meningitis (B45.1)

herpesviral [herpes simplex] meningitis (B00.3)

infectious mononucleosis complicated by meningitis (B27.- with fourth character 2)

measles complicated by meningitis (B05.1)

meningoencephalitis and meningomyelitis in other infectious and parasitic diseases classified elsewhere (G05)

mumps meningitis (B26.1)

rubella meningitis (B06.02)

varicella [chickenpox] meningitis (B01.0)

zoster meningitis (B02.1)

G03 Meningitis due to other and unspecified causes

Includes arachnoiditis NOS

leptomeningitis NOS

meningitis NOS

pachymeningitis NOS

Excludes1 meningoencephalitis (G04.-)

meningomyelitis (G04.-)

G03.0 Nonpyogenic meningitis

Aseptic meningitis

Nonbacterial meningitis

G03.1 Chronic meningitis

G03.2 Benign recurrent meningitis [Mollaret]

G03.8 Meningitis due to other specified causes

G03.9 Meningitis, unspecified

Arachnoiditis (spinal) NOS

G04 Encephalitis, myelitis and encephalomyelitis

Includes acute ascending myelitis

meningoencephalitis

meningomyelitis

Excludes1 encephalopathy NOS (G93.40)

other noninfectious acute disseminated encephalomyelitis (noninfectious ADEM) (G04.81)

Excludes2 acute transverse myelitis (G37.3-)

alcoholic encephalopathy (G31.2)

benign myalgic encephalomyelitis (G93.3)

multiple sclerosis (G35)

subacute necrotizing myelitis (G37.4)

toxic encephalitis (G92)

toxic encephalopathy (G92)

G04.0 Acute disseminated encephalitis and encephalomyelitis (ADEM)

Excludes1 acute necrotizing hemorrhagic encephalopathy (G04.3-)

G04.00 Acute disseminated encephalitis and encephalomyelitis, unspecified

G04.01 Postinfectious acute disseminated encephalitis and encephalomyelitis (postinfectious ADEM)

Excludes1 post chickenpox encephalitis (B01.1)

post measles encephalitis (B05.0)

post measles myelitis (B05.1)

G04.02 Postimmunization acute disseminated encephalitis, myelitis and encephalomyelitis

Encephalitis, post immunization

Encephalomyelitis, post immunization

Use additional code to identify the vaccine (T50.A-, T50.B-, T50.Z-)

G04.1 Tropical spastic paraplegia

G04.2 Bacterial meningoencephalitis and meningomyelitis, not elsewhere classified

G04.3 Acute necrotizing hemorrhagic encephalopathy

Sudden and severe CNS disease with pathology of hemorrhages and necrosis of white matter

Excludes1 acute disseminated encephalitis and encephalomyelitis (G04.0-)

G04.30 Acute necrotizing hemorrhagic encephalopathy, unspecified

G04.31 Postinfectious acute necrotizing hemorrhagic encephalopathy

G04.32 Postimmunization acute necrotizing hemorrhagic encephalopathy

Use additional code to identify vaccine (T50.A-, T50.B-, T50.Z-)

G04.39 Other acute necrotizing hemorrhagic encephalopathy

Code also underlying etiology, if applicable

G04.8 Other encephalitis, myelitis and encephalomyelitis

Code also any associated seizure (G40.-, R56.9)

G04.81 Other encephalitis and encephalomyelitis

Noninfectious acute disseminated encephalomyelitis (noninfectious ADEM)

G04.89 Other myelitis

G04.9 Encephalitis, myelitis and encephalomyelitis, unspecified

G04.90 Encephalitis and encephalomyelitis, unspecified

Ventriculitis (cerebral) NOS

G04.91 Myelitis, unspecified

Figure 5-2, cont'd

4. Place an X in front of each of the following diagnostic statements included in category code G04 and its subcategories.

_______________ meningymyelitis

_______________ meningoencphalitis

_______________ pyogenic meningitis

_______________ epidemic meningitis

_______________ tuberculous meningitis

_______________ acute ascending myelitis

5. Write the code numbers for category G04.0 that require fifth digits.

____

DIAGNOSTIC CODING ASSIGNMENTS

In this chapter, the points awarded for assignments that require diagnostic codes are 1 point for each correct digit.

ASSIGNMENT 5-4 OBTAIN GENERAL DIAGNOSTIC CODES FOR CONDITIONS

Performance Objective

Task: Locate the correct diagnostic code for each diagnosis listed.

Conditions: Use pen or pencil and ICD-10-CM diagnostic code book.

Standards: Time: ________________ minutes

Accuracy: ________________

(Note: The time element and accuracy criteria may be given by your instructor.)

Directions: Using the *International Classification of Diseases, Tenth Revision, Clinical Modification* (ICD-10-CM) code book, read each diagnosis and locate the condition in Volume 2, the Alphabetic Index. Then go to Volume 1, to the Tabular List of Diseases. Match the definition as closely as possible to the written description and assign the correct code, entering it on the blank line.

Problems	ICD-10-CM Codes
1. Breast mass	________________
2. *Klebsiella* pneumonia	________________
3. Acute lateral wall myocardial infarction; initial episode	________________
4. Acute cerebrovascular accident	________________
5. Atherosclerotic cardiovascular disease	________________
6. Dyspnea, R/O cystic fibrosis	________________
7. Ileitis	________________
8. Osteoarthritis of elbow	________________
9. Tinnitus	________________
10. Acute exacerbation of chronic asthmatic bronchitis	________________

ASSIGNMENT 5-5 CODE DIAGNOSES FROM MEDICAL RECORDS

Performance Objective

Task: Locate the correct diagnostic code for each case scenario.

Conditions: Use pen or pencil and ICD-10-CM diagnostic code book.

Standards: Time: ______________ minutes

Accuracy: ______________

(Note: The time element and accuracy criteria may be given by your instructor.)

Directions: This exercise will give you experience in basic diagnostic coding for physicians' insurance claims. First list the ICD-10-CM code for the diagnosis, condition, problem, or other reason for the admission and/or encounter (visit) shown in the medical record to be chiefly responsible for the services provided. Then list additional diagnostic codes that describe any coexisting conditions that affect patient care. Always assign codes to their highest level of specificity—the more digits, the more specific. Do not code probable, rule out, suspected, or questionable conditions. Assign the correct code(s), entering it (them) on the blank line.

Problems — **ICD-10-CM Codes**

Problem 1. A patient, Mrs. Jennifer Hanson, calls Dr. Input's office stating she has blood in her stool. Dr. Input suspects a GI bleed and tells Mrs. Hanson to come in immediately. It is discovered that the reason for the blood in the stool is a bleeding duodenal ulcer. Code the diagnosis to be listed on the insurance claim for the office visit. ______________

Problem 2. a. Jason Belmen comes in with a fractured humerus. He also has chronic obstructive pulmonary disease (COPD), which is not treated. Code the diagnosis. ______________

b. Assume Mr. Belmen needs general anesthesia for open reduction of the fractured humerus. The COPD could now be considered a risk factor. List the diagnostic code in the second part of this scenario. ______________

Problem 3. Margarita Sanchez came into the office for removal of sutures. Code the diagnosis. ______________

Problem 4. A patient, George Martin, has benign prostatic hypertrophy (BPH). He is seen for catheterization because of urinary retention. Code the primary and secondary diagnoses for the office visit. (Note: BPH is an enlargement of the prostate gland, due to overgrowth of androgen-sensitive glandular elements, which occurs naturally with aging.) ______________

Problem 5. Mia Bartholomew is seen in the office complaining of a sore throat. A throat culture is done, and the specimen is sent to an outside laboratory for a culture and sensitivity study to determine the presence of *Streptococcus*. List the diagnostic code the physician would use if the insurance claim is submitted before the results are known. List the diagnostic code used if the physician submits the insurance claim after the laboratory report is received indicating *Streptococcus* is present. ______________

ASSIGNMENT 5-6 CODE DIAGNOSES USING Z CODES

Performance Objective

Task: Locate the correct diagnostic code for each case scenario.

Conditions: Use pen or pencil and ICD-10-CM diagnostic code book.

Standards: Time: ______________ minutes

Accuracy: ______________

(Note: The time element and accuracy criteria may be given by your instructor.)

Directions: In this exercise, you will be reviewing Z codes in the ICD-10-CM code book. Assign the correct code, entering it on the blank line. These are some key words under which Z codes may be located in Volume 2:

admission	checking/checkup	donor	insertion of	status post
aftercare	conflict	evaluation	maintenance	vaccination
attention to	contact	examination	observation	
border	contraception	fitting of	person with	
care of	counseling	follow-up	problem with	
carrier	dialysis	history of	screening	

Problems **ICD-10-CM Codes**

1. Kathy Osborn, a patient, is seen in the office for an annual checkup. ______________
2. Daniel Matsui is seen in the office for adjustment of a lumbosacral corset. ______________
3. Philip O'Brien comes into the office to receive a prophylactic flu shot. ______________
4. Bernadette Murphy is seen in the office for a pregnancy test; the result is positive. ______________
5. Michiko Fujita is seen in the office for a fractured rib. No x-rays are taken because Mrs. Fujita thinks she is pregnant. ______________
6. Dr. Perry Cardi sees Kenneth Pickford in the office for a cardiac pacemaker adjustment. The pacemaker was implanted because of sick sinus syndrome. ______________
7. Frank Meadows returns for follow-up, postoperative transurethral prostatic resection (TURP) for prostate cancer after treatment has been completed. ______________

ASSIGNMENT 5-7 CODE NEOPLASTIC DIAGNOSES

Performance Objective

Task: Locate the correct diagnostic code for each diagnosis listed.

Conditions: Use pen or pencil and ICD-10-CM diagnostic code book.

Standards: Time: ______________ minutes

Accuracy: ______________

(Note: The time element and accuracy criteria may be given by your instructor.)

Directions: In this exercise, you will be reviewing diagnostic codes in the ICD-10-CM code book involving neoplasms. Assign the correct code, entering it on the blank line.

Problems	ICD-10-CM Codes
1. Leiomyoma, uterus	______________
2. Ewing's sarcoma, forearm	______________
3. Adenocarcinoma, right breast, central portion, female	______________
4. Dyspnea resulting from carcinoma of the breast, female with metastasis to the upper lobe, right lung	______________
5. Patient is seen for a yearly examination 1 year after a mastectomy for breast cancer; she is disease-free at this time	______________

ASSIGNMENT 5-8 CODE DIAGNOSES FOR PATIENTS WITH DIABETES

Performance Objective

Task: Locate the correct diagnostic code for each diagnosis listed.

Conditions: Use pen or pencil and ICD-10-CM diagnostic code book.

Standards: Time: ______________ minutes

Accuracy: ______________

(Note: The time element and accuracy criteria may be given by your instructor.)

Directions: In this exercise, you will review diagnostic codes in the ICD-10-CM code book involving cases of patients with diabetes. The diabetes codes are combination codes that include the type of diabetes, the body system affected, and the complications affecting that body system. Use as many codes as are necessary to describe all of the complications of the disease. Assign as many codes from categories E08 through E13 as needed to identify all of the associated conditions that the patient has.

Example: If a patient with type 2 uncontrolled diabetes is treated for a skin ulcer on the lower extremity, look up "diabetes" in Volume 2 and find the subterm "with skin ulcer." The diabetes code listed is E11.622. Go to Volume 1 and verify. Volume 1 instructs you to *use additional code to identify site of ulcer* (L97.-, L98.-). The additional code L97.809 is selected as it describes *Non-pressure chronic ulcer of other part of unspecified lower leg with unspecified severity.*

Always verify all codes in Volume 1 before assigning them. Assign the correct code(s) for each case involving diabetes, entering it (them) on the blank line.

Problems	ICD-10-CM Codes
1. Diabetes mellitus	______________
2. Type 2, non–insulin-dependent diabetes mellitus with neuropathy.	______________
3. Diabetic gangrene (type 1 diabetes)	______________
4. Type 2 diabetes with cataract	______________
5. Type 1 diabetes with diabetic polyneuropathy and retinopathy	______________

ASSIGNMENT 5-9 CODE DIAGNOSES FOR PATIENTS WITH HYPERTENSION

Performance Objective

Task: Locate the correct diagnostic code for each diagnosis listed.

Conditions: Use pen or pencil and ICD-10-CM diagnostic code book.

Standards: Time: ________________ minutes

Accuracy: ________________

(Note: The time element and accuracy criteria may be given by your instructor.)

Directions: In this exercise, you will review diagnostic codes in the ICD-10-CM code book involving patients who have hypertension. To begin coding, look in Volume 2 under "hypertension."

Assign the correct code(s) for each case, entering it (them) on the blank line.

Problems	ICD-10-CM Codes
1. High blood pressure reading	________________
2. Malignant hypertension	________________
3. Hypertension complicating pregnancy	________________
4. Hypertension with kidney disease	________________
5. Hypertension due to arteriosclerotic cardiovascular disease (ASCVD) and systolic congestive heart failure (CHF)	________________
6. Myocarditis and CHF due to malignant hypertension	________________

ASSIGNMENT 5-10 CODE DIAGNOSES FOR INJURIES, FRACTURES, BURNS, LATE EFFECTS, AND COMPLICATIONS

Performance Objective

Task: Locate the correct diagnostic code for each diagnosis listed.

Conditions: Use pen or pencil and ICD—CM diagnostic code book.

Standards: Time: ______________ minutes

Accuracy: ______________

(Note: The time element and accuracy criteria may be given by your instructor.)

Directions: In this exercise, you will review diagnostic codes from the ICD-10-CM code book involving patients who have suffered injuries, burns, fractures, and late effects. Here are some guidelines for coding injuries, fractures, burns, late effects, and complications.

Injuries

When coding injuries, assign separate codes for each injury unless a combination code is provided, in which case the combination code is assigned. The code for the most serious injury, as determined by the provider and the focus of treatment, is sequenced first.

Fractures

Fractures are presumed to be closed unless otherwise specified. Fracture not indicated, whether displaced or not displaced, should be coded as displaced.

Burns

Multiple burns at the same site, but of different degrees, are coded to the most severe degree.

Code the extent of body surface involved (percentage of body surface), when specified, as an additional code.

Late Effects

A residual, late effect is defined as the current condition resulting from a previous acute illness or injury that is no longer the current problem. Late effects are coded using the residual or late effect as the primary diagnosis. The cause of the residual or late effect is coded second.

Complications

For conditions resulting from the malfunction of internal devices, use the subterm "mechanical" found under the main term "complication."

Postoperative complications are sometimes found under the subterm "postoperative," which appears under the main term identifying the condition. If not found there, look for a subterm identifying the type of procedure, type of complication, or surgical procedure under the main term "complication."

Problems — **ICD-10-CM Codes**

1. Supracondylar fracture of right femur with intracondylar extension of lower end; initial encounter ______________
2. Fracture of left humerus and left foot; subsequent encounter ______________
3. Comminuted fracture of left radius and ulna, not displaced; initial encounter ______________
4. Pathologic fracture of right hip due to drug-induced osteoporosis; initial encounter for fracture ______________
5. Lacerations of the upper arm with embedded glass; initial encounter ______________
6. Burns on the face and neck; sequela ______________
7. Second- and third-degree burns on chest wall; 20% of body involved, 10% third-degree; initial encounter ______________
8. Bursitis of the knee resulting from crushing injury to the knee 1 year ago ______________

ASSIGNMENT 5-11 CODE DIAGNOSES FOR PREGNANCY, DELIVERY, AND NEWBORN CARE

Performance Objective

Task: Locate the correct diagnostic code for each case scenario.

Conditions: Use pen or pencil and ICD-10-CM diagnostic code book.

Standards: Time: ______________ minutes

Accuracy: ______________

(Note: The time element and accuracy criteria may be given by your instructor.)

Directions: In this exercise, you will review diagnostic codes from the ICD-10-CM code book involving patients who have conditions involving pregnancy and delivery, and newborn infants.

For the supervision of a normal pregnancy, turn to Volume 2 and look up "pregnancy." This is a long category. Look up the subterm "supervision" and find the sub-subterm "normal" (NEC Z34.8-) and "first" (Z34.0-). Check Volume 1 to verify these codes. Also see code Z33.1 "pregnancy state, incidental." This code is used in the second position to tell the insurance carrier that the patient is pregnant in addition to any other diagnosis.

If a patient has complications, turn to Volume 2 and look under the main term "pregnancy." Find the subterm "complicated by" and find the sub-subterm stating the complication. These are codes from ICD-10-CM Chapter 15: "Pregnancy, Childbirth, and Puerperium" (O00-O9a).

Delivery in a completely normal case is coded O80 and is listed under the main term "delivery, uncomplicated." Normal is described as "delivery requiring minimal or no assistance, with or without episiotomy, without fetal manipulation (e.g., rotation version) or instrumentation (forceps) of a spontaneous, cephalic, vaginal, full-term, single, live-born infant." This code is for use as a single diagnosis code and is not to be used with any other code from Chapter 15.

When coding deliveries, always include a code for the status of the infant. Look up "outcome of delivery" in Volume 2 and you will find various Z37 codes listing possible outcomes. These codes would be listed as secondary codes on the insurance claim form for the delivery.

On the insurance claim form for the newborn, turn to "newborn" in Volume 2. You will find codes from Z38.0 to Z38.8 describing the birth of the newborn. Use these codes in the first position when billing for services for the newborn infant.

Assign the correct code(s) for each case, entering it (them) on the blank line.

Problems	ICD-10-CM Codes
1. A pregnant patient who is due to deliver in 6 weeks presents in the office with preeclampsia.	______________
2. A patient presents with a chief complaint of severe episodes of pain and vaginal hemorrhage. The physician determines that the patient has an incomplete spontaneous abortion complicated by excessive hemorrhage; she was 6 weeks pregnant.	______________
3. A patient comes in who is diagnosed with a kidney stone; the patient is pregnant.	______________
4. A patient is delivered of twins, both live born by cesarean section because of cephalopelvic disproportion, which caused an obstruction. Code the mother's chart.	______________

ASSIGNMENT 5-12 CODE DIAGNOSES USING TABLE OF DRUGS AND CHEMICALS

Performance Objective

Task: Locate the correct diagnostic code for each diagnosis listed.

Conditions: Use pen or pencil and the ICD-10-CM diagnostic code book.

Standards: Time: ____________ minutes

Accuracy: ____________

(Note: The time element and accuracy criteria may be given by your instructor.)

Directions: In this exercise, you will be reviewing diagnostic codes from the ICD-10-CM code book involving patients who may have had an adverse effect from ingesting a toxic substance. Read the definitions for poisoning and drug intoxication in the *Handbook.*

Injury codes T36 through T65 are combination codes that include the substances related to adverse effects, poisonings, toxic effects, and underdosing, as well as the external cause. No additional external cause code is required to report poisonings, toxic effects, adverse effects, or underdosing codes.

A code from categories T36 through T65 is sequenced first, followed by the code(s) that specify the nature of the adverse effect, poisoning, or toxic effect.

Assign the correct code(s) for each case and enter it (them) on the blank line.

Problems	ICD-10-CM Codes
1. Light-headedness caused by digitalis intoxication; initial encounter	____________
2. Treatment of a rash after an initial dose of penicillin is given	____________
3. Initial encounter for accidental overdose of meperidine (Demerol)	____________
4. A 20-month-old baby accidentally ingests approximately 15 aspirin and is severely nauseated.	____________
5. A patient presents in the physician's office with a vague complaint of not feeling well. The physician notices that the patient has ataxia (a staggering gait). After reviewing the patient's history, the physician determines the ataxia is due to the meprobamate the patient is taking.	____________
6. Initial visit for internal bleeding: abnormal reaction to a combination of chloramphenicol and warfarin (Coumadin)	____________

6 Procedural Coding

Karen Levein

KEY TERMS

Your instructor may wish to select some words pertinent to this chapter for a test. For definitions of the terms, further study, and/or reference, the words, phrases, and abbreviations may be found in the glossary at the end of the Handbook. *Key terms for this chapter follow.*

alternative billing codes
bilateral
bundled codes
comprehensive code
conversion factor
Current Procedural Terminology
customary fee
downcoding
fee schedule
global surgery policy
Healthcare Common Procedure Coding System
modifiers
never event
procedure code numbers
professional component
reasonable fee
relative value studies
relative value unit
resource-based relative value scale
surgical package
technical component
unbundling
upcoding
usual, customary, and reasonable

KEY ABBREVIATIONS

See how many abbreviations and acronyms you can translate and then use this as a handy reference list. Definitions for the key abbreviations are located near the back of the Handbook *in the glossary.*

ABCs ____________________

AHA ____________________

CF ____________________

CPT ____________________

DME ____________________

ECG ____________________

ED ____________________

E/M service ____________________

EMTALA ____________________

EOB ____________________

FTC ____________________

GAF ____________________

GPCIs ____________________

HCPCS ____________________

NCCI edits ____________________

PC ____________________

RBRVS ____________________

RVS ____________________

RVU ____________________

TC ____________________

UCR ____________________

PERFORMANCE OBJECTIVES

The student will be able to:

- Define and spell the key terms and key abbreviations for this chapter, given the information from the *Handbook* glossary, within a reasonable time period and with enough accuracy to obtain a satisfactory evaluation.
- Answer the fill-in-the-blank, mix and match, multiple choice, and true/false review questions after reading the chapter, with enough accuracy to obtain a satisfactory evaluation.
- Select the five-digit procedure code numbers, modifiers, and/or descriptors of each service, given a series of problems relating to various medical procedures and services and using the *Current Procedural Terminology* (CPT) code book or the Mock Fee Schedule in Appendix A of the *Workbook*, with enough accuracy to obtain a satisfactory evaluation.
- Fill in the correct meaning of each abbreviation given in a list of common medical abbreviations and symbols that appear in chart notes, with enough accuracy to obtain a satisfactory evaluation.

STUDY OUTLINE

Understanding the Importance of Procedural Coding Skills
  Current Procedural Terminology
Methods of Payment
  Fee Schedule
  Usual, Customary, and Reasonable
  Developing a Fee Schedule Using Relative Value Studies Conversion Factors
Format and Content of the CPT Code Book
  Category I, II, and III Codes
  Code Book Symbols
  Evaluation and Management Section
  Surgery Section
  Unlisted Procedures
  Coding Guidelines for Code Edits
  Code Monitoring
Helpful Hints in Coding
  Office Visits
  Drugs and Injections
  Adjunct Codes
  Basic Life or Disability Evaluation Services
Code Modifiers
  Correct Use of Common CPT Modifiers
  Comprehensive List of Modifier Codes
Procedure 6-1: Determine Conversion Factors
Procedure 6-2: Locate Correct Level II HCPCS Codes for Professional Services
Procedure 6-3: Choose Correct Procedural Codes for Professional Services

ASSIGNMENT 6-1 REVIEW QUESTIONS

Part I Fill in the Blank

Review the objectives, key terms, and chapter information before completing the following review questions.

1. The coding system used for billing professional medical services and procedures is found in a book titled ____________________.

2. The Medicare program uses a system of coding composed of two levels, and this is called ____________________.

3. A medical service or procedure performed that differs in some way from the code description may be shown by using a CPT code with a/an ____________________.

4. A relative value scale or schedule is a listing of procedure codes indicating the relative value of services performed, which is shown by ____________________.

5. Name three methods for basing payments adopted by insurance companies and by state and federal programs.

   a. ____________________

   b. ____________________

   c. ____________________

6. List four situations that can occur in a medical practice when referring to charges and payments from a fee schedule.

   a. ____________________

   b. ____________________

   c. ____________________

   d. ____________________

7. Name the six sections of Category I in the CPT code book published by the American Medical Association.

   a. ____________________

   b. ____________________

   c. ____________________

   d. ____________________

   e. ____________________

   f. ____________________

8. Name five hospital departments where critical care of a patient may take place.

a. ____________________

b. ____________________

c. ____________________

d. ____________________

e. ____________________

9. A surgical package includes

a. ____________________

b. ____________________

c. ____________________

d. ____________________

e. ____________________

f. ____________________

g. ____________________

10. Medicare global surgery policy includes

a. ____________________

b. ____________________

c. ____________________

d. ____________________

e. ____________________

f. ____________________

g. ____________________

11. A function of computer software that performs online checking of codes on an insurance claim to detect improper code submission is called a/an ____________________.

12. A single code that describes two or more component codes bundled together as one unit is known as a/an ____________________.

13. To group related codes together is commonly referred to as ____________________.

14. Use of many procedural codes to identify procedures that may be described by one code is termed ____________________.

15. A code used on a claim that does not match the code system used by the third-party payer and is converted to the closest code rendering less payment is termed

____________________.

16. Intentional manipulation of procedural codes to generate increased reimbursement is called ____________________.

17. Give eight reasons for using modifiers on insurance claims.

a. ____________________

b. ____________________

c. ____________________

d. ____________________

e. ____________________

f. ____________________

g. ____________________

h. ____________________

18. What modifier is usually used when billing for an assistant surgeon who is not in a teaching hospital?

____

19. Explain when to use the -99 modifier code.

____

____

Part II Mix and Match

20. Match the symbol in the first column with the definitions in the second column. Write the correct letters on the blanks.

________	▶◀	a. New code
________	●	b. Modifier -51 exempt
________	➲	c. Add-on code
________	⊘	d. New or revised text
________	+	e. Revised code
________	▲	f. Reference material
________	⊙	g. Moderate (conscious) sedation

21. Match the two-digit modifier in the first column with the definitions in the second column. Write the correct letters on the blanks.

________	-23	a. Increased procedural service
________	-22	b. Multiple procedures
________	-25	c. Staged or related procedure
________	-26	d. Decision for surgery
________	-51	e. Significant, separately identifiable E/M service by the same physician on the same day of the procedure or other service
________	-52	f. Unusual anesthesia
________	-57	g. Reduced services
________	-58	h. Professional component

Part III Multiple Choice Questions

Choose the best answer.

22. The codes used to bill ambulance services, surgical supplies, and durable medical equipment are
    a. CPT codes.
    b. alternative billing codes.
    c. Level I HCPCS CPT codes.
    d. Level II HCPCS national codes.

23. A complex reimbursement system in which three fees are considered in calculating payment is known as
    a. usual, customary, and reasonable (UCR).
    b. relative value studies (RVS).
    c. resource-based relative value scale (RBRVS).
    d. relative value unit (RVU).

24. Medicare defines the postoperative global periods as
    a. 0, 25, 50, or 100 days.
    b. 10 or 90 days.
    c. 0, 10, 20, or 50 days.
    d. 0, 20, 50, or 90 days.

25. To code a bilateral procedure as two separate codes that include the same surgical approach may be referred to as
    a. unbundling.
    b. downcoding.
    c. bundling.
    d. upcoding.

26. When two surgeons work together as primary surgeons performing distinct parts of a procedure and each doctor bills for performing their distinct part of the procedure, the CPT surgical code is listed with modifier
    a. -62.
    b. -66.
    c. -80.
    d. -82.

Part IV True/False

Write "T" or "F" in the blank to indicate whether you think the statement is true or false.

_______ 27. Procedure coding is the transformation of written descriptions of procedures and professional services into numeric designations (code numbers).

_______ 28. Category II codes describe clinical components that may be typically included in evaluation and management services or clinical services.

_______ 29. When multiple lacerations have been repaired using the same technique and are in the same anatomic category, each repair should be assigned a code when billing an insurance claim.

_______ 30. When listing a sterile tray for an in-office surgical procedure, the tray is bundled with the procedure unless additional supplies are needed in addition to those usually used.

_______ 31. HCPCS Level II modifiers consist of only two alphanumeric characters.

ASSIGNMENT 6-2 DEFINE MEDICAL ABBREVIATIONS

To reinforce abbreviations you have learned, let's review some of those encountered during the *Workbook* assignments presented in this chapter. You should be able to decode these abbreviations without a reference. However, if you have difficulty with one or two, simply refer to Appendix A of this *Workbook*.

I & D ______

IM ______

Pap ______

ER ______

EEG ______

DPT ______

ECG ______

IUD ______

OB ______

D & C ______

OV ______

KUB ______

GI ______

Hgb ______

new pt ______

rt ______

UA ______

est pt ______

ASHD ______

tet. tox. ______

CBC ______

E/M ______

CPT ______

Ob-Gyn ______

TURP ______

cm ______

T & A ______

mL ______

inj ______

hx ______

NC ______

PROCEDURE CODING ASSIGNMENTS

In this chapter, the points awarded for assignments that require procedure codes are 1 point for each correct digit.

ASSIGNMENT 6-3 INTRODUCTION TO CPT AND CODING EVALUATION AND MANAGEMENT SERVICES

Performance Objective

Task: Locate the correct information and/or procedure code for each question and/or case scenario.

Conditions: Use pen or pencil and the *Current Procedural Terminology* code book.

Standards: Time: ______________ minutes

Accuracy: ______________

(Note: The time element and accuracy criteria may be given by your instructor.)

1. To become acquainted with the sections of the *Current Procedural Terminology* code book, match the code number in the left column with the appropriate description in the right column by writing the letters in the blanks. Locate each code number in the *Current Procedural Terminology* code book. As you progress through the assignment, the problems get more difficult and complex.

99231	________	a.	Chest x-ray
59400	________	b.	Anesthesia for procedures on cervical spine and cord
71010	________	c.	Subsequent hospital care
00600	________	d.	Supplies and materials
85025	________	e.	Routine OB care, antepartum and postpartum
99070	________	f.	CBC

2. Name the section of the CPT where each of the following codes is located.

a. 65091 ______________________________

b. 86038 ______________________________

c. 92596 ______________________________

d. 75982 ______________________________

e. 0026T ______________________________

f. 01320 ______________________________

g. 99324 ______________________________

h. 0503F ______________________________

3. Evaluation and Management (E/M) codes are used by physicians to report a significant portion of their services. Remember, it is the physician's responsibility to assign E/M codes, and the exercises presented here are only for familiarization. The problems will acquaint you with terminology for this section of the CPT code book. Select the appropriate **new patient** office visit codes using the key components:

   a. This is a Level 3 case: Detailed history

      Detailed examination

      Low-complexity decision making ______________

   b. This is a Level 1 case: Problem-focused history

      Problem-focused examination

      Straightforward decision making ______________

   c. This is a Level 5 case: Comprehensive history

      Comprehensive examination

      High-complexity decision making ______________

4. Select the appropriate **established patient** office visit codes using the key components. Coding these cases illustrates consideration of two of three components.

   a. This is a Level 4 case: Detailed history

      Detailed examination

      Low-complexity decision making ______________

   b. This is a Level 5 case: Comprehensive history

      Comprehensive examination

      Moderate-complexity decision making ______________

   c. This is a Level 5 case: Detailed history

      Comprehensive examination

      High-complexity decision making ______________

5. Evaluation and management (E/M) codes **99201** to **99239** are used for services provided in the physician's office or in an outpatient or hospital facility. Read the brief statement and then locate the code number in the *Current Procedural Terminology* code book.

   a. Office visit of a 20-year-old patient seen within the past 3 years for instruction in diabetes injection sites by RN (minimal problem). Patient not seen by physician at this brief visit. ________________

   b. Office visit of a 30-year-old new patient with allergic rhinitis. This case had an expanded problem-focused hx & exam and straightforward decision making. ________________

   c. Discussion of medication with the son of an 80-year-old patient with dementia on discharge from the observation unit. ________________

   d. Admission to hospital of 60-year-old established patient in acute respiratory distress with bronchitis. Comprehensive hx & exam and medical decision making of moderate complexity. ________________

   e. Hospital visit of a 4-year-old boy, now stable, who will be discharged the next day. This is a problem-focused interval hx & exam and medical decision making of low complexity. ________________

   f. New patient seen in the office for chest pain, congestive heart failure, and hypertension. Comprehensive hx & exam and highly complex decision making. ________________

6. Evaluation and Management codes **99241** to **99255** are used for consultations provided in the physician's office or in an outpatient or inpatient hospital facility. A consultation is a service provided by a physician whose opinion about a case is requested by another physician. Read the brief statement and then locate the code number in the *Current Procedural Terminology* code book.

   a. Office consultation for a 30-year-old woman complaining of palpitations and chest pains. Her family physician described a mild systolic click. This is an expanded problem-focused hx & exam and straightforward decision making. ______________

   b. Subsequent inpatient consultation for a 54-year-old woman, who is now stable, admitted 2 days ago for a bleeding ulcer. This case requires a detailed hx & exam and low-complexity decision making. ______________

   c. Office consultation for a 14-year-old boy with poor grades in school and suspected alcohol abuse. This is a comprehensive hx & exam and medical decision making of moderate complexity. ______________

   d. Subsequent inpatient consultation for a 50-year-old man who is diabetic and is suffering with fever, chills, gangrenous heel ulcer, rhonchi, and dyspnea (difficulty breathing), an unstable condition. The patient appears lethargic and tachypneic (rapid breathing). This case is comprehensive hx & exam with highly complex medical decision making. ______________

   e. Initial emergency department consultation for a senior who presents with thyrotoxicosis, exophthalmos, cardiac arrhythmia, and congestive heart failure. This case is a comprehensive hx & exam with highly complex medical decision making. ______________

   f. Initial hospital consultation for a 30-year-old woman, post-abdominal surgery, who is exhibiting a fever. This case is an expanded problem-focused hx & exam and straightforward medical decision making. ______________

7. Evaluation and management codes **99281** to **99499** are used for emergency department, critical care, nursing facility, rest home, custodial care, home, prolonged, physician standby, and preventive medicine services. Read the brief statement and then locate the code number in the *Current Procedural Terminology* code book.

   a. First hour of critical care of a senior who, following major surgery, suffers a cardiac arrest from a pulmonary embolus. ____________

   b. A 40-year-old woman is admitted to the OB unit, and the primary care physician has requested the neonatologist to stand by for possible cesarean section and neonatal resuscitation. Code for a 1-hour standby. ____________

   c. A child is seen in the emergency department with a fever, diarrhea, abdominal cramps, and vomiting. This case had an expanded problem-focused hx & exam, and a moderately complex medical decision was made. ____________

   d. A patient is seen for an annual visit at a nursing facility for detailed hx & comprehensive exam and low-complexity medical decision making. ____________

   e. An initial visit is made to a domiciliary care facility for a developmentally disabled individual with a mild rash on hands and face. This case had an expanded problem-focused hx & exam and low-complexity medical decision making. ____________

   f. A 50-year-old man with a history of asthma comes into the office with acute bronchospasm and moderate respiratory distress. Office treatment is initiated. The case requires intermittent physician face-to-face time with the patient for 2 hours and prolonged services. Assume the appropriate E/M code has been assigned for this case. ____________

ASSIGNMENT 6-4 CODE ANESTHESIA PROBLEMS

Performance Objective

Task: Locate the correct procedure and modifier, if necessary, for each question and/or case scenario.

Conditions: Use pen or pencil and *Current Procedural Terminology* code book.

Standards: Time: ______________ minutes

Accuracy: ______________

(Note: The time element and accuracy criteria may be given by your instructor.)

Directions: Anesthesia codes **00100** to **01999** may be used by anesthesiologists and physicians. Some plastic surgeons, other medical specialists, and large clinics may have a room set aside to perform surgical procedures that might be performed in a hospital outpatient surgical department. For Medicare claims, some regions do not use the Anesthesia section of CPT for billing but use a surgical code with an HCPCS modifier appended. Read the brief statement and then locate the code number in the *Current Procedural Terminology* code book. Special modifiers **P1** through **P6** may be needed when coding for this section, as well as code numbers for cases that have difficult circumstances. Definitions for abbreviations may be found in Appendix A of this *Workbook.*

a. Cesarean delivery following neuraxial labor anesthesia, normal healthy patient ______________ ______________

______________ ______________

b. Reduction mammoplasty of a woman with mild systemic disease ______________ ______________

c. Total right hip replacement, 71-year-old patient, normal healthy patient ______________ ______________

____

d. Repair of cleft palate, newborn infant, normal healthy patient ______________ ______________

____

e. TURP, normal healthy male ______________ ______________

ASSIGNMENT 6-5 CODE SURGICAL PROBLEMS

Performance Objective

Task: Locate the correct procedure code and modifier, if necessary, for each question and/or case scenario.

Conditions: Use pen or pencil and *Current Procedural Terminology* code book.

Standards: Time: ________ minutes

Accuracy: ________

(Note: The time element and accuracy criteria may be given by your instructor.)

Directions: Surgery codes **10040** to **69979** are used for each anatomic part of the body. Read over each case carefully. It is preferable to use the *Current Procedural Terminology* code book, but if you do not have one, then refer to the Mock Fee Schedule found in Appendix A of this *Workbook* to obtain the correct code number for each descriptor given. Full descriptors for services rendered have been omitted in some instances to give you practice in abstracting the correct descriptor from the available information. Indicate the correct two-digit modifier if necessary. The skill of critical thinking enters this section of the assignment, in that you may have to use your own judgment to code because the cases do not contain full details. Definitions for abbreviations may be found in Appendix A of this *Workbook*. Remember to use the index at the back of the CPT code book.

a. Suppose you work in an office that has an encounter form listing code 36540. Check your edition of CPT and see whether you can locate this code number. If the code does not appear, what code number are you directed to use? ________

Integumentary System 10040-19499

b. Removal of benign lesion from the back (1.0 cm) and left foot (0.5 cm) ________

c. Drainage of deep breast abscess ________

d. Laser destruction of two benign facial lesions ________

Musculoskeletal System 20000-29909

Reminder: Be sure to read the "Application of casts and strapping" guidelines in your CPT code book that appears before the 29000 codes.

e. Aspiration of fluid (arthrocentesis) from right knee joint; not infectious ________

f. Deep tissue biopsy of left upper arm ________

g. Fracture of the left tibia, closed treatment ________

Does the procedural code include application and removal of the first cast? ________

If done as an office procedure, may supplies be coded? ________

If so, what is the code number from the Medicine section? ____________

Does the procedural code include subsequent replacement of a cast for follow-up care? ____________

If not, list the code number for application of a walking short leg cast. ____________

Respiratory System 30000-32999

h. Parietal pleurectomy ____________

i. Removal of two nasal polyps, simple ____________

j. Diagnostic bronchoscopy with bronchial biopsy ____________

Cardiovascular System 33010-37799

k. Pacemaker insertion with transvenous electrode, atrial ____________

l. Thromboendarterectomy with patch graft ____________

m. Introduction of intracatheter and injection procedure for contrast venography ____________

Hemic/Lymphatic/Diaphragm 38100-39599

n. Repair, esophageal/diaphragmatic hernia transthoracic ____________

o. Partial splenectomy ____________

p. Excision, two deep cervical nodes ____________

Digestive System 40490-49999

q. T & A, 12-year-old boy ____________

r. Balloon dilation of esophagus ____________

Urinary System/Male and Female Genital 50010-55980

s. Removal of urethral diverticulum from female patient ____________

t. Anastomosis of single ureter to bladder ____________

Laparoscopy/Peritoneoscopy/Hysteroscopy/Female Genital/Maternity 56300-59899

u. Routine OB care, antepartum and postpartum care ____________

v. Therapeutic D & C, nonobstetric ____________

ASSIGNMENT 6-6 CODE PROBLEMS FOR RADIOLOGY AND PATHOLOGY

Performance Objective

Task: Locate the correct procedure code and modifier, if necessary, for each question and/or case scenario.

Conditions: Use pen or pencil and *Current Procedural Terminology* code book.

Standards: Time: ______________ minutes

Accuracy: ______________

(Note: The time element and accuracy criteria may be given by your instructor.)

Radiologists, as well as other physicians in many specialties, perform these studies. A physician who interprets, dictates, and signs a report may not bill for the report separately because it is considered part of the radiology procedure.

Some medical practices perform basic laboratory tests under a waived test certificate that complies with the rules of the Clinical Laboratory Improvement Amendments (CLIA) of 1988, implemented in September 1992.

a. Upper GI x-ray study with films and KUB ______________

b. Ultrasound, pregnant uterus after first trimester, two gestations ______________ and ______________

c. Routine urinalysis with microscopy, nonautomated ______________

d. Hemoglobin (Hgb), electrophoretic method ______________

ASSIGNMENT 6-7 PROCEDURE CODE AND MODIFIER PROBLEMS

Performance Objective

Task: Locate the correct procedure code and modifiers, if necessary, for each case scenario.

Conditions: Use pen or pencil and *Current Procedural Terminology* code book.

Standards: Time: ____________ minutes

Accuracy: ____________

(Note: The time element and accuracy criteria may be given by your instructor.)

Directions: Find the correct procedure codes and modifiers, if necessary. This assignment will reinforce what you have already learned about procedural coding because code numbers for the case scenarios presented are located in all the sections of the CPT code book. Also search for codes in the Medicine section, if necessary. The CPT list of modifiers may be found in the *Handbook*.

1. A new patient had five benign skin lesions on the right arm destroyed with surgical curettement. Complete the coding for the surgery.

Code Number	*Description*
a. ____________	Level 3, detailed history and exam with low-complexity decision making, initial new pt office visit
b. ____________	Destruction of benign skin lesion rt arm
c. ____________	Destruction of second, third, fourth, and fifth lesions

2. Mrs. Stayman had four moles on her back. Dr. Davis excised the multiple nevi in one new patient office visit after an expanded problem-focused history and exam and straightforward medical decision making. The information on the pathology report stated nonmalignant lesions measuring 2.2 cm, 1.5 cm, 1 cm, and 0.75 cm.

Code Number		*Description*
a. ____________	________	Initial OV
b. ____________		Excision, benign lesion 2.2 cm
c. ____________	________	Excision, benign lesion 1.5 cm
d. ____________	________	Excision, benign lesion 1 cm
e. ____________	________	Excision, benign lesion 0.75 cm

In another case, if a patient required removal of a 1-cm lesion on the back and a 0.5-cm lesion on the neck, the procedural codes would be ____________ for the back lesion and ____________ for the neck lesion.

3. Dr. Davis stated on his operative report that Mr. Allen was suffering from a complex, complicated nasal fracture. Dr. Davis débrided the wound because it was contaminated and performed an open reduction with internal fixation in a complex and complicated procedure.

Code Number		*Description*
a. ________________	________	Initial OV, complex hx & exam, moderate-complexity decision making
b. ________________		Open tx nasal fracture, complicated
c. ________________	________	Débridement, skin, subcutaneous tissue, muscle, and bone

4. An RN, an established patient (est pt), age 40 years, sees the doctor for an annual physical. A Pap (Papanicolaou) smear is obtained and sent to an outside laboratory. The patient also has a furuncle on the right axilla at the time of the visit, which the doctor incises and drains (I & D).

Code Number	*Description*
a. ________________	Periodic physical examination
b. ________________	Handling of specimen
c. ________________	I & D, furuncle, right axilla
d. ________________	5-mL penicillin inj IM

5. While making his rounds in the hospital during the noon hour, Dr. James sees a new patient in the ED (emergency department) for a laceration of the forehead, 5 cm long. The doctor does a workup for a possible concussion.

Code Number		*Description*
a. ________________	________	ED care, expanded problem-focused history, expanded problem-focused examination, low-complexity decision making
b. ________________		Repair of laceration, simple, face

6. The physician sees a new patient in the office with the same condition as the patient in Problem 5; however, an infection has developed, and the patient is seen for daily dressing changes. On day 11, the sutures are removed, and on day 12, a final dressing change is made and the patient is discharged.

Code Number		*Description*
a. ________________	________	Level 3, detailed history and exam with low-complexity decision making, initial new patient office visit
b. ________________		Repair of laceration
c. ________________		Tet tox (tetanus toxoid) 0.5 mL
d. ________________		Administration intramuscular injection
e. ________________		Minimal service, OV (suture removal)
f. ________________		Minimal service, OV (dressing change)

Note: Some fee schedules allow no follow-up days; Medicare fee schedule allows 10 follow-up days for the procedural code number for repair of laceration.

7. The physician sees 13-year-old Bobby Jones (est pt) for a Boy Scout physical. Bobby is in good health and well groomed. His troop is going for a 1-week camping trip in 12 days. The physician reviewed safety issues with Bobby, talked to him about school, and counseled him about not getting into drugs or alcohol. Bobby denied any problems with that or of being sexually active. He said that he plays baseball. He has no allergies. The physician performed a detailed examination. The physician completed information for scouting papers and cleared him for camping activity.

Code Number	*Description*
a. ______________	Periodic preventive evaluation and management

8. A new patient, David Ramsey, age 15 years, was seen by Dr. Menter for lapses of memory and frequent headaches. The doctor performed an EEG (electroencephalogram) and some psychological tests (including a psychodiagnostic assessment using personality and psychopathology tests [Rorschach and MMPI]). Dr. Astro Parkinson was called in as a consultant. All the test results were negative, and the patient was advised to come in for weekly psychotherapy.

Code Number	*Description*
Dr. Menter's bill:	
a. ______________	OV, comp hx & exam, moderate-complexity decision making
b. ______________	EEG, extended monitoring (1 hour)
c. ______________	Psychological tests (Rorschach and MMPI)
d. ______________	Psychotherapy (50 minutes – done on a different day)
Dr. Parkinson's bill:	
e. ______________	Consultation, expanded problem-focused hx and exam, straightforward decision making

9. An est pt, age 70 years, requires repair of a bilateral initial inguinal hernia (reducible). The code for this initial procedure is

a. ______________ ______________

ASSIGNMENT 6-8 HCPCS/MODIFIER CODE MATCH

Performance Objective

Task: Locate the correct HCPCS code and modifier, if necessary, for each medical drug, supply item, or service presented.

Conditions: Use pen or pencil and HCPCS code reference list in Appendix B of this *Workbook*.

Standards: Time: ____________ minutes

Accuracy: ____________

(Note: The time element and accuracy criteria may be given by your instructor.)

Directions: Match the HCPCS code in the first or second column with the description of the drug, supply item, or service presented in the third or fourth column. Write the correct letters on the blanks.

E1280	______	J0760	______	a. Vitamin B_{12}, 1000 mg	k. Blood (whole) for transfusion/unit
E0141	______	A9150	______	b. Injection, insulin per 5 units	l. Heavy-duty wheelchair with detachable arms
J0290	______	J2001	______	c. Rigid walker, wheeled, without seat	m. Ampicillin inj, up to 500 mg
J3420	______	L0160	______	d. Waiver of liability statement on file	n. Dimethyl sulfoxide (DMSO) inj
J1815	______	L3100-RT	______	e. Nonemergency transportation, taxi	o. Urine strips
P9010	______	A4250	______	f. Inj of colchicine	p. Vancomycin (Vancocin) inj
J1212	______	J2590	______	g. Cervical occipital/ mandibular support	q. Oxytocin (Pitocin) inj
J3370	______	A4927	______	h. Inj of lidocaine (Xylocaine)	r. Wide, heavy-duty wheelchair with detachable arms and leg rests
E1092	______	A0100	______	i. Gloves, nonsterile	s. Rt hallux valgus night splint
A4211	______	-GA	______	j. Supplies for self-administered drug injections	t. nonprescription drug

ASSIGNMENT 6-9 PROCEDURAL CODING CASE SCENARIOS

Performance Objective

Task: Locate the correct procedure code and modifier, if necessary, for each case scenario.

Conditions: Use pen or pencil and *Current Procedural Terminology* code book.

Standards: Time: ______________ minutes

Accuracy: ______________

(Note: The time element and accuracy criteria may be given by your instructor.)

Directions: Find the correct procedure codes and modifiers, if necessary, for each case scenario.

1. The physician sees Horace Hart, a 60-year-old new patient, in the office for bronchial asthma, ASHD (arteriosclerotic heart disease), and hypertension. He performs an ECG (electrocardiogram) and UA (urinalysis) without microscopy, and obtains x-rays. Comprehensive metabolic and lipid panels and a CBC (complete blood count) are done by an outside laboratory.

Code Number	*Description*
Physician's bill:	
a. ______________	Initial OV, comp hx & exam, high-complexity decision making
b. ______________	ECG with interpret and report
c. ______________	UA, routine, nonautomated
d. ______________	Chest x-ray, two views
e. ______________	Routine venipuncture for handling of specimen
Laboratory's bill:	
f. ______________	Comprehensive metabolic panel: albumin, bilirubin, calcium, carbon dioxide, chloride, creatinine, glucose, phosphatase (alkaline), potassium, protein, sodium, ALT, AST, and urea nitrogen
g. ______________	Lipid panel
h. ______________	CBC, completely automated with complete automated differential

If the doctor decides to have the chest x-rays interpreted by a radiologist, the procedural code billed by the radiologist would be ______________.

2. Mr. Hart is seen again in the office on May 12. On May 25, he is seen at home at 2 AM with asthma exacerbation, possible myocardial infarct, and congestive heart failure. The doctor consulted with a thoracic cardiovascular surgeon by telephone. He also called to make arrangements for hospitalization. To complete the patient care, these services required 2 hours and 40 minutes of non–face-to-face time in addition to the time spent examining the patient during the house call.

Code Number	*Description*
a. ______________	OV, problem-focused hx & exam, straightforward decision making
b. ______________	Home visit, detailed interval hx & exam, high-complexity decision making
c. ______________	Detention time, prolonged (list time required)

3. On June 9, Horace Hart is seen again in the hospital. The thoracic cardiovascular surgeon who was telephoned the previous day was called in for consultation to formally examine the patient and says that surgery is necessary, which is scheduled the following day. The patient's physician sees the patient for his asthmatic condition and acts as assistant surgeon. The surgeon does the follow-up care and assumes care in the case.

Code Number	*Description*
Primary care physician/assistant surgeon's bill:	
a. ______________	Hospital visit, problem-focused hx & exam, low-complexity decision making
b. ______________	Pericardiotomy
Thoracic cardiovascular surgeon's bill:	
c. ______________	Consultation, comp hx & exam, moderate-complexity decision making
d. ______________	Pericardiotomy

ASSIGNMENT 6-10 CASE SCENARIO FOR CRITICAL THINKING

Performance Objective

Task: Locate the correct procedure codes and modifiers, if necessary, for a case scenario.

Conditions: Use pen or pencil and *Current Procedural Terminology* code book.

Standards: Time: ______________ minutes

Accuracy: ______________

(Note: The time element and accuracy criteria may be given by your instructor.)

Directions: Read through this progress note on Roy A. Takashima. Abstract information from the note about the subjective symptoms, objective findings, and diagnoses. List the diagnostic and procedure codes you think this case would warrant. If your instructor tells you to also find the ICD-10-CM codes, a draft version may be downloaded from the following website: http://www.cdc.gov/nchs/icd/icd10cm.htm#10update. The most recent version is available for download.

Takashima, Roy A.
October 5, 20xx

Pt. has many things going on. First, he's had no difficulties following the feral cat bite, and the cat was normal on quarantine.

He seemed to be recovering from the flu but is plagued with a persistent cough and pain down the center of his chest due to bronchitis without fever or grossly discolored phlegm.

Physical exam shows expiratory rhonchi and gross exacerbation of his cough on forced expiration. Spirometry before and after bronchodilator was remarkably good; he is symptomatically improved with a Proventil inhaler, which he is given as a sample. I don't think other antibiotics would help.

His reflux is under good control with proprietary antacids with a clear exam.

He has several areas of seborrheic keratoses on his face and head that need attention.

Finally, in follow-up of all the above, he needs a complete physical exam.

Ting Cho, MD

Diagnosis: Influenza and acute bronchitis

Subjective symptoms ____

____

Objective findings ____

____

____

Diagnosis and Dx code ______________________________ ______________

______________________________ ______________

E/M code ______________

Spirometry code ______________________________ ______________

7 The Paper Claim: CMS-1500 (02-12)

Linda Smith

KEY TERMS

Your instructor may wish to select some words pertinent to this chapter for a test. For definitions of the terms, further study, and/or reference, the words, phrases, and abbreviations may be found in the glossary at the end of the Handbook. *Key terms for this chapter follow.*

clean claim
deleted claim
dirty claim
durable medical equipment number
electronic claim
employer identification number
facility provider number
group National Provider Identifier (group NPI)
Health Insurance Claim Form (CMS-1500 [02-12])
incomplete claim
intelligent character recognition
invalid claim
National Provider Identifier
optical character recognition
paper claim
pending claim
physically clean claim
rejected claim
Social Security number
state license number

KEY ABBREVIATIONS

See how many abbreviations and acronyms you can translate and then use this as a handy reference list. Definitions for the key abbreviations are located near the back of the Handbook *in the glossary.*

ASCA ____________________

CMS-1500 ____________________

DME ____________________

DNA ____________________

EIN ____________________

EMG ____________________

EPSDT ____________________

ICR ____________________

LMP ____________________

MSP ____________________

NA, N/A ____________________

NPI ____________________

NUCC ____________________

OCR ____________________

SOF ____________________

SSN ____________________

PERFORMANCE OBJECTIVES

The student will be able to:

- Define and spell the key terms and key abbreviations for this chapter, given the information from the *Handbook* glossary, within a reasonable time period and with enough accuracy to obtain a satisfactory evaluation.
- After reading the chapter, answer the fill-in-the-blank, mix and match, multiple choice, and true/false review questions, with enough accuracy to obtain a satisfactory evaluation.
- Given a handwritten CMS-1500 (02-12) form, type a CMS-1500 (02-12) Health Insurance Claim Form and list the reasons why the claim was either rejected or delayed, within a reasonable time period and with enough accuracy to obtain a satisfactory evaluation.
- Given the patients' medical chart notes, ledger cards, encounter forms, and blank insurance claim forms, complete each CMS-1500 (02-12) Health Insurance Claim Form for billing, within a reasonable time period and with enough accuracy to obtain a satisfactory evaluation.
- Using the Mock Fee Schedule in Appendix A in this *Workbook*, correctly post payments, adjustments, and balances to the patients' ledger cards, within a reasonable time period and with enough accuracy to obtain a satisfactory evaluation.
- Given a list of common medical abbreviations and symbols that appear in chart notes, fill in the correct meaning of each abbreviation, within a reasonable time period and with enough accuracy to obtain a satisfactory evaluation.

STUDY OUTLINE

The Paper Claim CMS-1500 (02-12)
- National Uniform Claim Committee
- History of the Paper Claim CMS-1500

Types of Submitted Claims
- Claim Status

Abstracting From Medical Records
- Cover Letter Accompanying Insurance Claims

Health Insurance Claim Form (CMS-1500 [02-12])
- Basic Guidelines for Submitting a Claim
- Completion of Insurance Claim Forms

Common Reasons Why Claim Forms Are Delayed or Rejected

Additional Claim Submission Errors

Claim Completion Guidelines
- Optical Character Recognition
- Do's and Don'ts for Claim Completion

Instructions for the Health Insurance Claim Form (CMS-1500 [02-12])
- Block-by-Block Instructions for Completion of the CMS-1500 (02-12)

Insurance Program Templates

ASSIGNMENT 7-1 REVIEW QUESTIONS

Part I Fill in the Blank

Review the objectives, key terms, chapter information, glossary definitions of key terms, and figures before completing the following review questions.

1. What legislation required all claims sent to the Medicare Program be submitted electronically, effective October 16, 2003?

   ____

2. State the name of the health insurance claim form that was required for use effective October 1, 2013. ______________________________

3. Does Medicare accept the CMS-1500 (02-12) claim form?

   ____

4. What is a pended claim?

   ____

5. How many days will it take to process a Medicare claim that is submitted electronically?

   ____

6. If a claim is submitted on behalf of the patient, and coverage of the services is denied, what is the most effective way to present the situation to the patient?

   ____

7. What is dual coverage?

   ____

8. The insurance company with the first responsibility for payment of a bill for medical services is known as the ______________________________.

9. The CMS-1500 (02-12) claim form allows for reporting of a maximum of __________ __________________ diagnosis codes per claim form.

10. What Internet resource can be used to find physician provider numbers?

    ____

11. For electronic submission of claims, what allows the physician's name to be printed in the signature block where it would normally be signed?

    ____

12. When preparing a claim that is to be optically scanned, birth dates are keyed in with how many digits? ______________________________

Part II Mix and Match

13. Match the types of claims listed in the right column with their descriptions, and fill in the blanks with the appropriate letters.

________	Claim missing required information	a. Clean claim
________	Phrase used when a claim is held back from payment	b. Paper claim
________	Claim that is submitted and then optically scanned by the insurance carrier and converted to electronic form	c. Invalid claim
________	Claim that needs manual processing because of errors or to solve a problem	d. Dirty claim
________	Claim that needs clarification and answers to some questions	e. Electronic claim
________	Claim that is canceled or voided if incorrect claim form is used or itemized charges are not provided	f. Pending claim
________	Claim that is submitted via telephone line or computer modem	g. Rejected claim
________	Claim that is submitted within the time limit and correctly completed	h. Incomplete claim
________	Medicare claim that contains information that is complete and necessary but is illogical or incorrect	i. Deleted claim

14. Match the types of numbers listed in the right column with their descriptions, and fill in the blanks with the appropriate letters.

________	A number issued by the federal government to each individual for personal use	a. State license number
________	A Medicare lifetime provider number	b. Employer identification number
________	A number listed on a claim when submitting insurance claims to insurance companies under a group name	c. Social Security number
________	A number that a physician must obtain to practice in a state	d. Group national provider number
________	A number used when billing for supplies and equipment	e. National Provider Identifier
________	A number issued to a hospital	f. Durable medical equipment number
________	An individual physician's federal tax identification number issued by the Internal Revenue Service	g. Facility provider number

Part III Multiple Choice

Choose the best answer.

15. The basic paper claim form currently used by health care professionals and suppliers to bill insurance carriers for services provided to patients is the
    a. CMS-1500 (08-05) claim form.
    b. CMS-1500 (02-12) claim form.
    c. Attending Physician's Statement.
    d. COMB-1.

16. What is the exception to ASCA's requirement for providers to send claims to Medicare electronically?
    a. Chiropractors
    b. Providers who have more than 25 full-time employees
    c. Providers with fewer than 10 full-time employees
    d. Any provider who requests a financial hardship

17. Under ASCA, plans other than Medicare
    a. may allow submission of claims on paper.
    b. will never allow submission of claims on paper.
    c. only allow submission of claim on paper.
    d. must follow the claims submission guidance of the AMA.

18. The National Uniform Claim Committee (NUCC) is made up of
    a. AMA representatives.
    b. CMS representatives.
    c. providers.
    d. all of the above.

19. The first standardized insurance claim form developed in 1958 was known as the
    a. CMS-1500 (02-12) claim form.
    b. CMS-1500 (08-05) claim form.
    c. HCFA-1500 (12-90).
    d. COMB-1.

20. The most recently revised version of the 1500 Health Insurance Claim Form developed in 2012 accommodates
    a. the change in the names of the government agency from Health Care Finance Administration to Center for Medicare and Medicaid Services (CMS).
    b. requirements for allowing optical scanning of the claim.
    c. changes in the Electronic Claims Submission Version 5010 837P.
    d. changes to the CPT coding system.

21. If a patient has dual coverage,
    a. insurance information for the primary carrier should be obtained.
    b. insurance information for both the primary and the secondary carrier should be obtained.
    c. insurance information for the secondary carrier can be obtained after the primary insurance carrier processes the claim.
    d. the primary carrier has insurance information for the secondary carrier and will automatically forward the claim to the secondary carrier if necessary.

22. HIPAA laws required that the provider rendering the service be identified on the claim form by
    a. reporting of the correct provider number.
    b. reporting of the correct ICD-9 code.
    c. reporting of the correct CPT code.
    d. reporting of the correct facility code.

23. The Omnibus Budget Reconciliation Act (OBRA) requires Medicare administrative contractors to
    a. deny all claims received after 1 year from date of service.
    b. pay all clean claims that are submitted within 1 year from date of service.
    c. investigate all clean claims not paid on time.
    d. pay interest on all clean claims not paid on time.

24. A claim that is investigated on a postpayment basis that is found to be "not due" will require
    a. resubmission of a claim.
    b. manual review of the claim.
    c. refund of the monies paid.
    d. additional medical records.

25. If there is a balance remaining on a patient's account after the patient's primary insurance has paid, and the patient has secondary coverage, the billing specialist should
    a. send a bill to the patient for the remaining balance.
    b. send a claim form to the secondary insurance for the remaining balance.
    c. send a claim form to the secondary insurance with a copy of the explanation of benefits from the primary carrier.
    d. monitor the claim to determine if the patient has sent a claim to the secondary carrier.

26. The maximum number of diagnostic codes that can be submitted on the CMS-1500 (02-12) claim form is
    a. four.
    b. six.
    c. eight.
    d. twelve.

27. National Provider Identification (NPI) numbers are used to report
    a. referring physicians.
    b. ordering physicians.
    c. performing physicians.
    d. all of the above.

28. National Provider Identification (NPI) numbers are assigned
    a. once in a lifetime, per health care provider.
    b. annually, per health care provider.
    c. once in a lifetime, per payer.
    d. each time the provider moves to another state.

29. To correct a claim that has been denied because of an invalid procedure code, the billing specialist should
    a. check the patient registration form to ensure all data were reported accurately.
    b. confirm the code in the CPT manual to ensure it is valid for the date of service.
    c. confirm the code in the ICD-9 manual to ensure it is valid for the date of service.
    d. confirm the provider's NPI number to make sure it was reported accurately.

30. To correct a claim that was denied because more than six lines were entered on the claim,
    a. readjust the printer so all claim lines fit on the form; reprint and send.
    b. reenter data with the appropriate code range for the dates of service and bill on one line.
    c. bill six claim lines on one claim and complete an additional paper claim for the additional claim lines.
    d. write off the additional claim lines that have been denied.

Part IV True/False

Write "T" or "F" in the blank to indicate whether you think the statement is true or false.

_______ 31. The insurance billing specialist does not need to know how to complete a paper claim because most claims are submitted electronically.

_______ 32. Physicians who experience downtimes of Internet services, which are out of their control for more than 2 days, may submit claims to Medicare on paper.

_______ 33. The goal of the NUCC is to provide a warehouse for providers to purchase CMS-1500 claim forms.

_______ 34. Effective June 1, 2013, providers were required to use only the CMS-1500 claim form (02-12).

_______ 35. Use of the standardized CMS-1500 claim form has simplified processing of paper claims.

_______ 36. Quantities of the CMS-1500 (02-12) claim form can be purchased through CMS or downloaded from the CMS website and used for submission.

_______ 37. Interest rates that apply to the Prompt Payment Interest Rate can be located on the Treasury's Financial Management Service page.

_______ 38. Medicare claims that require further investigation prior to being processed are referred to as "other" claims.

_______ 39. A diagnosis should never be submitted without supporting documentation in the medical record.

_______ 40. Claims for dates of services in two different years may be submitted on the same claim form.

_______ 41. Services that are inclusive in the global surgical package that have no charge associated with them should not be submitted on the CMS-1500 claim form.

_______ 42. Proofreading claims prior to submission can prevent denials and delay of claim processing.

_______ 43. When submitting supplemental documentation for processing of a claim, the patient's name and date of service needs only be on the front of a two-sided document.

_______ 44. Handwriting is permitted on optically scanned paper claims.

_______ 45. Use the abbreviation "DNA" when information is not applicable.

ASSIGNMENT 7-2 COMPLETE A HEALTH INSURANCE CLAIM FORM FOR A PRIVATE CASE

Performance Objective

Task: Complete a health insurance claim form and post the information to the patient's financial account record/statement.

Conditions: Use Merry M. McLean's E/M code slip (Figure 7-1), patient record (Figure 7-2), and financial account record/statement (Figure 7-3); one health insurance claim form (print from Evolve website); a computer or pen; procedural and diagnostic code books; and Appendixes A and B in the *Workbook.*

Standards: Claim Productivity Measurement

Time: ______________ minutes

Accuracy: ______________

(Note: The time element and accuracy criteria may be given by your instructor.)

E/M Code Slip

Patient *McLean, Merry M.*

Date *5-6-XX*

CPT Code ______

Dx Code ______

HISTORY

- ☐ Problem Focused
  Chief complaint; Brief history of present illness
- ☐ Expanded Problem Focused
  Chief complaint; Brief history of present illness; Problem pertinent system review
- ☑ Detailed
  Chief complaint: Extended history of present illness; Extended system review; Pertinent past family, social history
- ☐ Comprehensive
  Chief complaint; Extended history of present illness; Complete system review; Complete past family, social history

EXAMINATION

- ☐ Problem Focused
  Exam limited to affected body area or organ system
- ☐ Expanded Problem Focused
  Exam extended to other symptomatic or related organ systems
- ☑ Detailed
  Extended exam of affected area(s) and other symptomatic or related systems
- ☐ Comprehensive
  Complete single system specialty exam or complete multi-system exam

MEDICAL DECISION MAKING

	Medical Decision	Number of Dx Options	Amount of Data	Risk M and M
☐	Straightforward	minimal 1 dx	minimal	minimal
☑	Low Complexity	limited 1-2 dx	limited	low
☐	Moderate Complexity	multiple 1-2 dx	moderate	moderate
☐	High Complexity	extensive 2-3 dx	extensive	high

☐ Counseling ☐ Time ______

☐ Consult ☐ Referring Dr. *Emdee Fine*

Diagnosis *See Pt record*

NP ✓ Est pt ______

Figure 7-1

Directions: Complete the Health Insurance Claim Form,* using NUCC guidelines, and send the form to the Prudential Insurance Company for Mrs. Merry M. McLean by referring to her E/M code slip, patient record, and financial account record/statement. Date the claim June 15. Refer to Appendix A in this *Workbook* to fill in the fees on the financial account record/statement.

1. Use your CPT code book or Appendix A in this *Workbook* to determine the correct five-digit code number and modifiers for each professional service rendered. To determine diagnostic codes, refer to ICD-10-CM code books.

2. Record on the financial account record/statement when you have billed the insurance company.

3. A Performance Evaluation Checklist may be reproduced from the "Instruction Guide to the Workbook" chapter if your instructor wishes you to submit it to assist with scoring and comments.

4. After the instructor has returned your work to you, either make the necessary corrections and place your work in a three-ring notebook for future reference, or, if you received a high score, place it in your portfolio for reference when applying for a job.

Abbreviations pertinent to this record:

NP ______	LC ______
UA ______	MDM ______
Dx ______	HV ______
ptr ______	PF ______
Cysto ______	SF ______
pt ______	RTO ______
Cont ______	postop ______
adm ______	OV ______
hosp ______	lb ______
C ______	adv ______
hx ______	retn ______
exam ______	est ______

*See Chapter 7 in the *Handbook* for help in completing the form.

PATIENT RECORD NO. 7-2

LAST NAME	FIRST NAME	MIDDLE NAME	BIRTH DATE	SEX	HOME PHONE
McLean	Merry	M.	02-02-48	F	555-486-1859

ADDRESS	CITY	STATE	ZIP CODE
4919 Dolphin Way	Woodland Hills,	XY	12345

CELL PHONE	PAGER NO.	FAX NO.	E-MAIL ADDRESS
555-430-7709	555-098-3456	555-486-1859	McLean@WB.net

PATIENT'S SOC. SEC. NO.	DRIVER'S LICENSE
459-XX-9989	M0039857

PATIENT'S OCCUPATION	NAME OF COMPANY
Secretary	Porter Company

ADDRESS OF EMPLOYER	PHONE
5490 Wilshire Blvd., Merck, XY 12346	555-446-7781

SPOUSE OR PARENT	OCCUPATION
Harry L. McLean	Computer programmer

EMPLOYER	ADDRESS	PHONE
IBM Corporation	5616 Wilshire Blvd., Merck, XY 12346	555-664-9023

NAME OF INSURANCE	INSURED OR SUBSCRIBER
Prudential Insurance Co., 5621 Wilshire Blvd., Merck, XY 12346	Harry L. McLean

POLICY/CERTIFICATE NO.	GROUP NO.
459-XX-9989	8832

REFERRED BY: Emdee Fine, MD, 5000 Wilshire Blvd., Merck, XY 12346 NPI # 73027175XX

DATE	PROGRESS NOTES No. 7-2
5-6-xx	NP presents in office with constant dribbling and wetting at night; uses 15 pads/day.
	Began March 10, 20xx. Pelvic exam done—normal findings. No bladder or uterine
	prolapse noted. UA dipstick performed (nonautomated with microscopy); few bacteria,
	few urates. Dx: urinary incontinence. ptr 4 days for cystourethroscopy.
	GU/llf Gene Ulibarri, MD
5-10-xx	Cysto performed—revealed vesico-vaginal fistula of bladder with an opening into urinary bladder
	and copious leakage into vagina. Schedule surgery to repair fistula. Pt cont to work.
	GU/llf Gene Ulibarri, MD
5-16-xx	Adm to College hosp. C hx/exam LC MDM. Dx: vesicovaginal fistula.
	GU/llf Gene Ulibarri, MD
5-17-xx	Closure of vesicovaginal fistula; abdominal approach.
	GU/llf Gene Ulibarri, MD
5-18-xx thru	Saw patient in hospital (HV) PF hx/exam SF MDM.
5-21-xx	GU/llf Gene Ulibarri, MD
5-22-xx	Discharge from hospital. RTO 2 weeks.
	GU/llf Gene Ulibarri, MD
6-5-xx	Post-op OV. Patient has no pain near operative site. Pt reports she has
	been walking daily and lifting more than 5 lb objects. Pt adv no excessive walking,
	no lifting, stooping, or bending until surgical site is completely healed. Retn to clinic in
	1 wk. Est return to work 7-1-xx. PF hx/exam SF MDM.
	GU/llf Gene Ulibarri, MD

Figure 7-2

Acct No. 7-2

STATEMENT
Financial Account

COLLEGE CLINIC
4567 Broad Avenue
Woodland Hills, XY 12345-0001
Tel. 555-486-9002
Fax No. 555-487-8976

Merry McLean
4919 Dolphin Way
Woodland Hills, XY 12345

Phone No. (H) (555) 486-1859 (W) (555) 446-7781 Birthdate 02-02-48

Primary Insurance Co. Prudential Insurance Co. Policy/Group No. 459-XX-9989/8832

	REFERENCE	DESCRIPTION	CHARGES	CREDITS PYMNTS.	CREDITS ADJ.	BALANCE
20XX		BALANCE FORWARD →				
05-06-xx		OV NP				
05-06-xx		UA				
05-10-xx		Cystourethroscopy				
5-16-xx		Initial hosp care				
05-17-xx		Repair vesicovaginal fistula				
05-18 to 05-22-xx		HV				
05-22-xx		Discharge				
06-05-xx		PO-OV				

PLEASE PAY LAST AMOUNT IN BALANCE COLUMN

THIS IS A COPY OF YOUR FINANCIAL ACCOUNT AS IT APPEARS ON OUR RECORDS

Figure 7-3

ASSIGNMENT 7-3 COMPLETE A HEALTH INSURANCE CLAIM FORM FOR A PRIVATE CASE

Performance Objective

Task: Complete a health insurance claim form and post the information to the patient's financial account record/statement.

Conditions: Use Billy S. Rubin's E/M code slip (Figure 7-4), patient record (Figure 7-5), and financial account record/statement (Figure 7-6); one health insurance claim form (print from Evolve website); a computer or pen; procedural and diagnostic code books; and Appendixes A and B in this *Workbook*.

Standards: Claim Productivity Measurement

Time: ______________ minutes

Accuracy: ______________

(Note: The time element and accuracy criteria may be given by your instructor.)

E/M Code Slip

Patient *Rubin, Billy S.*

Date *

CPT Code ______

Dx code ______

HISTORY

- [x] Problem Focused
  Chief complaint; Brief history of present illness
- [ ] Expanded Problem Focused
  Chief complaint; Brief history of present illness; Problem pertinent system review
- [ ] Detailed
  Chief complaint; Extended history of present illness; Extended system review; Pertinent past family, social history
- [ ] Comprehensive
  Chief complaint; Extended history of present illness; Complete system review; Complete past family, social history

EXAMINATION

- [x] Problem Focused
  Exam limited to affected body area or organ system
- [ ] Expanded Problem Focused
  Exam extended to other symptomatic or related organ systems
- [ ] Detailed
  Extended exam of affected area(s) and other symptomatic or related symptoms
- [ ] Comprehensive
  Complete single system specialty exam or complete multi-system exam

MEDICAL DECISION MAKING

	Medical Decision	Number of Dx Options	Amount of Data	Risk M and M
[ ]	Straightforward	minimal 1 dx	minimal	minimal
[x]	Low Complexity	limited 1-2 dx	limited	low
[ ]	Moderate Complexity	multiple 1-2 dx	moderate	moderate
[ ]	High Complexity	extensive 2-3 dx	extensive	high

- [ ] Counseling
- [ ] Time ______
- [ ] Consult
- [ ] Referring Dr. ______

Diagnosis *see pt. record*

NP ______ Est pt ✓

* For space constraints, this E/M code slip is being used for 8-7-00, 8-14-00, and 8-16-00

Figure 7-4

Directions: Complete the Health Insurance Claim Form* on Mr. Billy S. Rubin for processing and send it to Aetna Life and Casualty Company by referring to Mr. Rubin's E/M code slip, patient record, and financial account record/statement. Date the claim August 30. Refer to Appendix A in this *Workbook* to fill in the fees on the financial statement. Use NUCC guidelines.

1. Use your CPT code book or Appendix A in this *Workbook* to determine the correct five-digit code number and modifiers for each professional service rendered. Do not include no-charge entries on the claim form. To determine diagnostic codes, refer to ICD-10-CM code books.

2. Record when you have billed the insurance company on the financial account record/statement.

3. On September 1, Mr. Rubin sends you check No. 421 in the amount of $200 to apply to his account. Post this entry and calculate the balance due.

4. A Performance Evaluation Checklist may be reproduced from the "Instruction Guide to the Workbook" chapter if your instructor wishes you to submit it to assist with scoring and comments.

5. After the instructor has returned your work to you, either make the necessary corrections and place your work in a three-ring notebook for future reference, or, if you received a high score, place it in your portfolio for reference when applying for a job.

Abbreviations pertinent to this record:

est ______________________

pt ______________________

CBC ______________________

CC ______________________

diff ______________________

PSA ______________________

bx ______________________

STAT ______________________

PTR ______________________

CA ______________________

adm ______________________

surg ______________________

TURP ______________________

wks ______________________

HV ______________________

PF ______________________

hx ______________________

exam ______________________

SF ______________________

MDM ______________________

Disch ______________________

hosp ______________________

postop ______________________

*See Chapter 7 in the *Handbook* for help in completing the form.

Additional Coding

1. Determine CPT codes that you would use to bill for College Hospital from the following services mentioned in the patient's progress notes.

	CPT code
A. Blood draw (venipuncture)	________________
B. Complete blood cell (CBC) count (automated) with differential	________________
C. Prostate-specific antigen (PSA) (total)	________________
D. Ultrasonography with guided fine-needle biopsy	________________
	________________

PATIENT RECORD NO. 7-3

Rubin	Billy	S.	11-09-53	M	555-893-5770
LAST NAME	FIRST NAME	MIDDLE NAME	BIRTH DATE	SEX	HOME PHONE

547 North Oliver Rd.	Woodland Hills	XY	12345
ADDRESS	CITY	STATE	ZIP CODE

555-430-9080	555-987-7790	555-893-5770	Rubin@WB.net
CELL PHONE	PAGER NO.	FAX NO.	E-MAIL ADDRESS

505-XX-1159	R0398056
PATIENT'S SOC. SEC. NO.	DRIVER'S LICENSE

salesman	Nate's Clothier's
PATIENT'S OCCUPATION	NAME OF COMPANY

7786 East Chabner Blvd., Dorland, XY 12347	555-449-6605
ADDRESS OF EMPLOYER	PHONE

Lydia B. Rubin (wife)
SPOUSE OR PARENT

EMPLOYER	ADDRESS	PHONE

Aetna Life and Casualty Co., 3055 Wilshire Blvd., Merck, XY 12345	Billy S. Rubin
NAME OF INSURANCE	INSURED OR SUBSCRIBER

42107	2641
POLICY/CERTIFICATE NO.	GROUP NO.

REFERRED BY: U. R. Wright, MD, 5010 Wrong Road, Torres, XY 12349 555-907-5440 NPI # 271385554XX

DATE	PROGRESS NOTES No. 7-3
8-7-xx	Office exam est pt. CC: urinary hesitancy, frequency and posturinary dribbling since
	July 15 of this year. Exam revealed hard nodule in prostate. Sent pt to College Hospital for
	laboratory work; CBC (automated with diff) and PSA (total). PTR in 1 wk.
	GU/llf Gene Ulibarri, MD
8-14-xx	Office exam. PSA elevated (5.6), CBC normal. Explained to pt that biopsy is needed at this
	point; may be done as outpatient at College Hospital. Pt elected to have immediate
	bx; arrangements made for stat. Ultrasound with guided fine needle bx. PTR in 2 days for
	results.
	GU/llf Gene Ulibarri, MD
8-16-xx	Pt returns for bx report; positive for CA in situ of prostate. Advised patient that an
	operation is necessary and explained surgical procedure, risks, and complications.
	Arranged for adm to College Hospital on 8/22/xx.
	GU/llf Gene Ulibarri, MD
8-22-xx	Admit to College Hospital. Surg: TURP, complete. Pt tolerated surg well and is comfortable
	in the recovery room. Pt last worked 8/21/xx; est disability 6 to 8 wks. Est return to work
	on 10/22/xx.
	GU/llf Gene Ulibarri, MD
8-23-xx thru	HV (PF hx/exam SF MDM)
8-26-xx	GU/llf Gene Ulibarri, MD
8-27-xx	Disch from hosp. Pt confined at home for 1 week at which time patient will return to
	office for postop check.
	GU/llf Gene Ulibarri, MD

Figure 7-5

Acct No. 7-3

STATEMENT
Financial Account
COLLEGE CLINIC
4567 Broad Avenue
Woodland Hills, XY 12345-0001
Tel. 555-486-9002
Fax No. 555-487-8976

Billy S. Rubin
547 North Oliver Road
Woodland Hills, XY 12345

Phone No. (H) (555) 893-5770 (W) (555) 449-6605 Birthdate 11-09-53

Primary Insurance Co. Aetna Life and Casualty Co. Policy/Group No. 421074/2641

	REFERENCE	DESCRIPTION	CHARGES	CREDITS PYMNTS.	CREDITS ADJ.	BALANCE
20XX				BALANCE FORWARD →		
08-07-xx		OV Est Pt				
08-14-xx		OV Est Pt				
08-16-xx		OV Est Pt				
08-22-xx		TURP				
08-23 to 08-26-xx		HV				
08-27-xx		Discharge				

PLEASE PAY LAST AMOUNT IN BALANCE COLUMN

THIS IS A COPY OF YOUR FINANCIAL ACCOUNT AS IT APPEARS ON OUR RECORDS

Figure 7-6

ASSIGNMENT 7-4 COMPLETE ONE HEALTH INSURANCE CLAIM FORM FOR A PRIVATE CASE

Performance Objective

Task: Complete one health insurance claim form and post the information to the patient's financial account record/statement.

Conditions: Use Walter J. Stone's E/M code slip (Figure 7-7), patient record (Figure 7-8), and financial account record/statement (Figure 7-9); one health insurance claim form (print from Evolve website); a computer or pen; procedural and diagnostic code books; and Appendixes A and B in this *Workbook*.

Standards: Claim Productivity Measurement

Time: ______________ minutes

Accuracy: ______________

(Note: The time element and accuracy criteria may be given by your instructor.)

E/M Code Slip

Patient *Stone, Walter J.*

Date *5/12/XX*

CPT Code ________

Dx Code ________

HISTORY

☐ Problem Focused
Chief complaint; Brief history of present illness

☑ Expanded Problem Focused
Chief complaint; Brief history of present illness; Problem pertinent system review

☐ Detailed
Chief complaint; Extended history of present illness; Extended system review; Pertinent past family, social history

☐ Comprehensive
Chief complaint; Extended history of present illness; Complete system review; Complete past family, social history

EXAMINATION

☐ Problem Focused
Exam limited to affected body area or organ system

☑ Expanded Problem Focused
Exam extended to other symptomatic or related organ systems

☐ Detailed
Extended exam of affected area(s) and other symptomatic or related systems

☐ Comprehensive
Complete single system specialty exam or complete multi-system exam

MEDICAL DECISION MAKING

	Medical Decision	Number of Dx Options	Amount of Data	Risk M and M
☐	Straightforward	minimal 1 dx	minimal	minimal
☑	Low Complexity	limited 1-2 dx	limited	low
☐	Moderate Complexity	multiple 1-2 dx	moderate	moderate
☐	High Complexity	extensive 2-3 dx	extensive	high

☐ Counseling ☐ Time ________

☐ Consult ☐ Referring Dr. ________

Diagnosis *see pt. record*

NP ____ Est pt ✓

Figure 7-7

Directions: You will be billing for all services listed on the patient's progress notes for Dr. Clarence Cutler. Complete one Health Insurance Claim Form,* addressing it to Travelers Insurance Company for Mr. Walter J. Stone by referring to his E/M code slip, patient record, and financial account record/statement. Date the claim May 5. Refer to Appendix A in this *Workbook* to fill in the fees on the financial account record/statement. Use NUCC guidelines.

1. Use your CPT code book or Appendix A in this *Workbook* to determine the correct five-digit code number and modifiers for each professional service rendered. To determine diagnostic codes, refer to ICD-10-CM code books.

2. On May 14, the insurance company sends the physician a check, number 48572, for $25. Post this entry.

3. Record on the financial account record/statement when you have billed the insurance company.

4. A Performance Evaluation Checklist may be reproduced from the "Instruction Guide to the Workbook" chapter if your instructor wishes you to submit it to assist with scoring and comments.

5. After the instructor has returned your work to you, either make the necessary corrections and place your work in a three-ring notebook for future reference, or, if you received a high score, place it in your portfolio for reference when applying for a job.

Abbreviations pertinent to this record:

est ______	exam ______
pt ______	LC ______
ER ______	MDM ______
BP ______	EGD ______
Dx ______	bx ______
GI ______	ofc ______
HV ______	wk ______
PF ______	OV ______
hx ______	adv ______

Additional Coding

1. Refer to Mr. Stone's patient record, abstract information, and code the procedures for services that would be billed by the hospital.

Description of Service	*Code*
a. Cholecystography with oral contrast	______
b. Abdominal ultrasound (complete)	______
c. EGD with biopsy	______

*See Chapter 7 in the *Handbook* for help in completing the form.

PATIENT RECORD NO. 7-4

Stone	Walter	J.	03-14-49	M	555-345-0776
LAST NAME	FIRST NAME	MIDDLE NAME	BIRTH DATE	SEX	HOME PHONE

2008 Converse Street	Woodland Hills	XY	12345
ADDRESS	CITY	STATE	ZIP CODE

555-980-7750	555-930-5674	555-345-0776	Stone@WB.net
CELL PHONE	PAGER NO.	FAX NO.	E-MAIL ADDRESS

456-XX-9989	H9834706
PATIENT'S SOC. SEC. NO.	DRIVER'S LICENSE

advertising agent	R. V. Black and Associates
PATIENT'S OCCUPATION	NAME OF COMPANY

1267 Broad Street, Woodland Hills, XY 12345	555-345-6012
ADDRESS OF EMPLOYER	PHONE

widower
SPOUSE OR PARENT

EMPLOYER	ADDRESS	PHONE

Travelers Insurance Co., 5460 Olympic Blvd., Woodland Hills, XY 12345	Walter J. Stone
NAME OF INSURANCE	INSURED OR SUBSCRIBER

456-XX-9989	6754
POLICY/CERTIFICATE NO.	GROUP NO.

REFERRED BY: John B. Stone (brother), former patient of Dr. Input

DATE	PROGRESS NOTES
5-3-xx	Est pt presented in ER after experiencing sudden onset of profuse rectal bleeding with nausea and severe abdominal pain. BP 150/90. Dr. Cutler called to ER by Dr. Input who recommended pt be admitted for further evaluation and diagnostic workup. Dr. Cutler performed a comprehensive history and examination with moderate complexity decision making and admitted the pt to College Hospital. Dx: Unspecified GI hemorrhage. Pt disabled from work.
	CC/llf Clarence Cutler, MD
5-4-xx	Pt underwent upper GI endoscopy to control bleeding. Endoscopy procedure was performed by Dr. Cutler. In the radiology department, the pt had a cholecystography with oral contrast and complete abdominal ultrasound that confirmed inflammatory gallbladder with stones. EGD with bx confirmed prepyloric gastric ulcer with hemorrhage. BP of 150/90. Dr. Cutler performed a laparoscopic cholecystectomy. DX: Cholecystitis with cholelithiasis.
	CC/llf Clarence Cutler, MD
5-5-xx	Pt discharged to home. Pt placed on amoxicillin t.i.d. for 2 wks to prevent infection and Prilosec in A.M. for 2 weeks to control stomach acid. Pt to be seen in ofc in 1 wk. It is estimated pt will resume work on 6/22/xx.
	CC/llf
	Clarence Cutler, MD

Figure 7-8

Acct No. 7-4

STATEMENT
Financial Account

COLLEGE CLINIC
4567 Broad Avenue
Woodland Hills, XY 12345-001
Tel. 555-486-9002
Fax No. 555-487-8976

Walter J. Stone
2008 Converse Street
Woodland Hills, XY 12345

Phone No. (H) (555) 345-0776 (W) (555) 345-6012 Birthdate 03-14-49

Primary Insurance Co. Travelers Insurance Co. Policy/Group No. 456-XX9989/6754

	REFERENCE	DESCRIPTION	CHARGES		CREDITS PYMNTS.		CREDITS ADJ.		BALANCE	
20XX		BALANCE FORWARD →								
01-03-xx	99214	OV	61	51					61	51
01-15-xx	01-03-xx	Billed Travelers Ins.							61	51
03-02-xx	Ck 95268	ROA Travlers Ins.			49	21			12	30
03-03-xx	99213	OV	40	20					52	50
04-03-xx	3-3-xx	Billed Travelers Ins.							52	50
05-03-xx		Initial hosp care								
05-04-xx		Endoscopy								
05-04-xx		Cholecystectomy								

PLEASE PAY LAST AMOUNT IN BALANCE COLUMN

THIS IS A COPY OF YOUR FINANCIAL ACCOUNT AS IT APPEARS ON OUR RECORDS

Figure 7-9

ASSIGNMENT 7-5 LOCATE ERRORS ON A COMPLETED HEALTH INSURANCE CLAIM FORM

Performance Objective

Task: Locate errors on a completed health insurance claim form and post the information to the patient's ledger card.

Conditions: Use Tom N. Parkinson's completed insurance claim (Figure 7-10), one health insurance claim form (print from Evolve website), and a computer or a pen.

Standards: Time: ______________ minutes

Accuracy: ______________

(Note: The time element and accuracy criteria may be given by your instructor.)

Guidance: To alleviate frustration and ease the process of completing a claim form for the first time, you will be editing a claim and then taking the correct information and inserting it on a blank CMS-1500 (02-12) form. Refer to Chapter 7 in the *Handbook* for block-by-block private payer instructions for completing the CMS-1500 (02-12) insurance claim form. Refer to Figure 7-3 in the *Handbook* for visual placement of data. Refer to Appendix A in this *Workbook* for the physician/clinic information and the clinic's mock fee schedule. The billing physician is Gerald Practon. The name of the insurance carrier is ABC Insurance Company at 111 Main Street in Denver, CO 80210.

Directions: Study the completed claim form (see Figure 7-10) and search for missing or incorrect information. If possible, verify all information. Highlight or circle in red all incorrect or missing information. Insert the correct information on the claim form. Now transfer all the data to a blank CMS-1500 (02-12) claim form. If mandatory information is missing, insert the word "NEED" in the corresponding block of the claim form.

A Performance Evaluation Checklist may be reproduced from the "Instruction Guide to the Workbook" chapter if your instructor wishes you to submit it to assist with scoring and comments.

Optional: List, in block-by-block order, the reasons why the claim may be either rejected or delayed according to the errors found.

General Directions for Claim Form Completion

Assume that the Health Insurance Claim Form* CMS-1500 (02-12) is printed in red ink for processing by OCR or ICR. Complete the form using NUCC guidelines and send it to the proper insurance carrier. Refer to Chapter 7 in the *Handbook* for block instructions. Claim form templates have been completed to use as visual examples for placement of data; they may be found at the end of Chapter 7 in the *Handbook*. Screened areas on each form do not apply to the insurance program example shown and should be left blank.

Many physicians complete an evaluation and management (E/M) code slip for each patient encounter. Chapter 7 assignments feature this form as a reference for part of each exercise and are used to assist you with E/M CPT code selection. In future assignments, you will identify key components for E/M services in the medical record. All physicians in College Clinic accept assignment of benefits for all types of insurance that you will be billing for; indicate this by checking "yes" in Block 27. For each claim completed, be sure to insert your initials at the lower left corner of the claim form. When coding services from the Surgery section of CPT, be sure to check the Mock Fee Schedule in Appendix A in this *Workbook* to determine how many follow-up days are included in the surgical or global package. Services provided during the surgical/global package time frame should not be included on the claim form; however, such services should be documented on the financial accounting record, referenced with code 99024 (postoperative follow-up visit; included in global service), and listed as no charge (N/C). Refer to the *Handbook* for detailed information about surgical/global package and follow-up days.

A list of abbreviations pertinent to the medical record has been provided as an exercise to reinforce learning. Not all medical offices use abbreviations in medical record documentation. In the College Clinic scenario, abbreviations are used in patient progress notes to give you an opportunity to practice reading and interpreting them.

---

*See Chapter 7 in the *Handbook* for help in completing the form.

DRAFT - NOT FOR OFFICIAL USE

HEALTH INSURANCE CLAIM FORM

APPROVED BY NATIONAL UNIFOR MCLAIM COMMITTEE (NUCC) 02/12

PICA — PICA — CARRIER

1. MEDICARE (Medicare#) [ ] MEDICAID (Medicaid#) [ ] TRICARE (ID#DoD#) [ ] CHAMPVA (Member ID#) [ ] GROUP HEALTH PLAN (ID#) [X] FECA BLK LUNG (ID#) [ ] OTHER (ID#) [ ]

1a. INSURED'S I.D. NUMBER (For Program in Item 1): PX4278A

2. PATIENT'S NAME (Last Name, First Name, Middle Initial): Parkinson, Tom, N

3. PATIENT'S BIRTH DATE MM DD YY: 04 06 1993 SEX M [X] F [ ]

4. INSURED'S NAME (Last Name, First Name, Middle Initial): Parkinson, Jamie, B

5. PATIENT'S ADDRESS (No., Street): 4510 South A Street

CITY: Woodland Hills STATE: XY

ZIP CODE: 12345-0000 TELEPHONE (Include Area Code): (555) 7421580

6. PATIENT RELATIONSHIP TO INSURED: Self [ ] Spouse [ ] Child [X] Other [ ]

7. INSURED'S ADDRESS (No., Street): 4510 South A Street

CITY: Woodland Hills STATE: XY

ZIP CODE: 12345-0000 TELEPHONE (Include Area Code): (555) 7421560

8. RESERVED FOR NUCC USE

9. OTHER INSURED'S NAME (Last Name, First Name, Middle Initial)

a. OTHER INSURED'S POLICY OR GROUP NUMBER

b. RESERVED FOR NUCC USE

c. RESERVED FOR NUCC USE

d. INSURANCE PLAN NAME OR PROGRAM NAME

10. IS PATIENT'S CONDITION RELATED TO:

a. EMPLOYMENT? (Current or Previous) [ ] YES [X] NO

b. AUTO ACCIDENT? [ ] YES [X] NO PLACE (State)

c. OTHER ACCIDENT? [ ] YES [X] NO

10d. CLAIM CODES (Designated by NUCC)

11. INSURED'S POLICY GROUP OR FECA NUMBER

a. INSURED'S DATE OF BIRTH MM DD YY SEX M [ ] F [ ]

b. OTHER CLAIM ID (Designated by NUCC)

c. INSURANCE PLAN NAME OR PROGRAM NAME

d. IS THERE ANOTHER HEALTH BENEFIT PLAN? [ ] YES [X] NO *If yes*, complete items 9, 9a, and 9d.

READ BACK OF FORM BEFORE COMPLETING & SIGNING THIS FORM.

12. PATIENT'S OR AUTHORIZED PERSON'S SIGNATUREI authorize the release of any medical or other information necessary to process this claim. I also request payment of government benefits either to myself or to the party who accepts assignment below.

SIGNED ____ DATE ____

13. INSURED'S OR AUTHORIZED PERSON'S SIGNATURE I authorize payment of medical benefits to the undersigned physician or supplier for services described below.

SIGNED ____

PATIENT AND INSURED INFORMATION

14. DATE OF CURRENT: ILLNESS, INJURY, or PREGNANCY(LMP) MM DD YY QUAL.

15. OTHER DATE QUAL. MM DD YY

16. DATES PATIENT UNABLE TO WORK IN CURRENT OCCUPATION MM DD YY FROM TO

17. NAME OF REFERRING PROVIDER OR OTHER SOURCE 17a. 17b. NPI

18. HOSPITALIZATION DATES RELATED TO CURRENT SERVICES MM DD YY FROM TO

19. ADDITIONAL CLAIM INFORMATION (Designated by NUCC)

20. OUTSIDE LAB? [ ] YES [X] NO $ CHARGES

21. DIAGNOSIS OR NATURE OF ILLNESS OR INJURY Relate A-L to service line below (24E) ICD Ind. 0

A. ____ B. ____ C. ____ D. ____
E. ____ F. ____ G. ____ H. ____
I. ____ J. ____ K. ____ L. ____

22. RESUBMISSION CODE ORIGINAL REF. NO.

23. PRIOR AUTHORIZATION NUMBER

	24. A. DATE(S) OF SERVICE From MM DD YY	To MM DD YY	B. PLACE OF SERVICE	C. EMG	D. PROCEDURES, SERVICES, OR SUPPLIES (Explain Unusual Circumstances) CPT/HCPCS	MODIFIER	E. DIAGNOSIS POINTER	F. $ CHARGES	G. DAYS OR UNITS	H. EPSDT Family Plan	I. ID. QUAL.	J. RENDERING PROVIDER ID. #
1	07 14 20XX				99242			80 24	1		NPI	
2	07 14 20XX				71020		A	38 96	1		NPI	4627889700
3											NPI	
4											NPI	
5											NPI	
6											NPI	

25. FEDERAL TAX I.D. NUMBER SSN EIN: 7034597 [ ] [ ]

26. PATIENT'S ACCOUNT NO.

27. ACCEPT ASSIGNMENT? (For govt. claims, see back) [X] YES [ ] NO

28. TOTAL CHARGE $ 119 20

29. AMOUNT PAID $

30. Rsvd for NUCC Use $

31. SIGNATURE OF PHYSICIAN OR SUPPLIER INCLUDING DEGREES OR CREDENTIALS (I certify that the statements on the reverse apply to this bill and are made a part thereof.)

Gerald Practon 071420XX

SIGNED *Gerald Practon* DATE

32. SERVICE FACILITY LOCATION INFORMATION

a. NPI b.

33. BILLING PROVIDER INFO & PH # (555) 4869002
College Clinic
4567 Broad Avenue
Woodland Hills XY 12345-0001

a. 3664021CC b.

PHYSICIAN OR SUPPLIER INFORMATION

NUCC Instruction Manual available at: www.nucc.org *PLEASE PRINT OR TYPE* OMB APPROVAL PENDING

Figure 7-10

ASSIGNMENT 7-6 REVIEW PATIENT RECORD ABBREVIATIONS

Performance Objective

Task: Insert meanings of abbreviations.

Conditions: Use a pencil or pen.

Standards: Time: ____________ minutes

Accuracy: ____________

(Note: The time element and accuracy criteria may be given by your instructor.)

Directions: After completing all the patient records in the *Workbook* that are pertinent to this chapter, you will be able to answer the next two questions.

1. What do these abbreviations mean?

   a. PTR ____________________

   b. TURP ____________________

   c. hx ____________________

   d. IVP ____________________

   e. $\bar{c}$ ____________________

   f. Dx ____________________

   g. BP ____________________

   h. CC ____________________

   i. UA ____________________

   j. PE ____________________

2. Give the abbreviations for the following terms.

   a. return ____________________

   b. cancer, carcinoma ____________________

   c. patient ____________________

   d. established ____________________

   e. discharged ____________________

   f. gallbladder ____________________

   g. initial ____________________

ASSIGNMENT 7-7 STUDENT SOFTWARE CHALLENGE: ASSIGNMENTS FOR CASES 1 THROUGH 6 ONSCREEN COMPLETION OF CMS-1500 (02-12) INSURANCE CLAIM FORMS FOR PRIVATE INSURANCE

Performance Objective

Task: Enter transactions from patients' onscreen encounter forms (superbills) and complete block-by-block onscreen health insurance claim forms.

Conditions: Onscreen encounter forms (superbills), patient records, and health insurance claim forms, and computer; procedural and diagnostic code books

Standards: Time: ______________ minutes

Accuracy: ______________

(Note: The time element and accuracy criteria may be given by your instructor.)

Directions: Log on to your Evolve account at *http://evolve.elsevier.com* and access the student resources for Fordney: *Insurance Handbook for the Medical Office,* 13th edition. Then choose Student Software Challenge.

1. For these assignments, follow the instructions for entering data into the onscreen CMS-1500 (02-12) health insurance claim form completing Blocks 1 through 33 for Cases 1 through 6.
2. Use your CPT code book or Appendix A in this *Workbook* to determine the correct five-digit code number and modifiers for each professional service rendered. To determine diagnostic codes, refer to diagnosis code books (ICD-9-CM or ICD-10-CM, as directed by your instructor).
3. Print a hard copy of the completed health insurance claim form for each case.
4. After the instructor has returned your work to you, either make the necessary corrections and place your work in a three-ring notebook for future reference, or, if you received a high score, place it in your portfolio for reference when applying for a job.

8 The Electronic Claim

Linda Smith

KEY TERMS

Your instructor may wish to select some words pertinent to this chapter for a test. For definitions of the terms, further study, and/or reference, the words, phrases, and abbreviations may be found in the glossary at the end of the Handbook. *Key terms for this chapter follow.*

Accredited Standards Committee X12
Accredited Standards Committee X12 Version 5010
application service provider
backup
batch
business associate agreement
cable modem
claim attachments
clearinghouse
code sets
covered entity
data elements
digital subscriber line
direct data entry
electronic data interchange
electronic funds transfer
electronic remittance advice
encoder
encryption
HIPAA Transaction and Code Set Rule
National Standard Format
password
real time
standard transactions
T-1
taxonomy codes
trading partner
trading partner agreement

KEY ABBREVIATIONS

See how many abbreviations and acronyms you can translate and then use this as a handy reference list. Definitions for the key abbreviations are located near the back of the Handbook *in the glossary.*

ANSI ____________________

ASC X12 ____________________

ASET ____________________

ASP ____________________

ATM ____________________

DDE ____________________

DHHS ____________________

DSL ____________________

EDI ____________________

EFT ____________________

EHR ____________________

EMC ____________________

EOMB ____________________

ePHI ____________________

ERA ____________________

HPID ____________________

IRS ____________________

MTS ____________________

NDC ____________________

NSF ____________________

PMS ____________________

TCS rule ____________________

UPS ____________________

PERFORMANCE OBJECTIVES

The student will be able to:

- Define and spell the key terms and key abbreviations for this chapter, given the information from the *Handbook* glossary, within a reasonable time period and with enough accuracy to obtain a satisfactory evaluation.
- After reading the chapter, answer the fill-in-the-blank, multiple choice, and true/false review questions with enough accuracy to obtain a satisfactory evaluation.
- Decide whether keyed medical and nonmedical data elements are required, situational, or not used when electronically submitting the 837P health care claim.
- State which medical and nonmedical code sets for 837P electronic claims are required, situational, or not used.
- Input data into the element for place of service codes for 837P electronic claims submission.
- Indicate the patient's relationship to the insured by using the individual relationship code numbers for 837P electronic claims submission.
- Select the correct taxonomy codes for the specialists for submission of 837P electronic claims submission.
- Locate errors, given computer-generated insurance forms, within a reasonable time period and with enough accuracy to obtain a satisfactory evaluation.
- Fill in the correct meaning of each abbreviation, given a list of common medical abbreviations and symbols that appear in chart notes, with enough accuracy to obtain a satisfactory evaluation.

STUDY OUTLINE

Electronic Data Interchange
Electronic Claims
Advantages of Electronic Claim Submission
Clearinghouses
Transaction and Code Set Regulations: Streamlining Electronic Data Interchange
- Transaction and Code Set Standards

Electronic Standard HIPAA 837P
- Levels of Information for 837P Standard Transaction Format
- Accredited Standards Committee X12 (ASC X12) Version 5010

Claims Attachments Standards
Standard Unique Identifiers
- Standard Unique Employer Identifier
- Standard Unique Health Care Provider Identifier
- Standard Unique Health Plan Identifier
- Standard Unique Patient Identifier

Practice Management System
Building the Claim
- Encounter or Multipurpose Billing Forms
- Scannable Encounter Form
- Keying Insurance Data for Claim Transmission
- Encoder
- Clean Electronic Claims Submission

Putting HIPAA Standard Transactions to Work
- Interactive Transactions
- Electronic Funds Transfer (EFT)

Electronic Remittance Advice
Driving the Data
Methods for Sending Claims
Computer Claims Systems
- Payer or Carrier-Direct
- Clearinghouse

Transmission Reports
- Electronic Processing Problems
- Solutions to Electronic Processing Problems
- Billing and Account Management Schedule
- Administrative Simplification Enforcement Tool (ASET)
- The Security Rule: Administrative, Physical, and Technical Safeguards

HIPAA: Application to the Practice Setting
Records Management
- Data Storage
- Data Disposal
- Electronic Power Protection
- Selection of an Office Computer System

ASSIGNMENT 8-1 REVIEW QUESTIONS

Part I Fill in the Blank

Review the objectives, key terms, glossary definitions of key terms, chapter information, and figures before completing the following review questions.

1. Exchange of data in a standardized format through computer systems is a technology known as ____________________.

2. The act of converting computerized data into a code so that unauthorized users are unable to read it is a security system known as ____________________.

3. Payment to the provider of service of an electronically submitted insurance claim may be received in approximately ____________________.

4. Medical practices that do not use the services of clearinghouses submit claims through a ____________________ to the insurance company.

5. Refer to Table 8-1 in the *Handbook* to list benefits of using HIPAA standard transactions and code sets.

   a. ____________________

   b. ____________________

   c. ____________________

   d. ____________________

   e. ____________________

   f. ____________________

6. Dr. Morgan has 10 or more full-time employees and submits insurance claims for his Medicare patients. Is his medical practice subject to the HIPAA transaction rules?

   ____

7. Dr. Maria Montez does not submit insurance claims electronically and has five full-time employees. Is she required to abide by HIPAA transaction rules? ____________________

8. Refer to Table 8-2 in the *Handbook* to name the standard code sets used for the following:

   a. Physician services ____________________

   b. Diseases and injuries ____________________

   c. Pharmaceuticals and biologics ____________________

9. Refer to Table 8-3 in the *Handbook* to complete these statements.

   a. The staff at College Clinic submits professional health care claims for each of their providers and must use the industry standard electronic format called ____________________ to transmit them electronically.

   b. The billing department at College Hospital must use the industry standard electronic format called ____________________ to transmit health care claims electronically.

c. The Medicare fiscal intermediary (insurance carrier) uses the industry standard electronic format called ______________________________ to transmit payment information to the College Clinic and College Hospital.

d. It has been 3 weeks since Gordon Marshall's health care claim was transmitted to the XYZ insurance company and you wish to inquire about the status of the claim. The industry standard electronic format that must be used to transmit this inquiry is called ______________________________.

e. Dr. Practon's insurance billing specialist must use the industry standard electronic format called ______________ to obtain information about Beatrice Garcia's health policy benefits and coverage from the insurance plan.

10. The family practice taxonomy code is ______________________________.

11. The Amercian National Standards Institute formed the ____________________, which developed the electronic data exchange standards.

12. Refer to Table 8-4 in the *Handbook* to name the levels for data collected to construct and submit an electronic claim.

a. ______________________________

b. ______________________________

c. ______________________________

d. ______________________________

e. ______________________________

f. ______________________________

13. HIPAA electronic standards for claim submission were upgraded to Version __________, and all providers, payers, and clearinghouses were required to use it effective January 1, 2012.

14. The Claims Attachments Standards have not yet been adopted; however, the health insurance specialist should prepare for the final rule that is expected to be published no later than ____________________ as required under the Affordable Care Act.

15. The ____________________ is an all numeric 10-character number assigned to each provider and required for all transactions with health plans effective May 23, 2007.

16. The most important function of a practice management system is ________________.

17. To look for and correct all errors before the health claim is transmitted to the insurance carrier, you may print an insurance billing worksheet or perform a front-end edit or ______________________________.

18. Much of the patient and insurance information required to complete the CMS-1500 form can be found on the ____________________ form that is used to post charges.

19. Add-on software to a practice management system that can reduce the time it takes to build or review a claim before batching is known as a/an ____________________.

20. Software that is used in a network that serves a group of users working on a related project allowing access to the same data is called a/an ____________________.

21. Many insurance companies, such as Medicare, provide instant access to information about pending claims through online ________________________________.

22. An electronic funds transfer agreement may allow for health plans to ____________ overpayments from a provider's bank account.

23. The Medicare electronic remittance advice was previously referred to as a/an

____.

24. On completion of a signed agreement and approval of enrollment with a third-party payer for electronic claims submission, the provider will be assigned a __________ number.

25. When computer software is upgraded, the physician must submit a batch of ____________________ to the insurance carrier to determine if claims can be transmitted successfully.

26. Under HIPAA transaction standard ASC X12 Version 5010, a ________________ digit ZIP code is required to report service facility locations.

27. The ____________________________________ is an electronic tool that enables organizations to file a complaint against a noncompliant covered entity that is negatively impacting the efficient processing of claims.

28. Access controls allow organizations to create ________________ for each job category that will restrict access to certain data.

29. Under HIPAA, ________________ efforts must be made to limit the use and disclosure of PHI.

Part II Multiple Choice

Choose the best answer.

30. Electronic claims are submitted by means of
    a. U.S. Postal Service.
    b. fax transmission.
    c. phone transmission.
    d. EDI.

31. Today, most claims are submitted by means of
    a. U.S. Postal Service.
    b. fax transmission.
    c. phone transmission.
    d. EDI.

32. The online error-edit process allows providers to
    a. correct claim errors prior to transmission of the claim.
    b. decrease labor costs by freeing staff to do other duties.
    c. reduce postage fees and trips to the post office.
    d. reduce storage of claims.

33. Under HIPAA, data elements that are used uniformly to document why patients are seen (diagnosis) and what is done to them during their encounter (procedure) are known as
    a. medical code sets.
    b. information elements.
    c. TCS standards.
    d. National Standard Format (NSF).

34. The standard transaction that replaces the paper CMS-1500 (02-12) claim form and more than 400 versions of the electronic National Standard Format is called the
    a. 270.
    b. 837I.
    c. 837P.
    d. 837D.

35. The next version of the electronic claims submission that will be proposed for consideration once lessons are learned from implementation of Version 5010 will be
    a. Version 5011.
    b. Version 5012.
    c. Version 6001.
    d. Version 6020.

36. A standard unique number that will be assigned to identify individual health plans under the Affordable Care Act is referred to as a
    a. EIN.
    b. ERA.
    c. HIPD.
    d. NPI.

37. Uniform patient identifiers
    a. were required on all claims effective May 23, 2007.
    b. were required on all claims effective October 1, 2012.
    c. will be required on all claims effective October 1, 2014.
    d. are not yet required, and the proposal is on hold for implementation of the standard.

38. Encounter forms should be reviewed annually for changes that may have been made to
    a. diagnosis codes.
    b. procedure codes.
    c. HCPCS codes.
    d. all of the above.

39. A technique for entry of data, which can save time and key strokes by recording commands into memory, is referred to as use of
    a. automated billing.
    b. templates.
    c. macros.
    d. encryption.

40. An authorization and assignment of benefits signature for a patient who was treated in the hospital but has never been to the provider's office
    a. should be obtained by the provider when he or she sees the patient in the hospital.
    b. must be mailed to the patient for signature prior to submission of a claim.
    c. can be obtained from the patient at his or her first office visit.
    d. is not required; the authorization obtained by the hospital applies to that provider's claim filing.

41. A paperless computerized system that enables payments to be transferred automatically to a physician's bank account by a third-party payer may be done via
    a. electronic savings account.
    b. electronic remittance advice (ERA).
    c. electronic funds transfer (EFT).
    d. electronic data interchange (EDI).

42. An electronic Medicare remittance advice that takes the place of a paper Medicare explanation of benefits (EOB) is referred to as
    a. ANSI 277.
    b. ANSI 820.
    c. ANSI 830.
    d. ANSI 835.

43. A method for submitting claims electronically by keying information into the payer system for processing is accomplished through use of
    a. a clearinghouse.
    b. direct data entry.
    c. an application service provider.
    d. DSL.

44. A report that is generated by a payer and sent to the provider to show how many claims were received as electronic claims and how many of the claims were automatically rejected and will not be processed is called a
    a. send-and-receive file report.
    b. scrubber report.
    c. transaction transmission summary.
    d. rejection analysis report.

45. The HIPAA transaction standard ASC X12 Version 5010 requires that anesthesia services be reported
    a. per day.
    b. per unit.
    c. per second.
    d. per minute.

46. Which section of the HIPAA Security Rule recommends unique "usernames" and passwords to log on to any computer with access to PHI?
    a. Administrative safeguards
    b. Technical safeguards
    c. Physical safeguards

47. Which section of the HIPAA Security Rule recommends use of screensavers that will activate after 1 to 60 minutes of inactivity?
    a. Administrative safeguards
    b. Technical safeguards
    c. Physical safeguards

48. Verification of successful backups by comparing original records with copied records should be performed
    a. once a day.
    b. once a week.
    c. once a month.
    d. once a year.

49. An acceptable method for ensuring that ePHI cannot be recovered from a hard drive that is being disposed of is by
    a. deletion of files.
    b. formatting drives.
    c. incineration.
    d. all of the above.

Part III True/False

Write "T" or "F" in the blank to indicate whether you think the statement is true or false.

________ 50. Like paper claims, electronic claims require the performing physician's signature.

________ 51. Claims can be submitted to various insurance payers in a single-batch electronic transmission.

________ 52. Under HIPAA, insurance payers can require health care providers to use the payer's own version of local code sets.

________ 53. As ICD and CPT codes are deleted and become obsolete, they should immediately be removed from the practice's computer system.

________ 54. HIPAA has brought forth electronic formats for determination of eligibility for a health insurance plan.

________ 55. HIPAA's electronic standard transactions are identified by a four-digit number that precedes "ASC X12N."

________ 56. Implementation of ICD-10 resulted in the upgrade to HIPAA transaction standard ASC X12 Version 6010.

________ 57. HIPAA requires that the NPI number be used to identify employers rather than inputting the actual name of the company when submitting claims.

________ 58. HIPAA limits how computer systems may transmit data and formats for storage of data.

________ 59. A paper remittance advice is generated by Medicare when using ANSI 835 Version 5010.

________ 60. HIPAA transaction standard ASC X12 Version 5010 allows employer identification numbers to be used to report as a primary identifier.

________ 61. When transmitting electronic claims, inaccuracies that violate the HIPAA standard transaction format are known as syntax errors.

________ 62. An organization may file a complaint online against someone whose actions impact the ability of a transaction to be accepted or efficiently processed by using the Administration Simplification Enforcement Tool (ASET).

________ 63. Incidental uses and disclosures of protected health information (PHI) are permissible under HIPAA when reasonable safeguards have been used to prevent inappropriate revelation of PHI.

________ 64. Deleting files or formatting the hard drive is sufficient to keep electronic protected health information from being accessed.

ASSIGNMENT 8-2 CRITICAL THINKING FOR MEDICAL AND NONMEDICAL CODE SETS FOR 837P ELECTRONIC CLAIMS SUBMISSION

Performance Objective

Task: Decide whether keyed medical and nonmedical data elements are required, situational, or not used when electronically submitting the 837P health care claim.

Conditions: List of keyed data elements (Table 8-5 in *Handbook*) and pen or pencil.

Standards: Time: ______________ minutes

Accuracy: ______________

(Note: The time element and accuracy criteria may be given by your instructor.)

Directions: When submitting the 837P health care claim, supporting code sets of medical and nonmedical data are composed of "Required" and "Situational" data elements. Read each keyed data element and answer whether you think it is **R** for required, **S** for situational, or **N** for not used.

a. Patient's last menstrual period ______________________________

b. Patient's telephone number ______________________________

c. Insured's name ______________________________

d. Diagnosis code ______________________________

e. Provider's NPI ______________________________

f. Procedure code ______________________________

g. Provider's signature ______________________________

h. Employer's name ______________________________

i. Place of service ______________________________

j. Procedure modifier ______________________________

ASSIGNMENT 8-3 INPUT DATA INTO ELEMENT FOR PLACE OF SERVICE CODES FOR 837P ELECTRONIC CLAIMS SUBMISSIONS

Performance Objective

Task: Insert the correct place of service code for each location description where medical professional service was rendered.

Conditions: Place of service codes reference (Figure 8-1), list of places where medical care was rendered, and pen or pencil.

Standards: Time: ______________ minutes

Accuracy: ______________

(Note: The time element and accuracy criteria may be given by your instructor.)

Directions: When submitting the 837P electronic claim, place of service codes must be entered in data element 1331. Refer to the place of service codes reference list and insert the correct code for each place of service for the following locations.

a. Inpatient psychiatric facility ______________________________

b. Doctor's office ______________________________

c. Outpatient hospital ______________________________

d. Intermediate nursing facility ______________________________

e. Independent clinic ______________________________

f. Independent laboratory ______________________________

g. Birthing center ______________________________

h. End-stage renal disease treatment facility ______________________________

i. Inpatient hospital ______________________________

j. Hospice ______________________________

PLACE OF SERVICE CODES	
Codes	**Place of Service**
01	Pharmacy
00-02	Unassigned
03	School
04	Homeless shelter
05	Indian health service free-standing facility
06	Indian health service provider-based facility
07	Tribal 638 free-standing facility
08	Tribal 638 provide r-based facility
09	Prison/correctional facility
10	Unassigned
11	Doctor's office
12	Patient's home
13	Assisted living facility
14	Group home
15	Mobile unit
16	Temporary lodging
17-19	Unassigned
20	Urgent care facility
21	Inpatient hospital
22	Outpatient hospital or urgent care center
23	Emergency department—hospital
24	Ambulatory surgical center
25	Birthing center
26	Military treatment facility/uniformed service treatment facility
27-30	Unassigned
31	Skilled nursing facility (s wing bed visits)
32	Nursing facility (intermediate/long-term care facilities)
33	Custodial care facility (domiciliary or rest home services)
34	Hospice (domiciliary or rest home services)
35-40	Unassigned
41	Ambulance—land
42	Ambulance—air or water
43-48	Unassigned
49	Independent clinic
50	Federally qualified health center
51	Inpatient psychiatric facility
52	Psychiatric facility—partial hospitalization
53	Community mental health care (outpatient, twenty-four-hours-a-day services, admission screening, consultation, and educational services)
54	Intermediate care facility/mentally retarded
55	Residential substance abuse treatment facility
56	Psychiatric residential treatment center
57	Non-residential substance abuse treatment facility
58-59	Unassigned
60	Mass immunization center
61	Comprehensive inpatient rehabilitation facility
62	Comprehensive outpatient rehabilitation facility
63-64	Unassigned
65	End-stage renal disease treatment facility
66-70	Unassigned
71	State or local public health clinic
72	Rural health clinic
73-80	Unassigned
81	Independent laboratory
82-98	Unassigned
99	Other unlisted facility

Figure 8-1

ASSIGNMENT 8-4 SELECT THE CORRECT INDIVIDUAL RELATIONSHIP CODE NUMBER FOR 837P ELECTRONIC CLAIMS SUBMISSION

Performance Objective

Task: Insert the correct individual relationship code for the patient's relationship to the insured.

Conditions: Individual relationship code number reference (Figure 8-2), list of individuals or entities, and pen or pencil.

Standards: Time: ______________ minutes

Accuracy: ______________

(Note: The time element and accuracy criteria may be given by your instructor.)

Directions: Refer to the individual relationship code number list, choose the correct code for the patient's relationship to the insured for the following persons, and insert it on the lines.

a. Mother ____________________________

b. Spouse ____________________________

c. Child ____________________________

d. Father ____________________________

e. Stepdaughter ____________________________

f. Emancipated minor ____________________________

g. Adopted child ____________________________

h. Handicapped dependent ____________________________

i. Stepson ____________________________

j. Sponsored dependent ____________________________

Individual Relationship Code	
Code	**Relationship**
01	Spouse
04	Grandfather or grandmother
05	Grandson or granddaughter
07	Nephew or niece
09	Adopted child
10	Foster child
15	Ward
17	Stepson or stepdaughter
19	Child
20	Employee
21	Unknown
22	Handicapped dependent
23	Sponsored dependent
24	Dependent of a minor dependent
29	Significant other
32	Mother
33	Father
34	Other adult
36	Emancipated minor
39	Organ donor
40	Cadaver donor
41	Injured plaintiff
43	Child where insured has no financial responsibility
53	Life partner
G8	Other relationship

Figure 8-2

ASSIGNMENT 8-5 SELECT THE CORRECT TAXONOMY CODES FOR MEDICAL SPECIALISTS FOR 837P ELECTRONIC CLAIMS SUBMISSION

Performance Objective

Task: Choose the correct taxonomy code for each specialist for submission of 837P electronic claims by referring to the Health Care Provider Taxonomy code list.

Conditions: Health Care Provider Taxonomy code list (Figure 8-3), list of providers of service, and pen or pencil.

Standards: Time: ______________ minutes

Accuracy: ______________

(Note: The time element and accuracy criteria may be given by your instructor.)

Directions: Refer to the Health Care Provider Taxonomy code list, choose the correct code for each of the following specialists, and insert the code numbers on the lines.

a. Raymond Skeleton, MD, orthopedist ______________________

b. Gaston Input, MD, gastroenterologist ______________________

c. Vera Cutis, MD, dermatologist ______________________

d. Gene Ulibarri, MD, urologist ______________________

e. Bertha Caesar, MD, obstetrician/gynecologist ______________________

f. Gerald Practon, MD, general practitioner ______________________

g. Pedro Atrics, MD, pediatrician ______________________

h. Astro Parkinson, MD, neurosurgeon ______________________

i. Brady Coccidioides, MD, pulmonary disease ______________________

j. Max Gluteus, RPT, physical therapist ______________________

College Clinic Staff		
Health Care Provider Taxonomy Codes		
Name	**Speciality**	**Taxonomy Code**
Concha Antrum, MD	Otolaryngologist	207Y00000X
Pedro Atrics, MD	Pediatrician	208000000X
Bertha Caesar, MD	Obstetrician/Gynecologist	207V00000X
Perry Cardi, MD	Cardiologist	207RC0000X
Brady Coccidioides, MD	Pulmonary disease	207RP1001X
Vera Cutis, MD	Dermatologist	207N00000X
Clarence Cutler, MD	General surgeon	208600000X
Dennis Drill, DDS	Dentist	122300000X
Max Gluteus, RPT	Physical therapist	208100000X
Cosmo Graff, MD	Plastic surgeon	208200000X
Malvern Grumose, MD	Pathologist	207ZP0105X
Gaston Input, MD	Gastroenterologist	207RG0100X
Adam Langerhans, MD	Endocrinologist	207RE0101X
Cornell Lenser, MD	Ophthalmologist	207W00000X
Michael Menter, MD	Psychiatrist	2084P0800X
Arthur O. Dont, DDS	Orthodontist	1223X0400X
Astro Parkinson, MD	Neurosurgeon	207T00000X
Nick Pedro, MD	Podiatrist	213E00000X
Gerald Practon, MD	General practitioner	208D00000X
Walter Radon, MD	Radiologst	2085R0202X
Rex Rumsey, MD	Proctologist	208C00000X
Sensitive E. Scott, MD	Anesthesiologist	207L00000X
Raymond Skeleton, MD	Orthopedist	207X00000X
Gene Ulibarri, MD	Urologist	208800000X

Figure 8-3

ASSIGNMENT 8-6 COMPOSE ELECTRONIC MAIL MESSAGES

Performance Objective

Task: Compose brief messages for electronic mail transmission after reading each scenario.

Conditions: List of scenarios, one sheet of 8½ × 11-inch plain typing paper, and a computer or a pen.

Standards: Time: _______________ minutes

Accuracy: _______________

(Note: The time element and accuracy criteria may be given by your instructor.)

Directions: Read each scenario. Compose polite, effective, and brief messages that, on the job, would be transmitted via electronic mail (e-mail). Use the guidelines for electronic mail presented on the Evolve website. Be sure to list a descriptive subject line as the first item in each composition. Single-space the message. Insert a short signature at the end of the message to include your name and affiliation, and create an e-mail address for yourself if you do not have one. Print hard copies of e-mail messages for Scenarios 1 through 5 to give to your instructor. After the instructor has returned your work, either make the necessary corrections and place your work in a three-ring notebook for future reference, or, if you received a high score, place it in your portfolio for use when applying for a job.

Scenario 1:

Ask an insurance biller, Mary Davis, in a satellite office to locate and fax you a copy of the billing done on account number 43500 for services rendered to Margarita Sylva on March 2, 20xx. Explain that you must telephone the patient about her account. Mary Davis' e-mail address is mdavis@aal.com.

Scenario 2:

Patient Ellen Worth was recently hospitalized; her hospital number is 20-9870-11. Compose an e-mail message to the medical record department at College Hospital (collegehospmedrecords@rrv.net) for her final diagnosis and the assigned diagnostic code needed to complete the insurance claim form.

Scenario 3:

You are working for a billing service and receive an encounter form that is missing the information about the patient's professional service received on August 2, 20xx. The patient's account number is 45098. You have the diagnosis data. Compose an e-mail message to Dr. Mason (pmason@email.mc.com) explaining what you must obtain to complete the billing portion of the insurance claim form.

Scenario 4:

A new patient, John Phillips, has e-mailed your office to ask what the outstanding balance is on his account. The account number is 42990. You look up the financial record and note the service was for an office visit on June 14, 20xx. The charge was $106.11. Compose an e-mail response to Mr. Phillips, whose e-mail address is jphillips@hotmail.com.

Scenario 5:

You are having difficulty deciding whether the codes 13101, 13102, and 13132 with modifier -51 selected for a case are appropriate. Compose an e-mail message that will be posted on the Part B News Internet listserv (PartB-L@usa.net) asking for comments. The case involves a 12-year-old boy who fell against a bicycle, lacerating the left side of his chest to the pectoralis muscle through a 12-cm gaping wound. He also sustained a 5-cm laceration to his left cheek. Complex repairs were required for these two wounds and totaled 17 cm. Find out whether modifier -15 should be appended to the second code or to the third code.

For each message, check for concise composition, single-spaced message, closing signature, and accuracy and effectiveness of message in terms of scenario presented. E-mail may contain abbreviations. On the job, a biller would compose a message quickly, so the instructor might want to award additional points for the speed with which this assignment is done.

ASSIGNMENT 8-7 PROOFREAD A COMPUTER-GENERATED HEALTH INSURANCE CLAIM FORM AND LOCATE INCORRECT AND MISSING DATA

Performance Objective

Task: Locate and designate blocks on the computer-generated insurance claim form that have incorrect or missing information; correct or add data before submission to the insurance company.

Conditions: Use Brad E. Diehl's patient record (Figure 8-4), completed insurance claim (Figure 8-5), and a highlighter and a red ink pen.

Standards: Time: ______________ minutes

Accuracy: ______________

(Note: The time element and accuracy criteria may be given by your instructor.)

Directions: Proofread the insurance claim form (see Figure 8-5) and locate blocks that need correction or completion before submission to the insurance company. Highlight all errors you discover. Refer to the patient's record (see Figure 8-4) to verify pertinent demographic and insurance information. Refer to the progress notes to verify procedures and determine diagnoses. Verify all entries on the claim form, including dates, codes, rounded-out fees, and physician identification numbers. Insert all corrections and missing information in red. If you cannot locate the necessary information but know it is mandatory, write "NEED" in the corresponding block.

Optional: Retype a blank CMS-1500 (02-12) claim form with all corrections and changes. Or, if you have access to a computer, log on to your Evolve account at http://evolve.elsevier.com and access the student resources for Fordney: *Insurance Handbook for the Medical Office,* 13th edition. There you can fill out a CMS-1500 PDF file and print it or save it.

Additional Coding

1. Assume that Mr. Diehl followed Dr. Input's treatment plan. Refer to his record, abstract information, and locate procedure codes that would be billed by providers outside of the office.

Site	*Description of Service*	*Code*
a. ABC Radiology	______________	______________
b. College Hospital	______________	______________
c. Surgeon	______________	______________

2. Code the symptoms Mr. Diehl was complaining about when he presented for the January 6, 20xx, office visit.

Symptom	*ICD-10-CM Code*
a. ______________	______________
b. ______________	______________
c. ______________	______________
d. ______________	______________
e. ______________	______________

PATIENT RECORD NO. 8-7

Diehl	Brad	E.	09-21-46	M	555-222-0123
LAST NAME	FIRST NAME	MIDDLE NAME	BIRTH DATE	SEX	HOME PHONE

3975 Hills Road	Woodland Hills	XY	12345
ADDRESS	CITY	STATE	ZIP CODE

555-703-6600	555-321-0988	555-222-0123	Diehl@WB.net
CELL PHONE	PAGER NO.	FAX NO.	E-MAIL ADDRESS

561-XX-1501	M0983457
PATIENT'S SOC. SEC. NO.	DRIVER'S LICENSE

radio advertising salesman	KACY Radio
PATIENT'S OCCUPATION	NAME OF COMPANY

4071 Mills Road, Woodland Hills, XY 12335	555-201-6666
ADDRESS OF EMPLOYER	PHONE

Tak E. Diehl (birthdate 4-7-45)	legal secretary
SPOUSE OR PARENT	OCCUPATION

Attys. Dilman, Forewise & Gilson,	12 West Dix Street, Woodland Hills, XY 12345	555-222-6432
EMPLOYER	ADDRESS	PHONE

Aetna Insurance Co., 2412 Main Street, Woodland Hills, XY 12345	Brad E. Diehl
NAME OF INSURANCE	INSURED OR SUBSCRIBER

403119	
POLICY/CERTIFICATE NO.	GROUP NO.

REFERRED BY: Raymond Skeleton, MD

DATE	PROGRESS NOTES No. 8-7
1-6-20xx	NP pt comes in complaining of coughing and sneezing; some difficulty breathing.
	Occasional dizziness and epigastric abdominal pain with cramping. Symptoms started in
	July of last year. Performed a detailed history and physical examination with low
	complexity medical decision making. AP & lat chest x-rays taken; neg findings. BP 178/98.
	Pt to have cholecystography with oral contrast at ABC Radiology. Diagnostic colonoscopy
	(flexible) to be scheduled at College Hospital. Dx: hypertension and respiratory distress;
	R/O irritable colon. No disability at this time.
	GI/llf Gaston Input, MD
1-20-xx	Pt retns for a EPF hx/exam LC MDM. Oral cholecystography reveals a single 1.5 cm
	radiolucent calculus within the cholecyst. Colonoscopy confirmed irritable bowel
	syndrome. Blood drawn and CBC (auto with diff) performed in office indicates
	WBC 10,000. DX: cholecystitis with cholelithiasis. Adv. cholecystectomy
	(abdominal approach) as soon as possible; to be scheduled at College Hospital.
	GI/llf Gaston Input, MD

Figure 8-4

DRAFT - NOT FOR OFFICIAL USE

HEALTH INSURANCE CLAIM FORM

APPROVED BY NATIONAL UNIFOR MCLAIM COMMITTEE (NUCC) 02/12

PICA | PICA | CARRIER

1. MEDICARE (Medicare#) ☐ MEDICAID (Medicaid#) ☐ TRICARE (ID#DoD#) ☐ CHAMPVA (Member ID#) ☐ GROUP HEALTH PLAN (ID#) [X] FECA BLK LUNG (ID#) ☐ OTHER (ID#) ☐

1a. INSURED'S I.D. NUMBER (For Program in Item 1): 403119

2. PATIENT'S NAME (Last Name, First Name, Middle Initial): Diehl, Brad, E

3. PATIENT'S BIRTH DATE MM DD YY: 09 21 1946 SEX M ☐ F ☐

4. INSURED'S NAME (Last Name, First Name, Middle Initial): Same

5. PATIENT'S ADDRESS (No., Street): 3975 Hills Road

6. PATIENT RELATIONSHIP TO INSURED: Self [X] Spouse ☐ Child ☐ Other ☐

7. INSURED'S ADDRESS (No., Street):

CITY: Woodland Hills STATE: XY

8. RESERVED FOR NUCC USE

CITY STATE

ZIP CODE: 12345-0000 TELEPHONE (Include Area Code): (555) 2220123

ZIP CODE TELEPHONE (Include Area Code) ( )

9. OTHER INSURED'S NAME (Last Name, First Name, Middle Initial)

10. IS PATIENT'S CONDITION RELATED TO:

11. INSURED'S POLICY GROUP OR FECA NUMBER

a. OTHER INSURED'S POLICY OR GROUP NUMBER

a. EMPLOYMENT? (Current or Previous) ☐ YES [X] NO

a. INSURED'S DATE OF BIRTH MM DD YY SEX M ☐ F ☐

b. RESERVED FOR NUCC USE

b. AUTO ACCIDENT? ☐ YES [X] NO PLACE (State)

b. OTHER CLAIM ID (Designated by NUCC)

c. RESERVED FOR NUCC USE

c. OTHER ACCIDENT? ☐ YES [X] NO

c. INSURANCE PLAN NAME OR PROGRAM NAME

d. INSURANCE PLAN NAME OR PROGRAM NAME

10d. CLAIM CODES (Designated by NUCC)

d. IS THERE ANOTHER HEALTH BENEFIT PLAN? ☐ YES [X] NO *If yes*, complete items 9, 9a, and 9d.

READ BACK OF FORM BEFORE COMPLETING & SIGNING THIS FORM.

12. PATIENT'S OR AUTHORIZED PERSON'S SIGNATUREI authorize the release of any medical or other information necessary to process this claim. I also request payment of government benefits either to myself or to the party who accepts assignment below.

SIGNED Signature on file DATE

13. INSURED'S OR AUTHORIZED PERSON'S SIGNATURE I authorize payment of medical benefits to the undersigned physician or supplier for services described below.

SIGNED Signature on file

PATIENT AND INSURED INFORMATION

14. DATE OF CURRENT: ILLNESS, INJURY, or PREGNANCY(LMP) MM DD YY QUAL.

15. OTHER DATE QUAL. MM DD YY

16. DATES PATIENT UNABLE TO WORK IN CURRENT OCCUPATION FROM MM DD YY TO MM DD YY

17. NAME OF REFERRING PROVIDER OR OTHER SOURCE: DN Raymond Skeleton Md

17a.

17b. NPI 12678547XX

18. HOSPITALIZATION DATES RELATED TO CURRENT SERVICES FROM MM DD YY TO MM DD YY

19. ADDITIONAL CLAIM INFORMATION (Designated by NUCC)

20. OUTSIDE LAB? ☐ YES ☐ NO $ CHARGES

21. DIAGNOSIS OR NATURE OF ILLNESS OR INJURY Relate A-L to service line below (24E) ICD Ind. 0

A. R06.00 B. I10 C. K80.60 D.

E. F. G. H.

I. J. K. L.

22. RESUBMISSION CODE ORIGINAL REF. NO.

23. PRIOR AUTHORIZATION NUMBER

	24. A. DATE(S) OF SERVICE From MM DD YY	To MM DD YY	B. PLACE OF SERVICE	C. EMG	D. PROCEDURES, SERVICES, OR SUPPLIES (Explain Unusual Circumstances) CPT/HCPCS	MODIFIER	E. DIAGNOSIS POINTER	F. $ CHARGES	G. DAYS OR UNITS	H. EPSDT Family Plan	I. ID. QUAL.	J. RENDERING PROVIDER ID. #
1	01 06 20XX		11		99203		A,B	70 92	1		NPI	32783127XX
2	01 06 20XX		11		71020		A	40 97	1		NPI	32783127XX
3	01 20 20XX		11		99213		C	40 20	1		NPI	32783127XX
4	01 20 20XX		11		85025		C	25 00	1		NPI	32783127XX
5	01 20 20XX		11				C		1		NPI	32783127XX
6											NPI	

PHYSICIAN OR SUPPLIER INFORMATION

25. FEDERAL TAX I.D. NUMBER SSN ☐ EIN ☐

26. PATIENT'S ACCOUNT NO.: 8

27. ACCEPT ASSIGNMENT? (For govt. claims, see back) [X] YES ☐ NO

28. TOTAL CHARGE $

29. AMOUNT PAID $

30. Rsvd for NUCC Use $

31. SIGNATURE OF PHYSICIAN OR SUPPLIER INCLUDING DEGREES OR CREDENTIALS (I certify that the statements on the reverse apply to this bill and are made a part thereof.)

012520XX

SIGNED DATE

32. SERVICE FACILITY LOCATION INFORMATION: Same

a. NPI b.

33. BILLING PROVIDER INFO & PH # (555) 4869002
College Clinic
4567 Broad Avenue
Woodland Hills XY 12345-0001

a. 3664021CC b.

NUCC Instruction Manual available at: www.nucc.org *PLEASE PRINT OR TYPE* OMB APPROVAL PENDING

Figure 8-5

ASSIGNMENT 8-8 PROOFREAD A COMPUTER-GENERATED HEALTH INSURANCE CLAIM FORM AND LOCATE INCORRECT AND MISSING DATA

Performance Objective

Task: Locate and designate blocks on the computer-generated insurance claim form that have incorrect information or need completion; correct or add data before submission to the insurance company.

Conditions: Use Evert I. Strain's patient record (Figure 8-6), completed insurance claim (Figure 8-7), and a highlighter and a red ink pen.

Standards: Time: ______________ minutes

Accuracy: ______________

(Note: The time element and accuracy criteria may be given by your instructor.)

Directions: Proofread the insurance claim form (see Figure 8-7) and locate blocks that need correction or completion before submission to the insurance company. Highlight all errors you discover. Refer to the patient's record (see Figure 8-6) to verify pertinent demographic and insurance information. Refer to the progress notes to verify procedures and determine diagnoses. Verify all entries on the claim form, including dates, codes, rounded-out fees, and physician identification numbers. Insert all corrections and missing information in red. If you cannot locate the necessary information but know it is mandatory, write "NEED" in the corresponding block.

Optional: Retype a blank CMS-1500 (02-12) claim form with all corrections and changes. Or, if you have access to a computer, log on to your Evolve account at http://evolve.elsevier.com and access the student resources for Fordney: *Insurance Handbook for the Medical Office,* 12th edition. There you can fill out a CMS-1500 claim form and print it or save it.

Additional Coding

1. Refer to Mr. Strain's medical record, abstract information, and code procedures that would be billed by outside providers.

Site	*Description of Service*	*Code*
a. ABC Laboratory	______________________	____________
b. ABC Radiology	______________________	____________

PATIENT RECORD NO. 8-8

LAST NAME	FIRST NAME	MIDDLE NAME	BIRTH DATE	SEX	HOME PHONE
Strain,	Evert	I	09-11-46	M	555-678-0211

ADDRESS	CITY	STATE	ZIP CODE
7650 None Such Road	Woodland Hills	XY	12345

CELL PHONE	PAGER NO.	FAX NO.	E-MAIL ADDRESS
555-430-2101	555-320-9980	555-678-0211	Strain@WB.net

PATIENT'S SOC. SEC. NO.	DRIVER'S LICENSE
453-XX-4739	Y0923658

PATIENT'S OCCUPATION	NAME OF COMPANY
mechanical engineer	R & R Company

ADDRESS OF EMPLOYER	PHONE
2400 Davon Road, Woodland Hills, XY 12345	555-520-8977

SPOUSE OR PARENT	OCCUPATION
Ester I. Strain (wife)	administrative assistant

EMPLOYER	ADDRESS	PHONE
University College, 4021 Book Road, Woodland Hills, XY 12345		555-450-9908

NAME OF INSURANCE	INSURED OR SUBSCRIBER
ABC Insurance Co., P.O. Box 130, Woodland Hills, XY 12345	Evert I. Strain

POLICY/CERTIFICATE NO.	GROUP NO.
453-XX-4739	96476A

REFERRED BY: Gerald C. Jones, MD, 1403 Haven Street, Woodland Hills, XY 12345 NPI # 54754966XX

DATE	PROGRESS NOTES No. 8-8
1-8-20xx	Est pt comes in complaining of frequent urination, headaches, polyphagia; unable to
	remember current events. These problems have been present for almost a year.
	A comprehensive history is taken and compared to his last H & P 2 years ago.
	A com PX is performed. BP 160/110; pt was prescribed antihypertensive medication but
	discontinued it when the prescription ran out. Lab report, hand carried by pt from an
	urgent care center indicates SGOT in normal range and cholesterol elevated. Fasting blood
	sugar extremely high. Dx: diabetes mellitus, malignant hypertensive, and ASCVD.
	Pt to have 3 hour GTT tomorrow a.m. at ABC laboratory. STAT CT scan of head s̄ contrast
	ordered at ABC radiology to follow lab work. Arrangement will be made for pt to be
	admitted to College Hospital. Disability 1/9 through 1/31.
	GI/llf Gerald Practon, MD
1-9-xx	Admit to College Hospital (C hx/exam MC MDM).
	GI/llf Gerald Practon, MD
1-10-xx	Hosp visit (PF hx/exam SF MDM). CT scan of head reviewed, neg. findings. Pt alert and
	comfortable. If blood sugar and BP remain stable, discharge planned for tomorrow.
	BP 130/85.
	GI/llf Gerald Practon, MD
1-11-xx	DC from hosp. Pt to be seen in one week in ofc.
	GI/llf Gerald Practon, MD

Figure 8-6

DRAFT - NOT FOR OFFICIAL USE

HEALTH INSURANCE CLAIM FORM

APPROVED BY NATIONAL UNIFOR MCLAIM COMMITTEE (NUCC) 02/12

PICA | PICA

CARRIER

1. MEDICARE (Medicare#) [ ] MEDICAID (Medicaid#) [ ] TRICARE (ID#DoD#) [ ] CHAMPVA (Member ID#) [ ] GROUP HEALTH PLAN (ID#) [X] FECA BLK LUNG (ID#) [ ] OTHER (ID#) [ ]

1a. INSURED'S I.D. NUMBER (For Program in Item 1): 453 XX 4739 96476A

2. PATIENT'S NAME (Last Name, First Name, Middle Initial): Strain, Evert, I

3. PATIENT'S BIRTH DATE MM DD YY: 09 21 1946 SEX M [X] F [ ]

4. INSURED'S NAME (Last Name, First Name, Middle Initial): Same

5. PATIENT'S ADDRESS (No., Street): 7650 None Such Road

6. PATIENT RELATIONSHIP TO INSURED: Self [X] Spouse [ ] Child [ ] Other [ ]

7. INSURED'S ADDRESS (No., Street)

CITY: Woodland Hills STATE: XY

8. RESERVED FOR NUCC USE

CITY STATE

ZIP CODE TELEPHONE (Include Area Code) ( )

ZIP CODE TELEPHONE (Include Area Code) ( )

9. OTHER INSURED'S NAME (Last Name, First Name, Middle Initial)

10. IS PATIENT'S CONDITION RELATED TO:

11. INSURED'S POLICY GROUP OR FECA NUMBER

a. OTHER INSURED'S POLICY OR GROUP NUMBER

a. EMPLOYMENT? (Current or Previous) [ ] YES [X] NO

a. INSURED'S DATE OF BIRTH MM DD YY SEX M [ ] F [ ]

b. RESERVED FOR NUCC USE

b. AUTO ACCIDENT? [ ] YES [X] NO PLACE (State)

b. OTHER CLAIM ID (Designated by NUCC)

c. RESERVED FOR NUCC USE

c. OTHER ACCIDENT? [ ] YES [X] NO

c. INSURANCE PLAN NAME OR PROGRAM NAME

d. INSURANCE PLAN NAME OR PROGRAM NAME

10d. CLAIM CODES (Designated by NUCC)

d. IS THERE ANOTHER HEALTH BENEFIT PLAN? [ ] YES [ ] NO *If yes*, complete items 9, 9a, and 9d.

READ BACK OF FORM BEFORE COMPLETING & SIGNING THIS FORM.

12. PATIENT'S OR AUTHORIZED PERSON'S SIGNATUREI authorize the release of any medical or other information necessary to process this claim. I also request payment of government benefits either to myself or to the party who accepts assignment below.

SIGNED Signature on file DATE

13. INSURED'S OR AUTHORIZED PERSON'S SIGNATURE I authorize payment of medical benefits to the undersigned physician or supplier for services described below.

SIGNED Signature on file

PATIENT AND INSURED INFORMATION

14. DATE OF CURRENT: ILLNESS, INJURY, or PREGNANCY(LMP) MM DD YY QUAL.

15. OTHER DATE QUAL. MM DD YY

16. DATES PATIENT UNABLE TO WORK IN CURRENT OCCUPATION FROM MM DD YY TO MM DD YY

17. NAME OF REFERRING PROVIDER OR OTHER SOURCE: DN Gerald C Jones

17a. 17b. NPI 54754966XX

18. HOSPITALIZATION DATES RELATED TO CURRENT SERVICES FROM 01 09 20XX TO 01 11 20XX

19. ADDITIONAL CLAIM INFORMATION (Designated by NUCC)

20. OUTSIDE LAB? [ ] YES [X] NO $ CHARGES

21. DIAGNOSIS OR NATURE OF ILLNESS OR INJURY Relate A-L to service line below (24E) ICD Ind. 0

A. E11.9 B. I10 C. I25.10 D.

E. F. G. H.

I. J K. L.

22. RESUBMISSION CODE ORIGINAL REF. NO.

23. PRIOR AUTHORIZATION NUMBER

	24. A. DATE(S) OF SERVICE From MM DD YY	To MM DD YY	B. PLACE OF SERVICE	C. EMG	D. PROCEDURES, SERVICES, OR SUPPLIES (Explain Unusual Circumstances) CPT/HCPCS	MODIFIER	E. DIAGNOSIS POINTER	F. $ CHARGES	G. DAYS OR UNITS	H. EPSDT Family Plan	I. ID. QUAL.	J. RENDERING PROVIDER ID. #
1	01 08 20XX		11		99215			96 97	1		NPI	46278897XX
2	01 09 20XX		21		99222			120 80	1		NPI	46278897XX
3	1 10 20XX		21		99231			37 74	1		NPI	46278897XX
4	01 11 20XX		21		99231			65 26	1		NPI	46278897XX
5											NPI	
6											NPI	

PHYSICIAN OR SUPPLIER INFORMATION

25. FEDERAL TAX I.D. NUMBER: 7034597 SSN [ ] EIN [X]

26. PATIENT'S ACCOUNT NO.: 8

27. ACCEPT ASSIGNMENT? (For govt. claims, see back) [X] YES [ ] NO

28. TOTAL CHARGE $ 320 77

29. AMOUNT PAID $

30. Rsvd for NUCC Use $ 320 77

31. SIGNATURE OF PHYSICIAN OR SUPPLIER INCLUDING DEGREES OR CREDENTIALS (I certify that the statements on the reverse apply to this bill and are made a part thereof.)

Gerald Practon MD 012520XX

SIGNED *Gerald Practon MD* DATE

32. SERVICE FACILITY LOCATION INFORMATION: Same

a. NPI b.

33. BILLING PROVIDER INFO & PH # (555) 4869002
College Clinic
4567 Broad Avenue
Woodland Hills XY 12345-0001

a. 3664021CC b.

NUCC Instruction Manual available at: www.nucc.org PLEASE PRINT OR TYPE OMB APPROVAL PENDING

Figure 8-7

ASSIGNMENT 8-9 DEFINE PATIENT RECORD ABBREVIATIONS

Performance Objective

Task: Insert definitions of abbreviations.

Conditions: Use pencil or pen.

Standards: Time: ______________ minutes

Accuracy: ______________

(Note: The time element and accuracy criteria may be given by your instructor.)

Directions: After completing the assignments in this chapter, you will be able to define the abbreviations shown here.

Abbreviations pertinent to the record of Brad E. Diehl:

NP ______________________________

LC ______________________________

pt ______________________________

MDM ______________________________

AP ______________________________

cm ______________________________

lat ______________________________

neg ______________________________

BP ______________________________

CBC ______________________________

R/O ______________________________

auto ______________________________

retn ______________________________

diff ______________________________

EPF ______________________________

WBC ______________________________

hx ______________________________

DX ______________________________

exam ______________________________

adv ______________________________

Abbreviations pertinent to the record of Evert I. Strain:

est ______________________________

CT ______________________________

pt ______________________________

C ______________________________

H & P ______________________________

hx ______________________________

comp ______________________________

exam ______________________________

PX ______________________________

MC ______________________________

BP ______________________________

MDM ______________________________

lab ______________________________

hosp ______________________________

SGOT ______________________________

PF ______________________________

Dx ______________________________

SF ______________________________

ASCVD ______________________________

neg ______________________________

GTT ______________________________

DC ______________________________

STAT ______________________________

ofc ______________________________

9 Receiving Payments and Insurance Problem Solving

Marilyn T. Fordney

KEY TERMS

Your instructor may wish to select some words pertinent to this chapter for a test. For definitions of the terms, further study, and/or reference, the words, phrases, and abbreviations may be found in the glossary at the end of the Handbook. *Key terms for this chapter follow.*

appeal
delinquent claim
denied paper or electronic claim
explanation of benefits
inquiry
lost claim
overpayment
peer review
rebill (resubmit)
rejected claim
remittance advice
review
suspended claim
suspense
tracer

KEY ABBREVIATIONS

See how many abbreviations and acronyms you can translate and then use this as a handy reference list. Definitions for the key abbreviations are located near the back of the Handbook *in the glossary.*

ALJ ______________________

CMS ______________________

DAB ______________________

EOB ______________________

ERISA ______________________

FTC ______________________

HIPAA ______________________

HMO ______________________

HO ______________________

NPI ______________________

RA ______________________

PERFORMANCE OBJECTIVES

The student will be able to:

- Define and spell the key terms and key abbreviations for this chapter, given the information from the *Handbook* glossary, within a reasonable time period and with enough accuracy to obtain a satisfactory evaluation.
- After reading the chapter, answer the fill-in-the-blank, multiple choice, and true/false review questions with enough accuracy to obtain a satisfactory evaluation.
- Complete the insurance claim tracer form, given a request for an insurance claim trace and the patient's insurance claim, within a reasonable time period and with enough accuracy to obtain a satisfactory evaluation.
- Locate the errors on each claim, given three returned insurance claims, within a reasonable time period and with enough accuracy to obtain a satisfactory evaluation.
- Complete form CMS-1965, Request for Medicare Hearing by an Administrative Law Judge, Part B, Medicare Claim, within a reasonable time period and with enough accuracy to obtain a satisfactory evaluation.
- File an appeal by composing and typing a letter with envelope, within a reasonable time period and with enough accuracy to obtain a satisfactory evaluation.

STUDY OUTLINE

Follow-Up after Claim Submission
Claim Policy Provisions
- Insured
- Payment Time Limits

Explanation of Benefits
- Components of an Explanation of Benefits
- Interpretation of an Explanation of Benefits
- Posting an Explanation of Benefits

Claim Management Techniques
- Insurance Claims Register
- Tickler File
- Aging Reports
- Insurance Company Payment History

Claim Inquiries
Problem Paper and Electronic Claims
- Types of Problems

Rebilling
Review and Appeal Process
Filing an Appeal
- Medicare Review and Redetermination Process
- TRICARE Review and Appeal Process

State Insurance Commissioner
- Commission Objectives
- Types of Problems

Commission Inquiries
Procedure 9-1: Trace an Unpaid Insurance Claim
Procedure 9-2: File an Appeal

ASSIGNMENT 9-1 REVIEW QUESTIONS

Part I Fill in the Blank

Review the objectives, key terms, and chapter information before completing the following review questions.

1. Name provisions seen in health insurance policies.

   a. ______________________________

   b. ______________________________

   c. ______________________________

   d. ______________________________

2. After an insurance claim is processed by the insurance carrier (paid, suspended, rejected, or denied), a document known as a/an ______________________________ is sent to the patient and to the provider of professional medical services.

3. Name other items that indicate the patient's responsibility to pay that may appear on the document explaining the payment and check issued by the insurance carrier.

   a. ______________________________

   b. ______________________________

   c. ______________________________

   d. ______________________________

   e. ______________________________

   f. ______________________________

4. After receiving an explanation of benefits (EOB) document and posting insurance payment, the copy of the insurance claim form is put into a file marked ______________________________.

5. To locate delinquent insurance claims on an insurance claims register quickly, which column should be looked at first?

   ____

   Would it appear blank or completed? ______________________________

6. Name some of the principal procedures that should be followed in good bookkeeping and record-keeping practice when a payment has been received from an insurance company.

   ____

   ____

   ____

7. In good office management, a manual method used to track submitted pending or resubmitted insurance claims, a/an ______________________________, is used.

8. Two procedures to include in a manual reminder system to track pending claims are

a. ______________________________.

b. ______________________________.

9. In making an inquiry about a claim by telephone, efficient secretarial procedure would be to

____

______________________________.

10. Denied paper or electronic claims are those denied because of

____

or ______________________________.

11. State the solution if a claim has been denied because the professional service rendered was for an injury that is being considered as compensable under workers' compensation.

____

____

____

12. At the time of his first office visit, Mr. Doi signed an Assignment of Benefits, and Dr. James' office submitted a claim to ABC Insurance Company. Mr. Doi received, in error, a check from the insurance company and cashed it. What steps should be taken by Dr. James' office after this error is discovered?

a. ______________________________

b. ______________________________

c. ______________________________

13. If an appeal of an insurance claim is not successful, the next step to proceed with is a/an

______________________________.

14. Name the five levels for appealing a Medicare claim.

a. ______________________________

b. ______________________________

c. ______________________________

d. ______________________________

e. ______________________________

15. Medicare reconsideration by the insurance carrier is usually completed within

______________ to ______________ days.

16. A Medicare patient has insurance with United American (a Medigap policy), and payment has not been received from the Medigap insurer within a reasonable length of time. State the action to take in this case.

____

____

____

17. A TRICARE EOB is received stating that the allowable charge for Mrs. Dayton's office visit is $30. Is it possible to appeal this for additional payment? Answer "yes" or "no," and explain.

____

____

18. A state department or agency that helps resolve complaints about insurance policies, medical claims, or insurance agents or brokers and that verifies that insurance contracts are carried out in good faith is known as a/an

____.

19. When an insurance company consistently pays slowly on insurance claims, it may help speed up payments if a formal written complaint is made to the

____.

Part II Multiple Choice

Choose the best answer.

20. If the insurance carrier is a self-insured plan, a Medicaid or Medicare health maintenance organization, or an Employee Retirement Income Security Act (ERISA)–based plan, the insurance commissioner
    a. is able to assist with carrier issues.
    b. is not able to assist with carrier issues.
    c. is able to assist on specific problem issues related to payment.
    d. is able to give help on denied insurance claims.

21. A written request made to an insurance company to locate the status of an insurance claim is often referred to as
    a. inquiry.
    b. follow-up.
    c. tracer.
    d. all of the above.

22. An insurance claim transmitted to the third-party payer that is rejected because it contains a technical error, such as missing insured's birth date, is also known as a
    a. soft denial.
    b. suspended claim.
    c. delinquent claim.
    d. downcoded claim.

23. When an electronic claim is transmitted for several services and one service is rejected for incomplete information, the solution is to
    a. resubmit a paper claim with the needed data for the rejected services only.
    b. add the required information in Field 19 that it is a retransmission.
    c. add the required information and retransmit the rejected claim.
    d. not retransmit a rejected claim.

24. A request for payment to a third-party payer asking for a review of an insurance claim that has been denied is referred to as a/an
    a. review.
    b. appeal.
    c. request.
    d. demand.

Part III True/False

Write "T" or "F" in the blank to indicate whether you think the statement is true or false.

_______ 25. If the provider has no contract with the insurance carrier, the provider is not obligated to the carrier's deadline.

_______ 26. A patient should be asked to sign an Advance Beneficiary Notice if he or she has decided to undergo plastic surgery that is not related to a medical condition.

_______ 27. An *overpayment* is receipt of less than the contract rate from a managed care plan for a patient who has received medical services.

_______ 28. In the Medicare reconsideration Level 2 process, the request must be within 9 months from the date of the original determination shown on the remittance advice.

_______ 29. A decision to appeal a claim should be based on whether there is sufficient data to back up the claim and if there is a large amount of money in question.

ASSIGNMENT 9-2 CRITICAL THINKING: LOCATE AND EXPLAIN CHOICE OF DIAGNOSTIC CODES

Performance Objective

Task: Locate the correct diagnostic code for the case scenario presented.

Conditions: Use a pen or pencil and the *International Classification of Diseases, Tenth Revision, Clinical Modification* (ICD-10-CM) diagnostic code book.

Standards: Time: ______________ minutes

Accuracy: ______________

(Note: The time element and accuracy criteria may be given by your instructor.)

Directions: Using your critical thinking skills, answer the following questions after reading the scenario. Record your answer on the blank lines. These questions are presented to enhance your skill in critical thinking.

Scenario: Using your code book, look up the ICD-10 -CM diagnostic code for a patient being treated for bacillary dysentery. How would you code this case and why?

1. Locate the main term or condition in the Alphabetic Index, Volume 2. What is the main term or condition? ______________
2. Refer to any notes under the main term. What is the subterm? ______________
3. Read any notes or terms enclosed in parentheses after the main term. What is the code number listed after the main term and subterm? ______________
4. What is the appropriate subterm after that? ______________
5. Look for the appropriate sub-subterm and follow any cross-reference instructions. What does it say?

   ____

   ____

6. Verify the code number in the Tabular List, Volume 1, and list it here. ______________
7. Read and be guided by any instructional terms in the Tabular List. It reads: ______________
8. Read the complete description and then code to the highest specificity. (Assign the code and write it here.) ______________
9. Write justification of chosen code(s).

   ____

   ____

ASSIGNMENT 9-3 POST TO A FINANCIAL ACCOUNTING RECORD (LEDGER) FROM AN EXPLANATION OF BENEFITS DOCUMENT

Performance Objective

Task: Post data from an EOB document to a patient's financial accounting record (ledger).

Conditions: Use a blank financial accounting record (ledger) (Figure 9-1), an EOB document (Figure 9-2), and a pen or computer.

Standards: Time: ______________ minutes

Accuracy: ______________

(Note: The time element and accuracy criteria may be given by your instructor.)

Directions: Post in ink the payment received and preferred provider organization (PPO) adjustment to a patient's financial accounting record (ledger) (see Figure 9-1) by referring to an EOB document (see Figure 9-2). An example of financial accounting record (ledger) entries is shown in Figure 3-14 in the *Handbook*. An EOB document is defined in Figure 9-1 in the *Handbook*.

After the instructor has returned your work to you, either make the necessary corrections and place your work in a three-ring notebook for future reference, or, if you received a high score, place it in your portfolio for reference when applying for a job.

1. Locate patient's financial accounting record (ledger) and EOB.

   (Note: Refer to the step-by-step procedures at the end of Chapter 3 in the *Handbook* and graphic examples in Figures 3-14 and 10-3.)

2. Ledger lines 6 and 7: Insert date of service (DOS), reference (CPT code number, check number, or dates of service for posting adjustments or when insurance was billed), description of the transaction, charge amounts, payments, adjustments, and running current balance. The posting date is the actual date the transaction is recorded. If the DOS differs from the posting date, list the DOS in the reference or description column.

   (Note: A good bookkeeping practice is to take a red pen and draw a line across the financial accounting record [ledger] from left to right to indicate the last entry billed to the insurance company.)

Acct No. 9-3

STATEMENT
Financial Account
COLLEGE CLINIC
4567 Broad Avenue
Woodland Hills, XY 12345-0001
Tel. 555-486-9002
Fax No. 555-487-8976

Mr. Jabe Bortolussi
989 Moorpark Road
Woodland Hills, XY 12345

Phone No. (H) (555) 230-8870 (W) (555) 349-6689 Birthdate 04-07-71

Primary Insurance Co. ABC Insurance Company Policy/Group No. 4206/010

DATE	REFERENCE	DESCRIPTION	CHARGES		CREDITS				BALANCE	
					PYMNTS.		ADJ.			
		BALANCE FORWARD →								
6-3-xx	99204	E/M NP Level 4	250	00					250	00
6-3-xx	94375	Respiratory flow vol loop	40	00					290	00
6-3-xx	94060	Spirometry	75	00					365	00
6-3-xx	94664	Aerosol inhalation	50	00					415	00
6-3-xx	94760	Pulse oximetry	50	00					465	00

PLEASE PAY LAST AMOUNT IN BALANCE COLUMN

THIS IS A COPY OF YOUR FINANCIAL ACCOUNT AS IT APPEARS ON OUR RECORDS

Figure 9-1

ABC Insurance Company
P.O. Box 4300
Woodland Hills, XY 12345-0001

Claim No.: 1-00-16987087-00-zmm
Group Name: COLLEGE CLINIC
Group No.: 010
Employee: JABE V. BORTOLUSSI
Patient: JABE V. BORTOLUSSI
SSN: 554-XX-8876
Plan No.: 4206
Prepared by: M. SMITH
Prepared on: 07/04/20XX

GERALD PRACTON MD
4567 BROAD AVENUE
WOODLAND HILLS XY 12345

Patient Responsibility	
Amount not covered:	00
Co-pay amount:	00
Deductible:	00
Co-insurance:	64.61
Patient's total responsibility:	64.61
Other insurance payment:	00

EXPLANATION OF BENEFITS

Treatment Dates	Service Code	CPT Code	Charge Amount	Not Covered	Reason Code	PPO Discount	Covered Amount	Deductible Amount	Co-pay Amount	Paid At	Payment Amount
06/03/xx	200	99204	250.00	00	48	136.00	114.00	00	00	80%	91.20
06/03/xx	540	94375	40.00	00	48	00	40.00	00	00	80%	32.00
06/03/xx	540	94060	75.00	00	48	00	75.00	00	00	80%	60.00
06/03/xx	200	94664	50.00	00	48	1.55	48.45	00	00	80%	38.76
06/03/xx	540	94760	50.00	00	48	4.40	45.60	00	00	80%	36.48
		TOTAL	465.00	00		141.95	323.05	00	00		258.44

Other Insurance Credits or Adjustments 00

Total Payment Amount 258.44

CPT Code
99204 OFFICE/OUTPT VISIT E&M NEW MOD-HI SEVERIT
94375 RESPIRATORY FLOW VOLUM LOOP
94060 BRONCHOSPSM EVAL SPIROM PRE & POST BRON
94664 AEROSOL/VAPOR INHALA; INIT DEMO & EVAL
94760 NONINVASIVE EAR/PULSE OXIMETRY-02 SAT

Reason Code
48 CON DISCOUNT/PT NOT RESPONSIBLE

Participant		Date
GERALD PRACTON MD		07-04-xx
Patient		ID Number
JABE V. BORTOLUSSI		554-XX-8876
Plan Number	Patient Number	Office No.
4206		010

GC 1234567890

258.44

PAY TO THE ORDER OF

COLLEGE CLINIC
4567 BROAD AVENUE
WOODLAND HILLS XY 12345

J M Smith
ABC Insurance Company

Figure 9-2

ASSIGNMENT 9-4 TRACE AN UNPAID INSURANCE CLAIM

Performance Objective

Task: Complete an insurance claim tracer form and attach to this document a photocopy of the claim.

Conditions: Use an Insurance Claim Tracer form (Figure 9-3), an insurance claim form from the *Handbook* (see Figure 7-3), and a computer.

Standards: Time: ______________ minutes

Accuracy: ______________

(Note: The time element and accuracy criteria may be given by your instructor.)

Directions: You discover that the insurance claim you submitted to ABC Insurance Company, 146 Main Street, Woodland Hills, XY 12345, on Harry N. Forehand 3 months ago was never paid. Complete an insurance claim tracer form (see Figure 9-3). Make a photocopy of Harry Forehand's insurance claim form from the *Handbook* in Chapter 7 to attach to the tracer form. Mr. Forehand's employer is Acme Electrical Company at 450 South Orange Street, Woodland Hills, XY 12345. Place your name on the tracer form as the person to contact at Dr. Antrum's office.

After the instructor has returned your work to you, either make the necessary corrections and place your work in a three-ring notebook for future reference, or, if you received a high score, place it in your portfolio for reference when applying for a job.

COLLEGE CLINIC
4567 Broad Avenue
Woodland Hills, XY 12345-0001
Telephone (555) 486-9002
Fax (555) 487-8976

INSURANCE CLAIM TRACER

INSURANCE COMPANY NAME ______________________ DATE: ______________.

ADDRESS ____.

Patient name: ______________________

Date of birth: ______________________

Employer: ______________________

Insured: ______________________

Policy/certificate No. ______________________

Group name/No. ______________________

Date of initial claim submission: ______________________

Date(s) of service: ______________________

Total charges submitted: ______________________

An inordinate amount of time has passed since submission of our original claim. We have not received a request for additional information and still await payment of this assigned claim. Please review the attached duplicate and process for payment within 7 days.

DETAILS OF INQUIRY

Please check the claim status and return this letter to our office. Thank you.

- ☐ No record of claim.
- ☐ Claim received and payment is in process.
- ☐ Claim is in suspense (comment please).
- ☐ Claim is in review (comment please).
- ☐ Additional information needed (comment please).
- ☐ Applied to deductible. Amount: $ ________
- ☐ Patient not eligible for benefits.
- ☐ Determination issued to beneficiary.
- ☐ Claim paid. Date: ______ Amount: $ _______ To whom: ______________________
- ☐ Claim denied (comment please).

Comments: ____

____

Thank you for your assistance in this important matter. Please contact the insurance specialist named below if you have any questions regarding this claim.

Insurance Specialist: ______________________ (555) 486-9002 Ext. ___________.

Treating Physician: ______________________ State license number ___________.

Provider Number: ______________________ Provider's IRS number ___________.

Figure 9-3

ASSIGNMENT 9-5 LOCATE ERRORS ON A RETURNED INSURANCE CLAIM

Performance Objective

Task: Highlight the blocks on the insurance claim form where errors are discovered.

Conditions: Use an insurance claim form (Figure 9-4) and a highlighter or red pen.

Standards: Time: ______________ minutes

Accuracy: ______________

(Note: The time element and accuracy criteria may be given by your instructor.)

Directions: An insurance claim (see Figure 9-4) was returned by the Prudential Insurance Company. Highlight or circle in red all blocks on the claim form where errors are discovered.

Option 1: Retype the claim and either insert the correction, if data are available to fix the error, or insert the word "NEED" in the block of the claim form.

Option 2: On a separate sheet of paper, list the blocks from 1 to 33 and state where errors occur.

A Performance Evaluation Checklist may be reproduced from the "Instruction Guide to the Workbook" chapter if your instructor wishes you to submit it to assist with scoring and comments.

After the instructor has returned your work to you, either make the necessary corrections and place your work in a three-ring notebook for future reference, or, if you received a high score, place it in your portfolio for reference when applying for a job.

DRAFT - NOT FOR OFFICIAL USE

HEALTH INSURANCE CLAIM FORM

APPROVED BY NATIONAL UNIFOR MCLAIM COMMITTEE (NUCC) 02/12

Prudential Insurance Company
500 South Bend Street
Woodland Hills XY 12345-0001

CARRIER

PICA | PICA

1. MEDICARE (Medicare#) ☐ MEDICAID (Medicaid#) ☐ TRICARE (ID#DoD#) ☐ CHAMPVA (Member ID#) ☐ GROUP HEALTH PLAN (ID#) ☐ FECA BLK LUNG (ID#) ☐ OTHER (ID#) ☒

1a. INSURED'S I.D. NUMBER (For Program in Item 1)

PATIENT AND INSURED INFORMATION

2. PATIENT'S NAME (Last Name, First Name, Middle Initial): Johnson, Emily B.	3. PATIENT'S BIRTH DATE MM DD YY: 02 12 1963; SEX M ☐ F ☐
4. INSURED'S NAME (Last Name, First Name, Middle Initial): Johnson, Erron T.	
5. PATIENT'S ADDRESS (No., Street): 4391 Everett Street	6. PATIENT RELATIONSHIP TO INSURED: Self ☐ Spouse ☒ Child ☐ Other ☐
7. INSURED'S ADDRESS (No., Street): Same	
CITY: Woodland Hills	STATE: XY
8. RESERVED FOR NUCC USE	CITY / STATE
ZIP CODE: 12345-0001	TELEPHONE (Include Area Code): ( )
ZIP CODE	TELEPHONE (Include Area Code): ( )
9. OTHER INSURED'S NAME (Last Name, First Name, Middle Initial)	10. IS PATIENT'S CONDITION RELATED TO:
11. INSURED'S POLICY GROUP OR FECA NUMBER	
a. OTHER INSURED'S POLICY OR GROUP NUMBER	a. EMPLOYMENT? (Current or Previous) ☐ YES ☐ NO
a. INSURED'S DATE OF BIRTH MM DD YY	SEX M ☐ F ☐
b. RESERVED FOR NUCC USE	b. AUTO ACCIDENT? ☐ YES ☐ NO PLACE (State)
b. OTHER CLAIM ID (Designated by NUCC)	
c. RESERVED FOR NUCC USE	c. OTHER ACCIDENT? ☐ YES ☐ NO
c. INSURANCE PLAN NAME OR PROGRAM NAME	
d. INSURANCE PLAN NAME OR PROGRAM NAME	10d. CLAIM CODES (Designated by NUCC)
d. IS THERE ANOTHER HEALTH BENEFIT PLAN? ☐ YES ☒ NO *If yes*, complete items 9, 9a, and 9d.	

READ BACK OF FORM BEFORE COMPLETING & SIGNING THIS FORM.

12. PATIENT'S OR AUTHORIZED PERSON'S SIGNATUREI authorize the release of any medical or other information necessary to process this claim. I also request payment of government benefits either to myself or to the party who accepts assignment below.

SIGNED *Emily B. Johnson* DATE 1/4/2020

13. INSURED'S OR AUTHORIZED PERSON'S SIGNATURE I authorize payment of medical benefits to the undersigned physician or supplier for services described below.

SIGNED *Emily B. Johnson*

PHYSICIAN OR SUPPLIER INFORMATION

14. DATE OF CURRENT: ILLNESS, INJURY, or PREGNANCY(LMP) MM DD YY QUAL.	15. OTHER DATE QUAL. MM DD YY
16. DATES PATIENT UNABLE TO WORK IN CURRENT OCCUPATION FROM MM DD YY TO MM DD YY	
17. NAME OF REFERRING PROVIDER OR OTHER SOURCE	17a. / 17b. NPI 67805027XX
18. HOSPITALIZATION DATES RELATED TO CURRENT SERVICES FROM MM DD YY TO MM DD YY	
19. ADDITIONAL CLAIM INFORMATION (Designated by NUCC)	20. OUTSIDE LAB? ☐ YES ☒ NO $ CHARGES
21. DIAGNOSIS OR NATURE OF ILLNESS OR INJURY Relate A-L to service line below (24E) ICD Ind. 0	22. RESUBMISSION CODE / ORIGINAL REF. NO.
A. B. C. D. E. F. G. H. I. J. K. L.	23. PRIOR AUTHORIZATION NUMBER

	24. A. DATE(S) OF SERVICE From MM DD YY	To MM DD YY	B. PLACE OF SERVICE	C. EMG	D. PROCEDURES, SERVICES, OR SUPPLIES (Explain Unusual Circumstances) CPT/HCPCS	MODIFIER	E. DIAGNOSIS POINTER	F. $ CHARGES	G. DAYS OR UNITS	H. EPSDT Family Plan	I. ID. QUAL.	J. RENDERING PROVIDER ID. #
1	01 04 20XX		11		99213		A	25 00	1		NPI	705687717XX
2	01 04 20XX		11		99213		A	25 00			NPI	
3											NPI	
4											NPI	
5											NPI	
6											NPI	

25. FEDERAL TAX I.D. NUMBER: 7180561XX SSN ☐ EIN ☐	26. PATIENT'S ACCOUNT NO.: 9	27. ACCEPT ASSIGNMENT? (For govt. claims, see back) ☒ YES ☐ NO	28. TOTAL CHARGE $ 60 00	29. AMOUNT PAID $	30. Rsvd for NUCC Use $
31. SIGNATURE OF PHYSICIAN OR SUPPLIER INCLUDING DEGREES OR CREDENTIALS (I certify that the statements on the reverse apply to this bill and are made a part thereof.) SIGNED *Vera Cutis, MD* DATE 01/06/20XX	32. SERVICE FACILITY LOCATION INFORMATION a. NPI b.	33. BILLING PROVIDER INFO & PH # (555) 4869002 College Clinic 4567 Broad Avenue Woodland Hills XY 12345-0001 a. 3664021CC b.			

NUCC Instruction Manual available at: www.nucc.org *PLEASE PRINT OR TYPE* OMB APPROVAL PENDING

Figure 9-4

ASSIGNMENT 9-6 LOCATE ERRORS ON A RETURNED INSURANCE CLAIM

Performance Objective

Task: Highlight the blocks on the insurance claim form where errors are discovered.

Conditions: Use an insurance claim form (Figure 9-5) and a highlighter or red pen.

Standards: Time: ______________ minutes

Accuracy: ______________

(Note: The time element and accuracy criteria may be given by your instructor.)

Directions: An insurance claim was returned by the Healthtech Insurance Company. Highlight or circle in red all blocks on the claim form where errors are discovered.

Option 1: Retype the claim and either insert the correction if data are available to fix the error or insert the word "NEED" in the block of the claim form.

Option 2: On a separate sheet of paper, list the blocks from 1 to 33 and state where errors occur.

A Performance Evaluation Checklist may be reproduced from the "Instruction Guide to the Workbook" chapter if your instructor wishes you to submit it to assist with scoring and comments.

After the instructor has returned your work to you, either make the necessary corrections and place your work in a three-ring notebook for future reference, or, if you received a high score, place it in your portfolio for reference when applying for a job.

DRAFT - NOT FOR OFFICIAL USE

HEALTH INSURANCE CLAIM FORM

APPROVED BY NATIONAL UNIFOR MCLAIM COMMITTEE (NUCC) 02/12

Healthtech Insurance Company
4821 West Lake Avenue
Woodland Hills XY 12345-0001

CARRIER

PICA | PICA

1. MEDICARE (Medicare#) [ ] MEDICAID (Medicaid#) [X] TRICARE (ID#DoD#) [X] CHAMPVA (Member ID#) [ ] GROUP HEALTH PLAN (ID#) [ ] FECA BLK LUNG (ID#) [ ] OTHER (ID#) [X]

1a. INSURED'S I.D. NUMBER (For Program in Item 1): 433129870ANC

2. PATIENT'S NAME (Last Name, First Name, Middle Initial): Dugan, Charles C

3. PATIENT'S BIRTH DATE MM DD YY: 12 24 1968 SEX M [X] F [ ]

4. INSURED'S NAME (Last Name, First Name, Middle Initial): Same

5. PATIENT'S ADDRESS (No., Street): 5900 Elm Street

6. PATIENT RELATIONSHIP TO INSURED: Self [X] Spouse [ ] Child [ ] Other [ ]

7. INSURED'S ADDRESS (No., Street): Same

CITY: Woodland Hills STATE: XY

8. RESERVED FOR NUCC USE

CITY STATE

ZIP CODE: 12345-0001 TELEPHONE (Include Area Code): (555) 5593300

ZIP CODE TELEPHONE (Include Area Code) ( )

9. OTHER INSURED'S NAME (Last Name, First Name, Middle Initial)

10. IS PATIENT'S CONDITION RELATED TO:

11. INSURED'S POLICY GROUP OR FECA NUMBER

a. OTHER INSURED'S POLICY OR GROUP NUMBER

a. EMPLOYMENT? (Current or Previous) [ ] YES [X] NO

a. INSURED'S DATE OF BIRTH MM DD YY SEX M [ ] F [ ]

b. RESERVED FOR NUCC USE

b. AUTO ACCIDENT? [ ] YES [X] NO PLACE (State)

b. OTHER CLAIM ID (Designated by NUCC)

c. RESERVED FOR NUCC USE

c. OTHER ACCIDENT? [ ] YES [X] NO

c. INSURANCE PLAN NAME OR PROGRAM NAME

d. INSURANCE PLAN NAME OR PROGRAM NAME

10d. CLAIM CODES (Designated by NUCC)

d. IS THERE ANOTHER HEALTH BENEFIT PLAN? [ ] YES [ ] NO *If yes*, complete items 9, 9a, and 9d.

READ BACK OF FORM BEFORE COMPLETING & SIGNING THIS FORM.

12. PATIENT'S OR AUTHORIZED PERSON'S SIGNATUREI authorize the release of any medical or other information necessary to process this claim. I also request payment of government benefits either to myself or to the party who accepts assignment below.

SIGNED ______ DATE ______

13. INSURED'S OR AUTHORIZED PERSON'S SIGNATURE I authorize payment of medical benefits to the undersigned physician or supplier for services described below.

SIGNED ______

PATIENT AND INSURED INFORMATION

14. DATE OF CURRENT: ILLNESS, INJURY, or PREGNANCY(LMP) MM DD YY QUAL.

15. OTHER DATE QUAL. MM DD YY

16. DATES PATIENT UNABLE TO WORK IN CURRENT OCCUPATION FROM MM DD YY TO MM DD YY

17. NAME OF REFERRING PROVIDER OR OTHER SOURCE

17a.

17b. NPI 67805027XX

18. HOSPITALIZATION DATES RELATED TO CURRENT SERVICES FROM MM DD YY TO MM DD YY

19. ADDITIONAL CLAIM INFORMATION (Designated by NUCC)

20. OUTSIDE LAB? [ ] YES [X] NO $ CHARGES

21. DIAGNOSIS OR NATURE OF ILLNESS OR INJURY Relate A-L to service line below (24E) ICD Ind. 0

A. S51.801 B. C. D.
E. F. G. H.
I. J. K. L.

22. RESUBMISSION CODE ORIGINAL REF. NO.

23. PRIOR AUTHORIZATION NUMBER

	24. A. DATE(S) OF SERVICE From MM DD YY	To MM DD YY	B. PLACE OF SERVICE	C. EMG	D. PROCEDURES, SERVICES, OR SUPPLIES (Explain Unusual Circumstances) CPT/HCPCS	MODIFIER	E. DIAGNOSIS POINTER	F. $ CHARGES	G. DAYS OR UNITS	H. EPSDT Family Plan	I. ID. QUAL.	J. RENDERING PROVIDER ID. #
1	09 55 20XX		11		99203		A	70 92	1		NPI	46278897XX
2	09 55 20XX		11		12001		A				NPI	46278897XX
3											NPI	
4											NPI	
5											NPI	
6											NPI	

25. FEDERAL TAX I.D. NUMBER SSN EIN: 7034597XX [ ] [X]

26. PATIENT'S ACCOUNT NO.: 9-6

27. ACCEPT ASSIGNMENT? (For govt. claims, see back) [X] YES [ ] NO

28. TOTAL CHARGE $

29. AMOUNT PAID $

30. Rsvd for NUCC Use $

31. SIGNATURE OF PHYSICIAN OR SUPPLIER INCLUDING DEGREES OR CREDENTIALS (I certify that the statements on the reverse apply to this bill and are made a part thereof.)

SIGNED Gerald Practon, MD DATE 09/30/20XX

32. SERVICE FACILITY LOCATION INFORMATION
College Hospital
4500 Broad Avenue
Woodland Hills XY 12345-0001

a. 937310XX b.

33. BILLING PROVIDER INFO & PH # (555) 4869002
College Clinic
4567 Broad Avenue
Woodland Hills XY 12345-0001

a. 3664021CC b.

PHYSICIAN OR SUPPLIER INFORMATION

NUCC Instruction Manual available at: www.nucc.org *PLEASE PRINT OR TYPE* OMB APPROVAL PENDING

Figure 9-5

ASSIGNMENT 9-7 LOCATE ERRORS ON A RETURNED INSURANCE CLAIM

Performance Objective

Task: Highlight the blocks on the insurance claim form where errors are discovered.

Conditions: Use an insurance claim form (Figure 9-6) and a highlighter or red pen.

Standards: Time: ______________ minutes

Accuracy: ______________

(Note: The time element and accuracy criteria may be given by your instructor.)

Directions: An insurance claim (see Figure 9-6) was returned by an insurance plan. Highlight or circle in red all blocks on the claim form where errors are discovered.

Option 1: Retype the claim and either insert the correction if data are available to fix the error or insert the word "NEED" in the block of the claim form.

Option 2: On a separate sheet of paper, list the blocks from 1 to 33 and state where errors occur.

A Performance Evaluation Checklist may be reproduced from the "Instruction Guide to the Workbook" chapter if your instructor wishes you to submit it to assist with scoring and comments.

After the instructor has returned your work to you, either make the necessary corrections and place your work in a three-ring notebook for future reference, or, if you received a high score, place it in your portfolio for reference when applying for a job.

DRAFT - NOT FOR OFFICIAL USE

HEALTH INSURANCE CLAIM FORM

APPROVED BY NATIONAL UNIFOR MCLAIM COMMITTEE (NUCC) 02/12

American Insurance Company
509 Main Street
Woodland Hills XY 12345-0001

CARRIER

PICA

1. MEDICARE (Medicare#) [ ] MEDICAID (Medicaid#) [ ] TRICARE (ID#DoD#) [ ] CHAMPVA (Member ID#) [ ] GROUP HEALTH PLAN (ID#) [ ] FECA BLK LUNG (ID#) [ ] OTHER (ID#) [X]

1a. INSURED'S I.D. NUMBER (For Program in Item 1)

2. PATIENT'S NAME (Last Name, First Name, Middle Initial): Mary T Avery

3. PATIENT'S BIRTH DATE MM DD YY: 05 07 1980 SEX M [ ] F [ ]

4. INSURED'S NAME (Last Name, First Name, Middle Initial): Same

5. PATIENT'S ADDRESS (No., Street): 4309 Main Street

6. PATIENT RELATIONSHIP TO INSURED: Self [X] Spouse [ ] Child [ ] Other [ ]

7. INSURED'S ADDRESS (No., Street)

CITY: Woodland Hills STATE: XY

8. RESERVED FOR NUCC USE

CITY STATE

ZIP CODE: 12345-0001 TELEPHONE (Include Area Code): (555) 4509899

ZIP CODE TELEPHONE (Include Area Code) ( )

9. OTHER INSURED'S NAME (Last Name, First Name, Middle Initial)

10. IS PATIENT'S CONDITION RELATED TO:

11. INSURED'S POLICY GROUP OR FECA NUMBER

a. OTHER INSURED'S POLICY OR GROUP NUMBER

a. EMPLOYMENT? (Current or Previous) [ ] YES [X] NO

a. INSURED'S DATE OF BIRTH MM DD YY SEX M [ ] F [ ]

b. RESERVED FOR NUCC USE

b. AUTO ACCIDENT? [ ] YES [X] NO PLACE (State)

b. OTHER CLAIM ID (Designated by NUCC)

c. RESERVED FOR NUCC USE

c. OTHER ACCIDENT? [ ] YES [X] NO

c. INSURANCE PLAN NAME OR PROGRAM NAME

d. INSURANCE PLAN NAME OR PROGRAM NAME

10d. CLAIM CODES (Designated by NUCC)

d. IS THERE ANOTHER HEALTH BENEFIT PLAN? [ ] YES [ ] NO *If yes*, complete items 9, 9a, and 9d.

READ BACK OF FORM BEFORE COMPLETING & SIGNING THIS FORM.

12. PATIENT'S OR AUTHORIZED PERSON'S SIGNATUREI authorize the release of any medical or other information necessary to process this claim. I also request payment of government benefits either to myself or to the party who accepts assignment below.

SIGNED *Mary T. Avery* DATE 11/20/2007

13. INSURED'S OR AUTHORIZED PERSON'S SIGNATURE I authorize payment of medical benefits to the undersigned physician or supplier for services described below.

SIGNED *Mary T. Avery*

PATIENT AND INSURED INFORMATION

14. DATE OF CURRENT: ILLNESS, INJURY, or PREGNANCY(LMP) MM DD YY QUAL.

15. OTHER DATE QUAL. MM DD YY

16. DATES PATIENT UNABLE TO WORK IN CURRENT OCCUPATION FROM 11 09 20XX TO 11 30 20XX

17. NAME OF REFERRING PROVIDER OR OTHER SOURCE: Gerald Practon MD

17a. 17b. NPI

18. HOSPITALIZATION DATES RELATED TO CURRENT SERVICES FROM 11 11 20XX TO 11 12 20XX

19. ADDITIONAL CLAIM INFORMATION (Designated by NUCC)

20. OUTSIDE LAB? [ ] YES [X] NO $ CHARGES

21. DIAGNOSIS OR NATURE OF ILLNESS OR INJURY Relate A-L to service line below (24E) ICD Ind. 0

A. J03.90 B. C. D.
E. F. G. H.
I. J. K. L.

22. RESUBMISSION CODE ORIGINAL REF. NO.

23. PRIOR AUTHORIZATION NUMBER

	24. A. DATE(S) OF SERVICE From MM DD YY	To MM DD YY	B. PLACE OF SERVICE	C. EMG	D. PROCEDURES, SERVICES, OR SUPPLIES (Explain Unusual Circumstances) CPT/HCPCS	MODIFIER	E. DIAGNOSIS POINTER	F. $ CHARGES	G. DAYS OR UNITS	H. EPSDT Family Plan	I. ID. QUAL.	J. RENDERING PROVIDER ID. #
1	11 10 20XX		11		99203		A	50 00	1		NPI	43050047XX
2	11 11 20XX		21		99222		A	120 80			NPI	43050047XX
3	11 11 20XX		21		42821		A	410 73			NPI	43050047XX
4	11 22 20XX		21		99231		A	20 00			NPI	
5											NPI	
6											NPI	

25. FEDERAL TAX I.D. NUMBER: 715737291XX SSN [ ] EIN [X]

26. PATIENT'S ACCOUNT NO.: 9-7

27. ACCEPT ASSIGNMENT? (For govt. claims, see back) [ ] YES [ ] NO

28. TOTAL CHARGE $

29. AMOUNT PAID $

30. Rsvd for NUCC Use $

31. SIGNATURE OF PHYSICIAN OR SUPPLIER INCLUDING DEGREES OR CREDENTIALS (I certify that the statements on the reverse apply to this bill and are made a part thereof.)

SIGNED DATE 11/15/20XX

32. SERVICE FACILITY LOCATION INFORMATION
College Hospital
4500 Broad Avenue
Woodland Hills XY 12345-0001

a. X950731067 b.

33. BILLING PROVIDER INFO & PH # (555) 4869002
College Clinic
4567 Broad Avenue
Woodland Hills XY 12345-0001

a. 3664021CC b.

PHYSICIAN OR SUPPLIER INFORMATION

NUCC Instruction Manual available at: www.nucc.org PLEASE PRINT OR TYPE OMB APPROVAL PENDING

Figure 9-6

ASSIGNMENT 9-8 REQUEST FOR MEDICARE HEARING BY AN ADMINISTRATIVE LAW JUDGE

Performance Objective

Task: Insert information on a Request for Medicare Hearing by an Administrative Law Judge CMS-5011 A/B form.

Conditions: Request for Medicare Hearing by an Administrative Law Judge CMS-5011 A/B form (Figure 9-7), and a computer with printer.

Standards: Time: ______________ minutes

Accuracy: ______________

(Note: The time element and accuracy criteria may be given by your instructor.)

Directions: After Medicare processes the tracer on the insurance claim for Bill Hutch, you receive a Medicare EOB and payment check, but the amount is incorrect because of an excessive reduction in the allowed payment. An appeal was made in September and denied; the document control number assigned by Medicare Blue Shield is 240-577-9008. Dr. Brady Coccidioides believes that a mistake has been made and wishes to request a hearing.

Complete the Request for Medicare Hearing by an Administrative Law Judge CMS-5011 A/B form for this case (see Figure 9-7) by referring to the tracer form (Figure 9-8) and Figure 7-5 in the *Handbook*. Mr. Hutch's e-mail address is bhutch@gmail.net. Complete the form as the appellant and do not fill in the representative's portion. As you will learn in the chapter on Medicare, the Health Insurance Claim Number is the patient's Medicare identification number as shown in Figure 7-5, Block 1a. No additional evidence is to be presented, the doctor does not wish to appear for the hearing. Date the form December 5, 20xx. The beneficiary has assigned his appeal rights to the provider.

After the instructor has returned your work to you, either make the necessary corrections and place your work in a three-ring notebook for future reference, or, if you received a high score, place it in your portfolio for reference when applying for a job.

DEPARTMENT OF HEALTH AND HUMAN SERVICES
OFFICE OF MEDICARE HEARINGS AND APPEALS

REQUEST FOR MEDICARE HEARING BY AN ADMINISTRATIVE LAW JUDGE

❑ Part A
❑ Part B

Effective July 1, 2005. For use by party to a reconsideration/fair hearing determination issued by a Fiscal Intermediary (FI), Carrier, or Quality Improvement Organization (QIO)
(Amount in controversy must be $100 or more.)

Send copies of this completed form to:
Original *— The FI, Carrier, or QIO that issued the Reconsideration/Fair Hearing Notice*
Copy *— Appellant*

Appellant *(The party appealing the reconsideration determination)*

Beneficiary *(Leave blank if same as the appellant.)*	Provider or Supplier *(Leave blank if same as the appellant.)*
Address	Address
City / State / Zip Code	City / State / Zip Code
Area Code/Telephone Number / E-mail Address	Area Code/Telephone Number / E-mail Address
Health Insurance (Medicare) Claim Number	Document control number assigned by the FI, Carrier, or QIO

FI, Carrier, or QIO that made the reconsideration/fair hearing determination	Dates of Service From	To

I DISAGREE WITH THE DETERMINATION MADE ON MY APPEAL BECAUSE:

You have a right to be represented at the hearing. If you are not represented but would like to be, your Office of Medicare Hearings and Appeals Field Office will give you a list of legal referral and service organizations. *(If you are represented and have not already done so, complete form CMS-1696.)*

Check **Only One** Statement:
- ❑ I **wish** to have a hearing.
- ❑ I **do not wish** to have a hearing and I request that a decision be made on the basis of the evidence in my case. *(Complete form HHS-723, "Waiver of Right to an ALJ Hearing.")*

Check **Only One** Statement:
- ❑ I **have** additional evidence to submit.
- ❑ I **have no** additional evidence to submit.

The appellant should complete No. 1 and the representative, if any, should complete No. 2. If a representative is not present to sign, print his or her name in No. 2. Where applicable, check to indicate if appellant will accompany the representative at the hearing. ❑ Yes ❑ No

1. (Appellant's Signature) / Date	**2.** (Representative's Signature/Name) / Date
Address	Address ❑ Attorney ❑ Non-Attorney
City / State / Zip Code	City / State / Zip Code
Area Code/Telephone Number / E-mail Address	Area Code/Telephone Number / E-mail Address

Answer the following questions that apply:

A) Does request involve multiple claims? ❑ Yes ❑ No
(If yes, a list of all the claims must be attached.)

B) Does request involve multiple beneficiaries? ❑ Yes ❑ No
(If yes, a list of beneficiaries, their HICNs and the dates of the applicable reconsideration determinations must be attached.)

C) Did the beneficiary assign his or her appeal rights to you as the provider/supplier? ❑ Yes ❑ No
(If yes, you must complete and attach form CMS-20031. Failure to do so will prevent approval of the assignment.)

D) If there was no assignment, are you a physician being held liable pursuant to 1842(l)(1)(A) of the Social Security Act? ❑ Yes ❑ No

CMS-5011A/B U2 (08/05) EF 08/2005 ATTACH A COPY OF THE RECONSIDERATION/FAIR HEARING DETERMINATION (IF AVAILABLE) TO THIS COPY.

Figure 9-7

College Clinic
4567 Broad Avenue
Telephone (555) 486-9002 Woodland Hills, XY 12345-0001 Fax (555) 487-8976

INSURANCE CLAIM TRACER

INSURANCE COMPANY NAME Medicare Blue Shield DATE 06-10-20xx

ADDRESS 146 Main Street, Woodland Hills, XY 12345

Patient name: Bill Hutch
Date of birth: 02-17-1944
Employer: Retired
Insured: Bill Hutch
Policy/certificate no. 123XX6789A
Group name/no. None
Date of initial claim submission: 03-10-20XX
Date(s) of service: 03-10-20XX
Total charges submitted: $132.00

An inordinate amount of time has passed since submission of our original claim. We have not received a request for additional information and still await payment of this assigned claim. Please review the attached duplicate and process for payment within 7 days.

DETAILS OF INQUIRY

Please check the claim status and return this letter to our office. Thank you.

- ☐ No record of claim.
- ☐ Claim received and payment is in process.
- ☐ Claim is in suspense (comment please).
- ☐ Claim is in review (comment please).
- ☐ Additional information needed (comment please)
- ☐ Applied to deductible. Amount: $ _________
- ☐ Patient not eligible for benefits.
- ☐ Determination issued to beneficiary.
- ☐ Claim paid. Date: _______ Amount: $ ________ To whom: ________________________
- ☐ Claim denied (comment please).

Comments: ____

Thank you for your assistance in this important matter. Please contact the insurance specialist named below if you have any questions regarding this claim.

Insurance Specialist: Student's name (555) 486-9002 Ext. ____________
Treating Physician: Brady Coccidioides, MD State license number ____________
Provider Number: 64211067XX Provider's IRS number ____________

Figure 9-8

ASSIGNMENT 9-9 FILE AN APPEAL

Performance Objective

Task: Compose, format, key, proofread, and print a letter of appeal, and attach to this document photocopies of information to substantiate reimbursement requested.

Conditions: Computer, printer, letterhead paper, envelope, attachments, thesaurus, English dictionary, medical dictionary, and pen or pencil.

Standards: Time: ______________ minutes

Accuracy: ______________

(Note: The time element and accuracy criteria may be given by your instructor.)

Scenario: After retyping and resubmitting Mary T. Avery's insurance claim in Assignment 9-7, the insurance company sends an EOB/RA (health insurance claim number 123098) with a check in the amount of $300 to the College Clinic for payment of the claim. Dr. Cutler wishes an appeal to be made for an increase of the payment to an additional $100. (Note: This patient's marital status is single, and the insured's identification number is T45098.)

Directions: Use the retyped claim to Assignment 9-7 for Mary T. Avery. Follow these basic step-by-step procedures.

1. Refer to the end of Chapter 4 in the *Handbook* and follow the procedure to compose, format, key, proofread, and print a letter.
2. Include the beneficiary's name, health insurance claim number, dates of service in question, and items or services in question with name, address, and signature of the provider.
3. Compose a letter with an introduction that stresses the medical practice's qualifications, the physician's commitment to complying with regulations and providing appropriate services, and the importance of the practice to the payer's panel of physicians or specialists.
4. Provide a detailed account of the necessity of the treatment given and its relationship to the patient's problems and chief complaint. You might cross-reference the medical record and emphasize parts of it that the reviewer may have missed.
5. Explain the reason why the provider does not agree with the payment. Use a blank sheet labeling it "Explanation of Benefits" because you do not have this printed document to attach.
6. Abstract excerpts from the coding resource book if necessary.
7. Direct the correspondence to Mr. Donald Pearson, a claims adjuster at the American Insurance Company, 509 Main Street, Woodland Hills, XY 12345.
8. Type an envelope for the letter.
9. Retain copies of all data sent for the physician's files.

10 Office and Insurance Collection Strategies

Marilyn T. Fordney

KEY TERMS

Your instructor may wish to select some words pertinent to this chapter for a test. For definitions of the terms, further study, and/or reference, the words, phrases, and abbreviations may be found in the glossary at the end of the Handbook. *Key terms for this chapter follow.*

accounts receivable
age analysis
American Medical Association Code of Ethics
automatic stay
balance
bankruptcy
bonding
cash flow
Code of Medical Ethics
collateral
collection ratio
credit
credit card
creditor
cycle billing
debit card
debt
debtor
discount
dun messages
embezzlement
estate administrator
estate executor
fee schedule
financial accounting record
garnishment
insurance balance billing
itemized statement
lien
manual billing
netback
no charge
nonexempt assets
professional courtesy
reimbursement
secured debt
skip
statute of limitations
unsecured debt
write-off

KEY ABBREVIATIONS

See how many abbreviations and acronyms you can translate and then use this as a handy reference list. Definitions for the key abbreviations are located near the back of the Handbook *in the glossary.*

A/R ____________________
ATM ____________________
CMS ____________________
e-check ____________________
ERISA ____________________
FACT ____________________
FCBA ____________________
FCRA ____________________
FDCPA ____________________
FEHBA ____________________
FTC ____________________
HMO ____________________
N/A ____________________
NC ____________________
NSF ____________________
TILA ____________________
W2 ____________________

PERFORMANCE OBJECTIVES

The student will be able to:

- Define and spell the key terms and key abbreviations for this chapter, given the information from the *Handbook* glossary, within a reasonable time period and with enough accuracy to obtain a satisfactory evaluation.
- After reading the chapter, answer the fill-in-the-blank, mix and match, multiple choice, and true/false review questions with enough accuracy to obtain a satisfactory evaluation.
- Select an appropriate dun message for a patient's bill, given a patient's ledger/statement, within a reasonable time period and with enough accuracy to obtain a satisfactory evaluation.
- Post a courtesy adjustment, given a patient's ledger/statement, within a reasonable time period and with enough accuracy to obtain a satisfactory evaluation.
- Post a patient's charges and payment to the patient's financial accounting record, using the Mock Fee Schedule in Appendix A in this *Workbook*, within a reasonable time period and with enough accuracy to obtain a satisfactory evaluation.
- Compose a collection letter for a delinquent account, given letterhead stationery, within a reasonable time period and with enough accuracy to obtain a satisfactory evaluation.
- Complete a credit card voucher, given a patient's ledger/statement, within a reasonable time period and with enough accuracy to obtain a satisfactory evaluation.
- Complete a financial agreement, given a patient's ledger/statement, within a reasonable time period and with enough accuracy to obtain a satisfactory evaluation.

STUDY OUTLINE

Cash Flow Cycle
Accounts Receivable
Patient Education
- Patient Registration Form

Fees
- Fee Schedule
- Missed Appointments
- Fee Adjustments
- Communicating Fees
- Collecting Fees

Credit Arrangements
- Payment Options

Credit and Collection Laws
- Statute of Limitations

The Collection Process
- Telephone Collection Procedures
- Collection Letters
- Insurance Collection
- Collection Agencies
- Credit Bureaus
- Credit Counseling
- Small Claims Court
- Tracing a Skip
- Special Collection Issues

Procedure 10-1: Seven-Step Billing and Collection Guidelines
Procedure 10-2: Telephone Collection Plan
Procedure 10-3: Create a Financial Agreement With a Patient
Procedure 10-4: File a Claim in Small Claims Court
Procedure 10-5: File an Estate Claim

ASSIGNMENT 10-1 REVIEW QUESTIONS

Part I Fill in the Blank

Review the objectives, key terms, chapter information, glossary definitions of key terms, and figures before completing the following review questions.

1. Third-party payers are composed of

   a. ________________________________

   b. ________________________________

   c. ________________________________

   d. ________________________________

2. The unpaid balance due from patients for professional services rendered is known as a/an

   ________________________________.

3. An important document that provides demographic and identifying data for each patient and assists in billing and collection is called a/an ________________________________

   ________________________________.

4. A term preferable to "write-off" when used in a medical practice is ________________.

5. To verify a check, ask the patient for a/an ________________________________

   and ________________________________.

6. The procedure of systematically arranging the accounts receivable, by age, from the date of service is called ________________________________.

7. Write the formula for calculating the office accounts receivable (A/R) ratio.

   ____

   ____

   ____

8. What is the collection rate if a total of $40,300 was collected for the month and the total of the accounts receivable is $50,670? ________________________________

9. Are physicians' patient accounts single-entry accounts, open-book accounts, or written contract accounts? ________________________________

10. A court order attaching a debtor's property or wages to pay off a debt is known as ________________.

11. An individual who owes on an account and moves, leaving no forwarding address, is called a/an ________________________________.

12. Translate these credit and collection abbreviations.

NSF	____________	T	____________
WCO	____________	SK	____________
PIF	____________	FN	____________
NLE	____________	UE	____________

13. A straight petition in bankruptcy or absolute bankruptcy is also known as a/an ____________.

14. A wage earner's bankruptcy is sometimes referred to as a/an ____________.

15. State three bonding methods.

a. ____________

b. ____________

c. ____________

16. A system of billing accounts at spaced intervals during the month on the basis of a breakdown of accounts by alphabet, account number, insurance type, or date of service is known as ____________.

Part II Mix and Match

17. Match the credit and collection terms in the right column with the descriptions, and fill in the blank with the appropriate letter.

_______ Reductions of the normal fee based on a specific amount of money or a percentage of the charge

_______ Phrase to remind a patient about a delinquent account

_______ Item that permits bank customers to withdraw cash at any hour from an automated teller machine

_______ Individual owing money

_______ Claim on the property of another as security for a debt

_______ Individual record indicating charges, payments, adjustments, and balances owed for services rendered

_______ Detailed summary of all transactions of a creditor's account

_______ Person to whom money is owed

_______ Listing of accepted charges or established allowances for specific medical procedures

a. debtor
b. itemized statement
c. fee schedule
d. discounts
e. financial account record (ledger)
f. creditor
g. dun message
h. debit card
i. lien

18. Match the following federal acts with their descriptions, and fill in the blank with the appropriate letter.

________ Law stating that a person has 60 days to complain about an error from the date that a statement is mailed	a. Equal Credit Opportunity Act
________ Consumer protection act that applies to anyone who charges interest or agrees on payment of a bill in more than four installments, excluding a down payment	b. Fair Credit Reporting Act
________ Regulates collection practices of third-party debt collectors and attorneys who collect debts for others	c. Fair Credit Billing Act
________ Federal law prohibiting discrimination in all areas of granting credit	d. Truth in Lending Act
________ Regulates agencies that issue or use credit reports on consumers	e. Fair Debt Collection Practices Act

Part III Multiple Choice

Choose the best answer.

19. Signing another person's name on a check to obtain money or pay off a debt without permission is called
    a. embezzlement.
    b. stealing.
    c. garnishing.
    d. forgery.

20. When sending monthly statements to patients for balances due, the postal service can forward mail if the addressed envelopes contain the statement
    a. "Please Forward."
    b. "Forwarding Service Requested."
    c. "Forwarding and Return Receipt Requested."
    d. "Send Forward."

21. When accepting a credit card as payment on an account, the proper guideline(s) to follow is/are to
    a. ask for photo identification.
    b. accept a card only from the person whose name is on the card.
    c. get approval from the credit card company.
    d. all of the above.

22. A service offered by a nonprofit agency assisting people in paying off their debts is known as
    a. credit counseling.
    b. debt solutions.
    c. grant-in-aid under the Hill-Burton Act.
    d. small claims court.

23. Insurance payment checks should be stamped in the endorsement area on the back "For Deposit Only," which is called a/an
    a. conditional endorsement.
    b. qualified endorsement.
    c. special endorsement.
    d. restrictive endorsement.

Part IV True/False

Write "T" or "F" in the blank to indicate whether you think the statement is true or false.

________ 24. Insurance companies and the federal government do not recommend waiving copayments to patients.

________ 25. Regulation Z of the Truth in Lending Consumer Credit Cost Disclosure law applies if the patient is making three payments.

________ 26. Most state collection laws allow telephone calls to the debtor between 8 AM and 9 PM.

________ 27. When a patient has declared bankruptcy, it is permissible to continue to send monthly statements for a balance due.

________ 28. A collection agency must follow all the laws stated in the Fair Debt Collection Practices Act.

ASSIGNMENT 10-2 SELECT A DUN MESSAGE

Performance Objective

Task: Select an appropriate dun message and insert it on a patient's financial accounting record (ledger card).

Conditions: Use the patient's financial accounting record (Figure 10-1), computer, and a printer.

Standards: Time: ______________ minutes

Accuracy: ______________

(Note: The time element and accuracy criteria may be given by your instructor.)

Directions: Read the scenario and refer to the patient's financial accounting record (see Figure 10-1). Select appropriate dun messages for each month the patient has been billed. You may wish to refer to Figure 10-3 in the *Handbook.*

Scenario: Carrie Jones was on vacation in June and July and did not pay on her account. It is August (current year).

June 1, 20XX dun message ____

July 1, 20XX dun message ____

August 1, 20XX dun message ____

After the instructor has returned your work to you, either make the necessary corrections and place your work in a three-ring notebook for future reference, or, if you received a high score, place it in your portfolio for reference when applying for a job.

Acct No. 10-2

STATEMENT
Financial Account
COLLEGE CLINIC
4567 Broad Avenue
Woodland Hills, XY 12345-0001
Tel. 555-486-9002
Fax No. 555-487-8976

Carrie Jones
15543 Dean Street
Woodland Hills, XY 12345

Phone No. (H) (555) 439-8800 (W) (555) 550-8706 Birthdate 05-14-72

Primary Insurance Co. Prudential Insurance Company Policy/Group No. 450998

	REFERENCE	DESCRIPTION	CHARGES		CREDITS PYMNTS.		CREDITS ADJ.		BALANCE	
		BALANCE FORWARD →							20	00
4-16–xx	99215	C hx/exam HC DM DX 582							154	99
4-17–xx		Prudential billed (4-16-xx)							154	99
5-27–xx		Rec'd insurance ck #435			30	00			124	99
6-1-xx		Billed pt							124	99
7-1-xx		Billed pt							124	99
8-1-xx		Billed pt							124	99

PLEASE PAY LAST AMOUNT IN BALANCE COLUMN

THIS IS A COPY OF YOUR FINANCIAL ACCOUNT AS IT APPEARS ON OUR RECORDS

Figure 10-1

ASSIGNMENT 10-3 MANUALLY POST A COURTESY ADJUSTMENT

Performance Objective

Task: Post a courtesy adjustment to a patient's financial accounting record (ledger card).

Conditions: Use the patient's financial accounting record (Figure 10-2) and a pen.

Standards: Time: ______________ minutes

Accuracy: ______________

(Note: The time element and accuracy criteria may be given by your instructor.)

Directions: Read the case scenario and refer to the patient's financial accounting record (see Figure 10-2). You may wish to refer to Figure 10-3 in the *Handbook*. Post a courtesy adjustment to her financial accounting record.

Scenario: Maria Smith recently lost her job and is raising two children as a single parent. It is September 1 (current year). A discussion with Dr. Gerald Practon leads to a decision to write off the balance of the current charges on the account but not the balance forward.

After the instructor has returned your work to you, either make the necessary corrections and place your work in a three-ring notebook for future reference, or, if you received a high score, place it in your portfolio for reference when applying for a job.

Acct No. 10-3

STATEMENT
Financial Account
COLLEGE CLINIC
4567 Broad Avenue
Woodland Hills, XY 12345-0001
Tel. 555-486-9002
Fax No. 555-487-8976

Ms. Maria Smith
3737 Unser Road
Woodland Hills, XY 12345

Phone No. (H) (555) 430-8877 (W) (555) 908-1233 Birthdate 06-11-80

Primary Insurance Co. Metropolitan Insurance Company Policy/Group No. 4320870

	REFERENCE	DESCRIPTION	CHARGES	CREDITS PYMNTS.	CREDITS ADJ.	BALANCE
		BALANCE FORWARD →				20 00
5-19-xx	99214	OV DX 582	61 51			81 51
5-20-xx		Metropolitan billed (5-19-xx)				81 51
6-20-xx		Rec'd ins ck #6778		25 00		56 51
7-1-xx		Pt billed				56 51
8-1-xx		Pt billed				56 51

PLEASE PAY LAST AMOUNT IN BALANCE COLUMN

THIS IS A COPY OF YOUR FINANCIAL ACCOUNT AS IT APPEARS ON OUR RECORDS

Figure 10-2

ASSIGNMENT 10-4 MANUALLY POST A PATIENT'S CHARGES AND PAYMENT

Performance Objective

Task: Post a payment to a patient's financial accounting record (ledger card).

Conditions: Use the patient's financial accounting record (Figure 10-3), the Mock Fee Schedule in Appendix A in this *Workbook,* and a pen.

Standards: Time: ______________ minutes

Accuracy: ______________

(Note: The time element and accuracy criteria may be given by your instructor.)

Directions: Read the case scenario, refer to the patient's financial accounting record (see Figure 10-3), and refer to the Mock Fee Schedule in Appendix A in this *Workbook*. You may wish to refer to Figure 10-3 in the *Handbook*. Post the charges for the services rendered and payment to the patient's financial accounting record.

Scenario: On October 12 (current year), new patient Kenneth Brown came in for a Level III office visit and electrocardiogram (ECG). He has no insurance and paid $50 on his account with check number 3421.

After the instructor has returned your work to you, either make the necessary corrections and place your work in a three-ring notebook for future reference, or, if you received a high score, place it in your portfolio for reference when applying for a job.

Acct No. 10-4

STATEMENT

Financial Account

COLLEGE CLINIC
4567 Broad Avenue
Woodland Hills, XY 12345-0001
Tel. 555-486-9002
Fax No. 555-487-8976

Mr. Kenneth Brown
8896 Aster Drive
Woodland Hills, XY 12345

Phone No. (H) (555) 760-5211 (W) (555) 987-3355 Birthdate 01-15-82

Primary Insurance Co. none Policy/Group No.

	REFERENCE	DESCRIPTION	CHARGES	CREDITS PYMNTS.	CREDITS ADJ.	BALANCE
			BALANCE FORWARD →			

PLEASE PAY LAST AMOUNT IN BALANCE COLUMN

THIS IS A COPY OF YOUR FINANCIAL ACCOUNT AS IT APPEARS ON OUR RECORDS

Figure 10-3

ASSIGNMENT 10-5 COMPOSE A COLLECTION LETTER

Performance Objective

Task: Key a letter for the physician's signature and post the entry on the patient's financial accounting record (ledger card).

Conditions: Use the patient's financial accounting record (Figure 10-4), one sheet of letterhead (Figure 10-5), a number 10 envelope, English dictionary, thesaurus, medical dictionary, computer, printer, and a pen.

Standards: Time: ______________ minutes

Accuracy: ______________

(Note: The time element and accuracy criteria may be given by your instructor.)

Directions: Read the case scenario, refer to the patient's financial accounting record (see Figure 10-4), and compose a collection letter, using your signature and requesting payment. Type this letter on letterhead stationery in full block format (paragraphs to left margin). Include a paragraph stating that a copy of the delinquent statement is enclosed. You may wish to refer to Figure 10-15 in the *Handbook*. Post an entry on the patient's financial accounting record.

Scenario: It is December 1 (current year), and you have sent Mr. Ron Kelsey two statements with no response. You tried to reach him by telephone without success and have decided to send him a collection letter (see Figure 10-5).

After the instructor has returned your work to you, either make the necessary corrections and place your work in a three-ring notebook for future reference, or, if you received a high score, place it in your portfolio for reference when applying for a job.

Acct No. 10-5

STATEMENT
Financial Account
COLLEGE CLINIC
4567 Broad Avenue
Woodland Hills, XY 12345-0001
Tel. 555-486-9002
Fax No. 555-487-8976

Mr. Ron Kelsey
6321 Ocean Street
Woodland Hills, XY 12345

Phone No. (H) (555) 540-9800 (W) (555) 890-7766 Birthdate 03-25-75

Primary Insurance Co. XYZ Insurance Company Policy/Group No. 8503Y

	REFERENCE	DESCRIPTION	CHARGES		CREDITS PYMNTS.		CREDITS ADJ.		BALANCE	
		BALANCE FORWARD →								
07-09-xx	99283	ER new pt EPF hx/exam MC DM	66	23					66	23
07-10-xx		XYZ Insurance billed (3-9-xx)							66	23
09-20-xx		EOB rec'd pt has not met deductible							66	23
10-01-xx		Billed pt							66	23
11-01-xx		Billed pt							66	23

PLEASE PAY LAST AMOUNT IN BALANCE COLUMN

THIS IS A COPY OF YOUR FINANCIAL ACCOUNT AS IT APPEARS ON OUR RECORDS

Figure 10-4

COLLEGE CLINIC
4567 Broad Avenue
Woodland Hills, XY 12345-0001
Tel. (555) 486-9002
FAX (555) 487-8976

Figure 10-5

ASSIGNMENT 10-6 COMPLETE A CREDIT CARD VOUCHER

Performance Objective

Task: Complete a credit card voucher and post an entry on the patient's ledger.

Conditions: Use the completed credit card payment authorization (Figure 10-6), patient's ledger card (Figure 10-7), a credit card voucher (Figure 10-8), and a pen.

Standards: Time: ______________ minutes

Accuracy: ______________

(Note: The time element and accuracy criteria may be given by your instructor.)

Directions: Read the case scenario and refer to the completed credit card payment authorization (see Figure 10-6) and patient's ledger/statement (see Figure 10-7). Fill in the credit card voucher (see Figure 10-8) and post an appropriate entry on the ledger/statement. You may wish to refer to Figure 10-12 in the *Handbook*.

Scenario: It is November 6 (current year), and you receive a telephone call at the College Clinic. It is Kevin Long, who has an unpaid balance, and it is up to you to discuss this delinquency with Mr. Long and come to an agreement on how the account can be paid. After discussion, Mr. Long decides to pay the total balance due by credit card, giving you his authorization. You call the bank, and the authorization number given is 534889.

After the instructor has returned your work to you, either make the necessary corrections and place your work in a three-ring notebook for future reference, or, if you received a high score, place it in your portfolio for reference when applying for a job.

Credit Card Payment Authorization

Patient name: Kevin O. Long ______ Account #: 10-06 ______

Type of card: ☒ MasterCard ☐ Visa ☐ Discover ☐ American Express

Credit card number: 567 1342 5437 XXX0 ______ Expiration date: 12-31-20XX ______

Billing address: 2443 Davis Street ______

Woodland Hills, XY 12345-0001 ______

3 digit security code on back of credit card: 090 ______

American Express cards only - 4 digit code on the front of the card: ______

Amount to be charged to the card: $ ______ Signature: *Kevin O. Long*

Figure 10-6

Acct No. 10-6

STATEMENT
Financial Account
COLLEGE CLINIC
4567 Broad Avenue
Woodland Hills, XY 12345-0001
Tel. 555-486-9002
Fax No. 555-487-8976

Mr. Kevin O. Long
2443 Davis Street
Woodland Hills, XY 12345

Phone No. (H) (555) 244-5600 (W) (555) 970-4466 Birthdate 08-15-76

Primary Insurance Co. Blue Cross Policy/Group No. 130-XX-0987

	REFERENCE	DESCRIPTION	CHARGES		CREDITS PYMNTS.		CREDITS ADJ.		BALANCE	
		BALANCE FORWARD →								
09-08-xx	99205	OV Level V DX 582	132	28					132	28
09-09-xx		Blue Cross billed (9-8-xx)							132	28
10-12-xx		BC EOB rec'd pt has not met deductible							132	28
10-23-xx		Not covered by insurance. Balance due							132	28

PLEASE PAY LAST AMOUNT IN BALANCE COLUMN

THIS IS A COPY OF YOUR FINANCIAL ACCOUNT AS IT APPEARS ON OUR RECORDS

Figure 10-7

BANKCARD SALES SLIP 3PT.

MOORE© SPEEDISET© MOORESCAN© PATENTED 205 PRINTED IN USA
FORM 50983C (12-08) P689

DO NOT WRITE ABOVE THIS LINE A555A

EXPIRATION DATE CHECKED

↑ PLEASE DO NOT WRITE ABOVE THIS LINE ↑

QTY.	CLASS	DESCRIPTION	PRICE	AMOUNT
DATE		AUTHORIZATION	SUB TOTAL	
		REG./DEPT. CLERK	TAX	
			TIPS / MISC.	
VISA MasterCard 5882352			TOTAL	

SIGN HERE

X

The issuer of the card identified on this item is authorized to pay the amount shown as TOTAL upon proper presentation. I promise to pay such TOTAL (together with any other charges due thereon) subject to and in accordance with the agreement governing the use of such card.

CUSTOMER: RETAIN THIS COPY FOR YOUR RECORDS

SALES SLIP
CUSTOMER COPY

Figure 10-8

ASSIGNMENT 10-7 COMPLETE A FINANCIAL AGREEMENT

Performance Objective

Task: Complete a financial agreement and post an entry on the patient's ledger.

Conditions: Use the patient's ledger card (Figure 10-9), a financial statement form (Figure 10-10), and a pen.

Standards: Time: ______________ minutes

Accuracy: ______________

(Note: The time element and accuracy criteria may be given by your instructor.)

Directions: Read the case scenario. Complete a financial agreement (see Figure 10-10) by subtracting the down payment from the total debt. Refer to the patient's ledger/statement (see Figure 10-9) and post an appropriate entry to the ledger/statement using a pen. You may wish to refer to Figure 10-7 in the *Handbook*. Review the completed financial agreement with the patient (role played by another student). Ask the patient (role played by another student) to sign the financial agreement. Make a photocopy of the form for the patient to retain. File the original financial agreement in the patient's financial files in the office.

Scenario: Mr. Joseph Small has a large balance due. Create a payment plan for this case. You have discussed the installment plan concerning the amount of the total debt, the down payment, amount and date of each installment, and the date of final payment. On June 1 (current year), Mr. Small is paying $500 cash as a down payment, and the balance is to be divided into five equal payments, due on the first of each month. There will be no monthly finance charge. Mr. Small's daytime telephone number is 555-760-5502. He is a patient of Dr. Brady Coccidioides.

After the instructor has returned your work to you, either make the necessary corrections and place your work in a three-ring notebook for future reference, or, if you received a high score, place it in your portfolio for reference when applying for a job.

Acct No. 10-7

STATEMENT
Financial Account
COLLEGE CLINIC
4567 Broad Avenue
Woodland Hills, XY 12345-0001
Tel. 555-486-9002
Fax No. 555-487-8976

Mr. Joseph Small
655 Sherry Street
Woodland Hills, XY 12345

Phone No. (H) (555) 320-8801 (W) (555) 760-5502 Birthdate 11-04-77

Primary Insurance Co. Blue Shield Policy/Group No. 870-XX-4398

	REFERENCE	DESCRIPTION	CHARGES		CREDITS PYMNTS.		CREDITS ADJ.		BALANCE	
		BALANCE FORWARD →							20	00
04-19-xx	99215	OV Level	96	97					116	97
04-30-xx	99218	Adm hosp	74	22					191	19
04-30-xx	32440	Pneumonectomy, total	1972	10					2163	29
05-20-xx		Blue Shield billed (1-19 to 30-xx)							2163	29
05-15-xx		BS EOB Pt deductible $2000 rec'd ck #544			163	29			2000	00

PLEASE PAY LAST AMOUNT IN BALANCE COLUMN

THIS IS A COPY OF YOUR FINANCIAL ACCOUNT AS IT APPEARS ON OUR RECORDS

Figure 10-9

College Clinic
4567 Broad Avenue
Woodland Hills, XY 12345-0001
Phone: 555/486-9002
Fax: 555/487-8976

FINANCIAL PAYMENT PLAN AGREEMENT

For medical professional services rendered to:

Patient Name ______________________ Account No. ______________

Responsible Party ______________________________

Address ______________________________

____

Telephones: Home ______________________________
Mobile ______________________________
Business ______________________________

1. Cash price of total medical treatment $ __________
2. Down payment (partial payment) $ __________
3. Amount covered by insurance plan $ __________
4. Unpaid balance due $ __________
5. **ANNUAL PERCENTAGE RATE** (interest rate) __________%
6. **FINANCE CHARGE** ($ amt of cost to patient) $ __________
7. Total amount of unpaid balance due __________
8. Monthly payment amount $ __________

TERMS:

1. ALL PAYMENTS ARE DUE ON OR BEFORE YOUR DUE DATE EACH MONTH.
2. The patient agrees to be fully responsible for the total payment of medical services performed in this office including any amounts not covered by any health insurance plan.
3. The patient has the right at any time to pay the unpaid balance due without penalty.
4. First payment due ____/____/____ and subsequent payments on the same day of each consecutive month until paid in full.

____

Signature of Patient/Responsible Party Date

____

Physician's signature or Authorized representative Date

Figure 10-10

11 The Blue Plans, Private Insurance, and Managed Care Plans

Marilyn T. Fordney

KEY TERMS

Your instructor may wish to select some words pertinent to this chapter for a test. For definitions of the terms, further study, and/or reference, the words, phrases, and abbreviations may be found in the glossary at the end of the Handbook. *Key terms for this chapter follow.*

ancillary services
buffing
capitation
carve outs
churning
claims-review type of foundation
closed panel program
comprehensive type of foundation
copayment
deductible
direct referral
disenrollment
exclusive provider organization
fee-for-service
formal referral
foundation for medical care
gatekeeper
health maintenance organization
in-area
independent (or individual) practice association
managed care organization
participating physician or provider
per capita
physician provider group
point-of-service plan
preferred provider organization
prepaid group practice model
primary care physician
self-referral
service area
staff model
stop loss
tertiary care
turfing
utilization review
verbal referral
withhold

KEY ABBREVIATIONS

See how many abbreviations and acronyms you can translate and then use this as a handy reference list. Definitions for the key abbreviations are located near the back of the Handbook *in the glossary.*

EBP ____________________

EPO ____________________

ERISA ____________________

FMC ____________________

HEDIS ____________________

HMO ____________________

IPA ____________________

MCO ____________________

NCQA ____________________

PCP ____________________

POS ____________________

PPG ____________________

PPO ____________________

QIO ____________________

QISMC ____________________

UR ____________________

PERFORMANCE OBJECTIVES

The student will be able to:

- Define and spell the key terms and key abbreviations for this chapter, given the information from the *Handbook* glossary, within a reasonable time period and with enough accuracy to obtain a satisfactory evaluation.
- After reading the chapter, answer the fill-in-the-blank, multiple choice, and true/false review questions with enough accuracy to obtain a satisfactory evaluation.
- Complete treatment authorization forms of managed care plans, given completed new patient information forms, within a reasonable time period and with enough accuracy to obtain a satisfactory evaluation.

STUDY OUTLINE

Private Insurance
- Blue Cross and Blue Shield Plans

Managed Care
- Prepaid Group Practice Health Plans
- Benefits

Managed Care Systems
- Health Maintenance Organizations
- Exclusive Provider Organizations
- Foundations for Medical Care
- Independent Practice Associations
- Preferred Provider Organizations
- Physician Provider Groups
- Point-of-Service Plans
- Triple-Option Health Plans
- Provider-Sponsored Organization
- Religious Fraternal Benefit Society
- Employee Retirement Income Security

Medical Review
- Quality Improvement Organization
- Utilization Review of Management

Management of Plans
- Contracts
- Carve Outs

Plan Administration
- Patient Information Letter
- Preauthorization or Prior Approval
- Diagnostic Tests
- Managed Care Guide

Financial Management
- Payment
- Statement of Remittance
- Accounting
- Fee-for-Service
- Year-End Evaluation
- Bankruptcy

ASSIGNMENT 11-1 REVIEW QUESTIONS

Part I Fill in the Blank

Review the objectives, key terms, glossary definitions of key terms, figures, and chapter information before completing the following review questions.

1. If a physician or hospital in a managed care plan is paid a fixed, per capita amount for each patient enrolled regardless of the type and number of services rendered, this is a payment system known as

   ______________________________.

2. When a prepaid group practice plan limits the patient's choice of personal physicians, this is termed a/an ______________________________ program.

3. In a managed care setting, a physician who controls patient access to specialists and diagnostic testing services is known as a/an ______________________________.

4. The oldest type of the prepaid health plans is ______________________________.

5. Name four types of health maintenance organization (HMO) models.

   a. ______________________________

   b. ______________________________

   c. ______________________________

   d. ______________________________

6. What is a foundation for medical care?

   ____

   ____

   ____

7. Name two types of operations used by foundations for medical care, and explain the main feature of each.

   a. ______________________________

   ____

   b. ______________________________

   ____

8. A health benefit program in which enrollees may choose any physician or hospital for services but obtain a higher level of benefits if preferred providers are used is known as a/an ______________________________.

9. HMOs and preferred provider organizations (PPOs) consisting of a network of physicians and hospitals that provide an insurance company or employer with discounts on their services are referred to collectively as a/an ______________________________.

10. An organization that reviews medical necessity, reasonableness, appropriateness, and completeness of inpatient hospital care is called a/an ______________________________.

11. To control health care costs, the process of reviewing and establishing medical necessity for services and providers' use of medical care resources is termed ______________________________
______________________________.

12. Explain the meaning of a "stop-loss" provision that might appear in a managed care contract.

____

____

13. When a certain percentage of the monthly capitation payment or a percentage of the allowable charges to physicians is set aside to operate a managed care plan, this is known as a/an

______________________________.

Part II Multiple Choice

Choose the best answer.

14. A Quality Improvement Organization (QIO)
    a. examines evidence for admission and discharge of a patient from the hospital.
    b. evaluates the quality and efficiency of services rendered by a practicing physician or physicians within a specialty group.
    c. settles disputes over fees.
    d. all of the above.

15. A type of managed care plan regulated under insurance statutes combining features of health maintenance organizations and preferred provider organizations that employers agree not to contract with any other plan is known as a/an
    a. independent practice association (IPA).
    b. exclusive provider organization (EPO).
    c. physician provider group (PPG).
    d. point-of-service (POS) plan.

16. Medical services that are not included in a managed care contract's capitation rate but that may be contracted for separately are referred to as
    a. carve outs.
    b. stop-loss limits.
    c. payment mechanisms.
    d. copayments.

17. When the primary care physician informs the patient and telephones the referring physician that the patient is being referred for an appointment, this is called a/an
    a. direct referral.
    b. formal referral.
    c. self-referral.
    d. verbal referral.

18. Plan-specified facilities listed in managed care plan contracts where patients are required to have laboratory and radiology tests performed are called
    a. hospital facilities.
    b. medical facilities.
    c. network facilities.
    d. outside facilities.

Part III True/False

Write "T" or "F" in the blank to indicate whether you think the statement is true or false.

________ 19. An HMO can be sponsored and operated by a foundation.

________ 20. A Quality Improvement Organization determines the quality and operation of health care.

________ 21. An employer may offer the services of an HMO clinic if he or she has five or more employees.

________ 22. Medicare and Medicaid beneficiaries may not join an HMO.

________ 23. Withheld managed care amounts that are not yet received from the managed care plan by the medical practice should be shown as a write-off in an accounts journal.

ASSIGNMENT 11-2 OBTAIN AUTHORIZATION FOR A CONSULTATION FROM A MANAGED CARE PLAN

Performance Objective

Task: Complete a treatment authorization form to obtain permission for an office consultation for a patient covered by a managed care plan.

Conditions: Use a treatment authorization form (Figure 11-1), a new patient information form (Figure 11-2), a computer, and a printer.

Standards: Time: ______________ minutes

Accuracy: ______________

(Note: The time element and accuracy criteria may be given by your instructor.)

Directions: Complete a treatment authorization form (see Figure 11-1) for Mrs. Cohn's managed care plan to obtain permission for the office consultation, and date it August 2 of the current year. To obtain information, refer to the New Patient Information form completed by Mrs. Cohn when she came into the office for her visit with Dr. Practon (see Figure 11-2). Dr. Practon's FHP provider number is FHP C01402X.

Scenario: Meriweather B. Cohn's primary care physician, Dr. Gerald Practon, took her clinical history. Physical examination revealed a normal blood pressure (120/80); however, abnormal heart sounds were heard and a diagnosis of a heart murmur was made. Dr. Practon decided to make a semi-urgent request to refer Mrs. Cohn for a cardiac consultation (other service) to Dr. Victor M. Salazar, whose office is located at 20 Excalibur Street, Woodland Hills, XY, 12345, and whose office telephone number is 555-625-7344. Dr. Salazar will take a detailed history, perform a detailed examination, and make low-complexity medical decisions to evaluate Mrs. Cohn's heart murmur.

After the instructor has returned your work to you, either make the necessary corrections and place your work in a three-ring notebook for future reference or, if you receive a high score, place it in your portfolio for reference when applying for a job.

FHP® HEALTH CARE

IPA TREATMENT AUTHORIZATION FORM

____ Referral
____ Participating
____ Non-Participating
____ Commercial
____ Senior

For Billing Instructions, Patient and Non-Affiliated Providers, and Consultants please see reverse side for instructions

THIS PORTION COMPLETED BY PHYSICIAN

Patient Name ______________________________ Date ____/____/____

M _____ F _____ Age _____ FHP # ______________ Home Phone ______________

Address ______________________________

Primary Care MD ______________ Primary Care MD's FHP # ______________

Referring MD ______________ Referring MD's FHP # ______________

Referred To ______________ Address ______________

______________ Office Phone ______________

Type of service: ☐ In-Patient ☐ Out-Patient Services ☐ Initial Visit ☐ Return Visit ☐ Other

Clinical History and Findings ______________________________

____

____

Diagnosis ______________________________

______________ **ICD-10-CM CODE** ______________

Evaluation and Treatment to Date ______________________________

____

____

Procedure ______________________________

____

______________ **RVS CPT-4 CODE** ______________

Reason for Referral/Consultation/Procedure ______________________________

____

____

Accident: ☐ Yes ☐ No Where Occurred: ☐ Home ☐ Work ☐ Auto ☐ Other

☐ Urgent ☐ Semi-Urgent ☐ Elective

Facility To Be Used: ______________ Estimated Length of Stay ______________

☐ Office ☐ Out-Patient ☐ In-Patient

THIS PORTION COMPLETED BY FHP UR

THIS AUTHORIZATION GOOD FOR 60 DAYS ONLY

Type of Contract: ☐ Capitation ☐ Fee For Service ☐ Per Diem

Projected Cost of Procedure ______________ Projected Cost of Facility ______________

HMO Verification: Effective ______________ Group # ______________

Benefits: Co-Pay Per Visit ______________ Hospital ______________

Limitations: ______________________________

_____ AuthorizedDate _____ Initials _____ Reason ______________ Authorization #______________

_____ Deferred Date _____ Initials _____ Reason ______________

_____ Denied Date _____ Initials _____ Reason ______________

_____ Modified Date _____ Initials _____ Reason ______________

WHITE – UR Copy CANARY – Hospital Copy PINK – Physician Copy GOLDENROD – Claims Copy

Figure 11-1

Welcome To Our Office

NEW PATIENT INFORMATION

DATE 8-2-20xx

PATIENT'S NAME (PLEASE PRINT)	S.S. #	MARITAL STATUS	SEX	BIRTH DATE	AGE	RELIGION (optional)
Meriweather B. Cohn	430-XX-0261	S [X]M W D SEP	M [X]F	11-14-65		

STREET ADDRESS PERMANENT TEMPORARY	CITY AND STATE	ZIP CODE	HOME PHONE #
267 Blake Street	Woodland Hills XY	12345	555-263-0911
PATIENT'S OR PARENT'S EMPLOYER	**OCCUPATION (INDICATE IF STUDENT)**	**HOW LONG EMPLOYED**	**BUS. PHONE # EXT #**
Sun Corporation	sales representative	5 yrs	555-263-0099
EMPLOYER'S STREET ADDRESS	**CITY AND STATE**		**ZIP CODE**
74 Rain Street	Woodland Hills XY		12345
DRUG ALLERGIES, IF ANY			
Penicillin			

SPOUSE OR PARENT'S NAME	S.S. #	BIRTH DATE	
Starkweather L. Cohn	273-XX-9961	7-9-63	
SPOUSE OR PARENT'S EMPLOYER	**OCCUPATION (INDICATE IF STUDENT)**	**HOW LONG EMPLOYED**	**BUS. PHONE #**
B & L Stormdrain Co.	accountant	10 yrs	555-421-0091
EMPLOYER'S STREET ADDRESS	**CITY AND STATE**		**ZIP CODE**
20 South Wind Road	Woodland Hills XY		12345
***SPOUSE'S STREET ADDRESS, IF DIVORCED OR SEPARATED**	**CITY AND STATE**	**ZIP CODE**	**HOME PHONE #**

PLEASE READ: ALL CHARGES ARE DUE AT THE TIME OF SERVICES. IF HOSPITALIZATION IS INDICATED, THE PATIENT IS RESPONSIBLE FOR FURNISHING INSURANCE CLAIM FORMS TO THE OFFICE PRIOR TO HOSPITALIZATION.

PERSON RESPONSIBLE FOR PAYMENT, IF NOT ABOVE	STREET ADDRESS, CITY, STATE		ZIP CODE	HOME PHONE #
BLUE SHIELD (GIVE NAME OF POLICYHOLDER) ☐	**EFFECTIVE DATE**	**CERTIFICATE #**	**GROUP #**	**COVERAGE CODE**
OTHER (WRITE IN NAME OF INSURANCE COMPANY) ☐ FHP Healthcare	**EFFECTIVE DATE** 1-1-8X		**POLICY #** FHP # A4932	
OTHER (WRITE IN NAME OF INSURANCE COMPANY) ☐	**EFFECTIVE DATE**		**POLICY #**	

MEDICARE (PLEASE GIVE NUMBER) ☐	RAILROAD RETIREMENT (PLEASE GIVE NUMBER) ☐

MEDICAID ☐	EFFECTIVE DATE	PROGRAM #	COUNTY #	CASE #	ACCOUNT #

INDUSTRIAL ☐	WERE YOU INJURED ON THE JOB? ☐ YES [X] NO	DATE OF INJURY	INDUSTRIAL CLAIM #
ACCIDENT ☐	WAS AN AUTOMOBILE INVOLVED? ☐ YES [X] NO	DATE OF ACCIDENT	NAME OF ATTORNEY
WERE X-RAYS TAKEN OF THIS INJURY OR PROBLEM?	☐ YES [X] NO	IF YES, WHERE WERE X-RAYS TAKEN? (HOSPITAL, ETC)	DATE X-RAYS TAKEN

HAS ANY MEMBER OF YOUR IMMEDIATE FAMILY BEEN TREATED BY OUR PHYSICIAN(S) BEFORE? INCLUDE NAME OF PHYSICIAN AND FAMILY MEMBER
No

REFERRED BY	STREET ADDRESS, CITY, STATE	ZIP CODE	PHONE #
BREEZIE N. CLOUD	521 N. Wind Rd., Woodland Hills XY	12345	555-721-9641

ALL PROFESSIONAL SERVICES RENDERED ARE CHARGED TO THE PATIENT, NECESSARY FORMS WILL BE COMPLETED TO HELP EXPEDITE INSURANCE CARRIER PAYMENTS. HOWEVER, THE PATIENT IS RESPONSIBLE FOR ALL FEES, REGARDLESS OF INSURANCE COVERAGE. IT IS ALSO CUSTOMARY TO PAY FOR SERVICES WHEN RENDERED UNLESS OTHER ARRANGEMENTS HAVE BEEN MADE IN ADVANCE WITH OUR OFFICE BOOKKEEPER.

INSURANCE AUTHORIZATION AND ASSIGNMENT

Name of Policy Holder Meriweather B. Cohn HC Number ________

I request that payment of authorized Medicare/Other Insurance company benefits be made either to me or on my behalf to College Clinic for any services furnished me by that party who accepts assignment/physcian. Regulations pertaining to Medicare assignment of benefits apply.

I authorize any holder of medical or other information about me to release to the Social Security Administration and Health Care Financing Administration or its intermediaries or carrier or any other insurance company any information needed for this or a related Medicare/Other Insurance company claim.

I understand my signature requests that payment be made and authorizes release of medical information necessary to pay the claim. If item 9 of the HCFA-1500 claim form is completed, my signature authorizes releasing of the information to the insurer or agency shown. In Medicare/Other Insurance company assigned cases, the physician or supplier agrees to accept the charge determination of the Medicare/Other Insurance company as the full charge, and the patient is responsible only for the deductible, coinsurance, and noncovered services. Coinsurance and the deductible are based upon the charge determination of the Medicare/Other Insurance company.

Signature Meriweather B. Cohn Date 8-2-20XX

NEW PATIENT INFORMATION

Figure 11-2

ASSIGNMENT 11-3 OBTAIN AUTHORIZATION FOR PHYSICAL THERAPY FROM A MANAGED CARE PLAN

Performance Objective

Task: Complete a treatment authorization form to obtain permission for physical therapy for a patient covered by a managed care plan.

Conditions: Use a treatment authorization form (Figure 11-3), computer, and printer.

Standards: Time: ______________ minutes

Accuracy: ______________

(Note: The time element and accuracy criteria may be given by your instructor.)

Directions: Complete the treatment authorization form for this patient (see Figure 11-3), date it July 7 of the current year, and submit it to the managed care plan. Refer to Figure 11-2 in the *Handbook* for visual guidance.

Scenario: Mrs. Rosario Jimenez comes into Dr. Gerald Practon's office complaining of neck pain. Mrs. Jimenez is a member of the managed care program HealthNet, and Dr. Practon is her primary care physician. Mrs. Jimenez lives at 350 South Carib Street, Woodland Hills, XY, 12345-0003. Her telephone number is 555-450-9987, and she was born April 6, 1960. Her plan identification number is JIM40896, and the effective date is January 1, 20xx. After taking a history, completing a physical examination, and taking and reviewing radiographs, Dr. Practon makes a diagnosis of cervical radiculitis. He gives Mrs. Jimenez a prescription for some medication and says it is necessary to order outpatient physical therapy (one area, for 15 minutes; therapeutic exercises to develop strength, motion, and flexibility) twice a week for 6 weeks at College Hospital. Authorization must be obtained for this treatment. Dr. Practon's HealthNet provider number is HN C01402X.

After the instructor has returned your work to you, either make the necessary corrections and place your work in a three-ring notebook for future reference or, if you receive a high score, place it in your portfolio for reference when applying for a job.

College Clinic
4567 Broad Avenue
Woodland Hills, XY 12345-0001
Telephone No. (555) 487-8976
Fax No. (555) 487-8976

MANAGED CARE PLAN AUTHORIZATION REQUEST

❑ Health Net ❑ Met Life
❑ Pacificare ❑ Travelers
❑ Secure Horizons ❑ Pru Care
❑ Other

Member/Group No.

TO BE COMPLETED BY PRIMARY CARE PHYSICIAN OR OUTSIDE PROVIDER

Patient Name__________ Date__________

❑ Male ❑ Female Birthdate__________ Home Telephone Number __________

Address __________

Primary Care Physician__________ NPI__________

Referring Physician __________ NPI__________

Referred to __________ NPI__________

Address __________ Telephone No. __________

Diagnosis Code __________ Diagnosis__________

Diagnosis Code __________ Diagnosis__________

Treatment Plan __________

Authorization requested for: ❑ Consult only ❑ Treatment only ❑ Consult/Treatment
❑ Consult/Procedure/Surgery ❑ Diagnostic Tests

Procedure Code: __________ Description: __________

Procedure Code: __________ Description: __________

Place of service ❑ Office ❑ Outpatient ❑ Inpatient ❑ Other Number of visits: __________

Facility: __________ Length of stay: __________

Physician's signature: __________

TO BE COMPLETED BY PRIMARY CARE PHYSICIAN

PCP Recommendations: __________ PCP Initials: __________

Date eligibility checked: __________

TO BE COMPLETED BY UTILIZATION MANAGEMENT

Authorized: __________ Auth. No: __________ Not Authorized __________

Deferred: __________ Modified: __________

Effective Date: __________ Expiration Date: __________ No. of visits: __________

Figure 11-3

ASSIGNMENT 11-4 OBTAIN AUTHORIZATION FOR DIAGNOSTIC ARTHROSCOPY FROM A MANAGED CARE PLAN

Performance Objective

Task: Complete a treatment authorization form to obtain permission for diagnostic arthroscopy with débridement for a patient covered by a managed care plan.

Conditions: Use a treatment authorization form (Figure 11-4), computer, and printer.

Standards: Time: ______________ minutes

Accuracy: ______________

(Note: The time element and accuracy criteria may be given by your instructor.)

Directions: Complete the treatment authorization form for this patient (see Figure 11-4), date it August 12 of the current year, and submit it to the managed care plan. Refer to Figure 11-2 in the *Handbook* for visual guidance.

Scenario: Daniel Chan has been referred by his primary care physician, Dr. Gerald Practon, to an orthopedic surgeon, Dr. Raymond Skeleton. Both physicians are members of his managed care plan, Metropolitan Life. The patient comes into Dr. Skeleton's office complaining of pain, swelling, and crepitus of the right knee. The patient is having difficulty walking but indicates no recent injury to the knee.

Mr. Chan lives at 226 West Olive Avenue, Woodland Hills, XY, 12345-0001, and his telephone number is 555-540-6700. His plan identification number is FTW90876, effective February 1, 20xx, and he was born February 23, 1971.

After taking a history, completing a physical examination, and taking and reviewing radiographs, Dr. Skeleton suspects the patient has a tear of the medial meniscus and may require débridement of articular cartilage. This procedure will be performed on an outpatient basis at College Hospital. Authorization must be obtained for the surgical arthroscopy with débridement of articular cartilage. Dr. Practon's Metropolitan Life provider number is ML C01402X and Dr. Skeleton's Metropolitan Life provider number is ML C4561X.

After the instructor has returned your work to you, either make the necessary corrections and place your work in a three-ring notebook for future reference or, if you received a high score, place it in your portfolio for reference when applying for a job.

College Clinic
4567 Broad Avenue
Woodland Hills, XY 12345-0001
Telephone No. (555) 487-8976
Fax No. (555) 487-8976

MANAGED CARE PLAN AUTHORIZATION REQUEST

❑ Health Net ❑ Met Life
❑ Pacificare ❑ Travelers
❑ Secure Horizons ❑ Pru Care
❑ Other

Member/Group No.

TO BE COMPLETED BY PRIMARY CARE PHYSICIAN OR OUTSIDE PROVIDER

Patient Name________ Date________
❑ Male ❑ Female Birthdate________ Home Telephone Number ________
Address ________
Primary Care Physician________ NPI________
Referring Physician ________ NPI________
Referred to ________ NPI________
Address ________ Telephone No. ________
Diagnosis Code ________ Diagnosis________
Diagnosis Code ________ Diagnosis________
Treatment Plan ________
Authorization requested for: ❑ Consult only ❑ Treatment only ❑ Consult/Treatment
❑ Consult/Procedure/Surgery ❑ Diagnostic Tests
Procedure Code: ________ Description: ________
Procedure Code: ________ Description: ________
Place of service ❑ Office ❑ Outpatient ❑ Inpatient ❑ Other Number of visits: ________
Facility: ________ Length of stay: ________
Physician's signature: ________

TO BE COMPLETED BY PRIMARY CARE PHYSICIAN

PCP Recommendations: ________ PCP Initials: ________
Date eligibility checked: ________

TO BE COMPLETED BY UTILIZATION MANAGEMENT
Authorized: ________ Auth. No: ________ Not Authorized ________
Deferred: ________ Modified: ________
Effective Date: ________ Expiration Date: ________ No. of visits: ________

Figure 11-4

ASSIGNMENT 11-5 OBTAIN AUTHORIZATION FOR CONSULTATION FROM A MANAGED CARE PLAN

Performance Objective

Task: Complete a treatment authorization form to obtain permission for consultation for a patient from a managed care plan.

Conditions: Use a treatment authorization form (Figure 11-5), computer, and printer.

Standards: Time: ______________ minutes

Accuracy: ______________

(Note: The time element and accuracy criteria may be given by your instructor.)

Directions: Complete the treatment authorization form for this patient (see Figure 11-5), date it September 3 of the current year, and submit it to the managed care plan. Refer to Figure 11-2 in the *Handbook* for visual guidance.

Scenario: Frederico Fellini, with a history of getting up four times during the night with a slow urinary stream, was seen by his primary care physician, Dr. Gerald Practon. An intravenous pyelogram yielded negative results except for distention of the urinary bladder. Physical examination of the prostate showed an enlargement. The preliminary diagnosis is benign prostatic hypertrophy (BPH).

The patient will be referred to Dr. Douglas Lee, a urologist, for consultation (Level 4) and cystoscopy. Transurethral resection of the prostate is possible at a future date. Dr. Lee's address is 4300 Cyber Street, Woodland Hills, XY, 12345, and his office telephone number is 555-675-3322. His NPI is 55026717XX.

Dr. Practon's managed care contract is with PruCare, identification number PC C01402X, of which this patient is a member.

Mr. Fellini lives at 476 Miner Street, Woodland Hills, XY, 12345, and his telephone number is 555-679-0098. His PruCare plan identification number is VRG87655, effective January 1, 20xx. His birth date is May 24, 1944.

After the instructor has returned your work to you, either make the necessary corrections and place your work in a three-ring notebook for future reference or, if you received a high score, place it in your portfolio for reference when applying for a job.

College Clinic
4567 Broad Avenue
Woodland Hills, XY 12345-0001
Telephone No. (555) 487-8976
Fax No. (555) 487-8976

MANAGED CARE PLAN AUTHORIZATION REQUEST

❑ Health Net
❑ Pacificare
❑ Secure Horizons
❑ Other
❑ Met Life
❑ Travelers
❑ Pru Care

Member/Group No.

TO BE COMPLETED BY PRIMARY CARE PHYSICIAN OR OUTSIDE PROVIDER

Patient Name________ Date________

❑ Male ❑ Female Birthdate________ Home Telephone Number ________

Address ________

Primary Care Physician________ NPI________

Referring Physician ________ NPI________

Referred to ________ NPI________

Address ________ Telephone No. ________

Diagnosis Code ________ Diagnosis________

Diagnosis Code ________ Diagnosis________

Treatment Plan ________

Authorization requested for: ❑ Consult only ❑ Treatment only ❑ Consult/Treatment ❑ Consult/Procedure/Surgery ❑ Diagnostic Tests

Procedure Code: ________ Description:________

Procedure Code: ________ Description:________

Place of service ❑ Office ❑ Outpatient ❑ Inpatient ❑ Other Number of visits:________

Facility: ________ Length of stay:________

Physician's signature: ________

TO BE COMPLETED BY PRIMARY CARE PHYSICIAN

PCP Recommendations: ________ PCP Initials: ________

Date eligibility checked:________

TO BE COMPLETED BY UTILIZATION MANAGEMENT

Authorized:________ Auth. No:________ Not Authorized ________

Deferred:________ Modified: ________

Effective Date:________ Expiration Date:________ No. of visits: ________

Figure 11-5

ASSIGNMENT 11-6 OBTAIN AUTHORIZATION FOR DIAGNOSTIC BODY SCAN FROM A MANAGED CARE PLAN

Performance Objective

Task: Complete a treatment authorization form to obtain permission for diagnostic complete body bone scan and mammogram for a patient covered by a managed care plan.

Conditions: Use a treatment authorization form (Figure 11-6), computer, and printer.

Standards: Time: ______________ minutes

Accuracy: ______________

(Note: The time element and accuracy criteria may be given by your instructor.)

Directions: Complete the treatment authorization form for this patient (see Figure 11-6), date it October 23 of the current year, and submit it to the managed care plan. Refer to Figure 11-2 in the *Handbook* for visual guidance.

Scenario: A patient, Debbie Dye, sees her primary care physician, Dr. Gerald Practon, for complaint of midback pain. She underwent a lumpectomy 2 years ago for a malignant neoplasm of the lower left breast; thus she has a history of breast cancer. She has been referred by Dr. Practon (PacifiCare identification number PC C01402X) to Dr. Donald Patos, an oncologist, for a complete workup. He finds that her complaint of midback pain warrants the need to refer her to XYZ Radiology for bilateral diagnostic mammography and a complete body bone scan.

Dr. Patos' address is 4466 East Canter Drive, Woodland Hills, XY, 12345, and his office telephone number is 555-980-5566. Dr. Patos' PacifiCare identification number is PC 5673X. His NPI is 6520101678XX.

Ms. Dye lives at 6700 Flora Road, Woodland Hills, XY, 12345, and her telephone number is 555-433-6755. Her PacifiCare plan identification number is SR45380, effective January 1, 20xx. Her birth date is August 6, 1952.

XYZ Radiology's address is 4767 Broad Avenue, Woodland Hills, XY, 12345-0001, and the office telephone number is 555-486-9162.

After the instructor has returned your work to you, either make the necessary corrections and place your work in a three-ring notebook for future reference or, if you received a high score, place it in your portfolio for reference when applying for a job.

College Clinic
4567 Broad Avenue
Woodland Hills, XY 12345-0001
Telephone No. (555) 487-8976
Fax No. (555) 487-8976

MANAGED CARE PLAN AUTHORIZATION REQUEST

❑ Health Net ❑ Met Life
❑ Pacificare ❑ Travelers
❑ Secure Horizons ❑ Pru Care
❑ Other

Member/Group No.

TO BE COMPLETED BY PRIMARY CARE PHYSICIAN OR OUTSIDE PROVIDER

Patient Name__________ Date__________

❑ Male ❑ Female Birthdate__________ Home Telephone Number __________

Address __________

Primary Care Physician__________ NPI__________

Referring Physician __________ NPI__________

Referred to __________ NPI__________

Address __________ Telephone No. __________

Diagnosis Code __________ Diagnosis__________

Diagnosis Code __________ Diagnosis__________

Treatment Plan __________

Authorization requested for: ❑ Consult only ❑ Treatment only ❑ Consult/Treatment
❑ Consult/Procedure/Surgery ❑ Diagnostic Tests

Procedure Code: __________ Description:__________

Procedure Code: __________ Description:__________

Place of service ❑ Office ❑ Outpatient ❑ Inpatient ❑ Other Number of visits:__________

Facility: __________ Length of stay:__________

Physician's signature: __________

TO BE COMPLETED BY PRIMARY CARE PHYSICIAN

PCP Recommendations: __________ PCP Initials: __________

Date eligibility checked:__________

TO BE COMPLETED BY UTILIZATION MANAGEMENT

Authorized:__________ Auth. No:__________ Not Authorized __________

Deferred:__________ Modified: __________

Effective Date:__________ Expiration Date:__________ No. of visits: __________

Figure 11-6

12 Medicare

Marilyn T. Fordney

KEY TERMS

Your instructor may wish to select some words pertinent to this chapter for a test. For definitions of the terms, further study, and/or reference, the words, phrases, and abbreviations may be found in the glossary at the end of the Handbook. *Key terms for this chapter follow.*

Advance Beneficiary Notice of Noncoverage
approved charges
assignment
benefit period
Centers for Medicare and Medicaid Services
Correct Coding Initiative
crossover claim
diagnostic cost groups
disabled
end-stage renal disease
formulary
hospice
hospital insurance
intermediate care facilities
limiting charge
medical necessity
Medicare
Medicare administrative contractors
Medicare Part A
Medicare Part B
Medicare Part C
Medicare Part D
Medicare/Medicaid
Medicare Secondary Payer
Medicare Summary Notice
Medigap
national alphanumeric codes
nonparticipating physician
nursing facility
participating physician
Physician Quality Reporting Initiative
premium
prospective payment system
Quality Improvement Organization
qui tam action
reasonable fee
Recovery Audit Contractor Initiative
relative value unit
remittance advice
resource-based relative value scale
respite care
Supplemental Security Income
supplementary medical insurance
volume performance standard
whistleblowers

KEY ABBREVIATIONS

See how many abbreviations and acronyms you can translate and then use this as a handy reference list. Definitions for the key abbreviations are located near the back of the Handbook *in the glossary.*

ABN ____________________

CAP ____________________

CCI ____________________

CLIA ____________________

CMS ____________________

COBRA ____________________

DC ____________________

DCGs ____________________

DEFRA ____________________

DME ____________________

EGHP ____________________

ERA ____________________

ESRD ____________________

GPCI ____________________

ICFs ____________________

ICU ____________________

LCD ____________________

LGHP ____________________

MAAC ________________________________

MACs ________________________________

Medi-Medi ________________________________

MG ________________________________

MMA ________________________________

MSA ________________________________

MSN ________________________________

MSP ________________________________

NCDs ________________________________

NEMB ________________________________

NF ________________________________

nonpar physician ________________________________

OASDI ________________________________

OBRA ________________________________

OCNA ________________________________

OIG ________________________________

OR ________________________________

par physician ________________________________

PAYRID ________________________________

PFFS plan ________________________________

PIN ________________________________

PPS ________________________________

PQRI ________________________________

PSO ________________________________

QIO ________________________________

RA ________________________________

RAC initiative ________________________________

RBRVS ________________________________

RFBS ________________________________

RVU ________________________________

SMI ________________________________

SOF ________________________________

SSI ________________________________

TEFRA ________________________________

VPS ________________________________

PERFORMANCE OBJECTIVES

The student will be able to:

- Define and spell the key terms and key abbreviations for this chapter, given the information from the *Handbook* glossary, within a reasonable time period and with enough accuracy to obtain a satisfactory evaluation.
- After reading the chapter, answer the fill-in-the-blank, multiple choice, and true/false review questions, with enough accuracy to obtain a satisfactory evaluation.
- Compute mathematical calculations, given Medicare problem situations, within a reasonable time period and with enough accuracy to obtain a satisfactory evaluation.
- Using the *Current Procedural Terminology* (CPT) code book or the Mock Fee Schedule in Appendix A in this *Workbook* and the Healthcare Common Procedure Coding System (HCPCS) list of codes in Appendix B in this *Workbook*, select the HCPCS and/or procedural code numbers, given a series of medical services, procedures, or supplies, within a reasonable time period and with enough accuracy to obtain a satisfactory evaluation.
- Fill in the correct meaning of each abbreviation, given a list of common medical abbreviations and symbols that appear in chart notes, within a reasonable time period and with enough accuracy to obtain a satisfactory evaluation.
- Complete each CMS-1500 (02-12) Health Insurance Claim Form for billing, given the patients' medical chart notes, ledger cards, and blank insurance claim forms, within a reasonable time period and with enough accuracy to obtain a satisfactory evaluation.
- Post payments, adjustments, and balances on the patients' ledger cards, using the Medicare Mock Fee Schedule in Appendix A in this *Workbook,* within a reasonable time period and with enough accuracy to obtain a satisfactory evaluation.

STUDY OUTLINE

Background
Policies and Regulations
- Eligibility Requirements
- Health Insurance Card
- Enrollment Status
- Benefits and Nonbenefits

Additional Insurance Programs
- Medicare/Medicaid
- Medicare/Medigap
- Medicare Secondary Payer
- Automobile or Liability Insurance Coverage

Medicare Managed Care Plans
- Health Maintenance Organizations
- Carrier Dealing Prepayment Organization

Utilization and Quality Control
- Quality Improvement Organizations
- Federal False Claims Amendment Act
- Clinical Laboratory Improvement Amendments

Payment Fundamentals
- Provider
- Prior Authorization
- Waiver of Liability Provision
- Elective Surgery Estimate
- Prepayment Screens
- Correct Coding Initiative

Medicare Reimbursement
- Chronology of Prospective Payment System
- Reasonable Fee
- Resource-Based Relative Value Scale
- Healthcare Common Procedure Coding System (HCPCS)
- Physician Quality Reporting Initiative

Claim Submission
- Local Coverage Determination
- Medicare Administrative Contractors and Fiscal Intermediaries
- Provider Identification Numbers
- Patient's Signature Authorization
- Time Limit
- Paper Claims
- Electronic Claims
- Medicare/Medicaid Claims
- Medicare/Medigap Claims
- Medicare/Employer Supplemental Insurance Claims
- Medicare/Supplemental and Medicare Supplementary Payer Claims
- Claims for Deceased Patients
- Physician Substitute Coverage

After Claim Submission
- Remittance Advice
- Medicare Summary Notice

Beneficiary Representative/Representative Payee
- Posting Payments
- Review and Redetermination Process

Procedure 12-1: Determine Whether Medicare Is Primary or Secondary and Determine Additional Benefits
Procedure 12-2: Complete an Advance Beneficiary Notice of Noncoverage (ABN) Form CMS-R-131

ASSIGNMENT 12-1 REVIEW QUESTIONS

Part I Fill in the Blank

Review the objectives, key terms, glossary definitions of key terms, chapter information, and figures before completing the following review questions.

1. An individual becomes eligible for Medicare Parts A and B at age ____________.

2. Medicare Part A is ____________ coverage, and

   Medicare Part B is ____________ coverage.

3. Name an eligibility requirement that would allow aliens to receive Medicare benefits.

   ____

4. Funding for the Medicare Part A program is obtained from

   ____

   and funding for the Medicare Part B program is obtained equally from

   ____________.

5. Define a Medicare Part A hospital benefit period.

   ____

   ____

   ____

6. A program designed to provide pain relief, symptom management, and supportive services to terminally ill individuals and their families is known as

   ____________.

7. Short-term inpatient medical care for terminally ill individuals to give temporary relief to the caregiver is known as ____________.

8. The frequency of Pap tests for Medicare patients is ____________, and that for mammograms is ____________.

9. Some third-party payers offer policies that fall under guidelines issued by the federal government and may cover prescription costs, Medicare deductibles, and copayments;

   these secondary or supplemental policies are known as ____________ insurance policies.

10. Name two types of health maintenance organization (HMO) plans that may have Medicare Part B contracts.

    a. ____________

    b. ____________

11. The federal laws establishing standards of quality control and safety measures in clinical laboratories are known as ____________.

12. Acceptance of assignment by a participating physician means that he or she agrees to

_______________ after the $ _______________
annual deductible has been met.

13. Philip Lenz is seen by Dr. Doe, who schedules an operative procedure in 1 month.

This type of surgery is known as _______________,
because it does not have to be performed immediately.

14. A Medicare insurance claim form showed an alphanumeric code, J0540, for an injection

of 600,000 U of penicillin G. This number is referred to as a/an _______________.

15. Organizations or claims processors under contract to the federal government that handle insurance claims and payments for hospitals under Medicare Part A are known as

_______________,

and those that process claims for physicians and other suppliers of services under Medicare

Part B are called _______________.

16. A Centers for Medicare and Medicaid Services (CMS)–assigned provider identification

number is known as a/an _______________.

Physicians who supply durable medical equipment must have a/an _______________
number.

17. If circumstances make it impossible to obtain a signature each time a paper claim is submitted or an electronic claim is transmitted, the Medicare patient's signature may

be obtained either _______________

or _______________, thus indicating the signature is on file.

18. The time limit for sending in a Medicare insurance claim is

_______________.

19. Mrs. Davis, a Medicare/Medicaid (Medi-Medi) patient, has a cholecystectomy. In completing the insurance claim form, the assignment portion is left blank in error. What will happen in this case?

____

____

20. If an individual is 65 years of age and is a Medicare beneficiary but is working and has a group insurance policy, where is the insurance claim form sent initially?

____

21. If a Medicare beneficiary is injured in an automobile accident, the physician submits the claim form to

_______________.

Part II Multiple Choice

Choose the best answer.

22. Medicare prescription drug benefits for individuals who purchase the insurance are available under
    a. Medicare Part A.
    b. Medicare Part B.
    c. Medicare Part C.
    d. Medicare Part D.

23. Medicare secondary payer (MSP) cases may involve
    a. Medicare-aged workers under group health plans of more than 20 covered employees.
    b. Medicare-aged or disabled individuals who also receive benefits under the Department of Veterans Affairs and Medicare.
    c. a Medicare patient who is involved in an automobile accident.
    d. all of the above.

24. If a Medicare patient is to receive a medical service that may be denied payment either entirely or partially, the provider should
    a. transmit a claim for adjudication to receive an official notice of denial.
    b. have the patient sign an Advance Beneficiary Notice of Noncoverage form.
    c. have the patient make a partial payment.
    d. ask the patient for payment.

25. A decision by a Medicare administrative contractor (MAC) whether to cover (pay) a particular medical service on a contractor-wide basis in accordance with whether it is reasonable and necessary is known as a/an
    a. Local Coverage Determination.
    b. Correct Coding Initiative edit.
    c. prepayment screen.
    d. redetermination process.

26. According to regulations, a Medicare patient must be billed for a copayment
    a. at least once before a balance is adjusted off as uncollectible.
    b. at least two times before a balance is adjusted off as uncollectible.
    c. at least three times before a balance is adjusted off as uncollectible.
    d. no more than four times before a balance is adjusted off as uncollectible.

Part III True/False

Write "T" or "F" in the blank to indicate whether you think the statement is true or false.

_______ 27. All patients who have a Medicare health insurance card have Part A hospital and Part B medical coverage.

_______ 28. Prescription drug plans refer to the drugs in their formularies by tier numbers.

_______ 29. Nonparticipating physicians may decide on a case-by-case basis whether to accept assignment when providing medical services to Medicare patients.

_______ 30. Medicare's Correct Coding Initiative was implemented by the Centers for Medicare and Medicaid Services to eliminate unbundling of CPT codes.

_______ 31. A Medicare/Medigap claim is not called a crossover claim.

ASSIGNMENT 12-2 CALCULATE MATHEMATICAL PROBLEMS

Performance Objective

Task: Calculate and insert the correct amounts for seven Medicare scenarios.

Conditions: Use a pen or pencil, the description of problem, and, for Problem 7, Figures 12-1 and 12-2.

Standards: Time: ______________ minutes

Accuracy: ______________

(Note: The time element and accuracy criteria may be given by your instructor.)

Directions: Submitting insurance claims, particularly Medicare claims, involves a bit of arithmetic. Several problems are given here so that you will gain experience with situations encountered daily in your work. The Medicare deductible is always subtracted from the allowed amount first before mathematical computations continue.

Problem 1: Mr. Doolittle has Medicare Parts A and B coverage. He was well during the entire past year. On January 1, Mr. Doolittle is rushed to the hospital, where Dr. Input performs an emergency gastric resection. The hospital bills Medicare under the Part A coverage, and under the Part B coverage, the physician bills $450 for surgical services. The doctor agrees to accept assignment. The patient has not paid any deductible. Complete the following statements by putting in the correct amounts.

Original Bill

a. Medicare allows $400. Medicare payment: ______________________________

b. Patient owes Dr. Input: ______________________________

c. Dr. Input's courtesy adjustment: ______________________________

Mathematical computations:

Problem 2: Mrs. James has Medicare Parts A and B coverage. She met her deductible when she was ill in March of this year. On November 1, Dr. Caesar performs a bilateral salpingo-oophorectomy. The hospital bills Medicare under the Part A coverage, and under Part B coverage, the physician bills $300 for surgical services. The doctor agrees to accept a Medicare assignment.

Original Bill

a. Medicare allows $275. Medicare payment: ______________________________

b. Patient owes Dr. Caesar: ______________________________

c. Dr. Caesar's courtesy adjustment: ______________________________

Mathematical computations for surgeon:

The assistant surgeon charged Mrs. James $60 (the Medicare limiting charge) and does not accept assignment. After receiving her check from Medicare, Mrs. James sends the surgeon his $60. Medicare has allowed $55 for the fee.

a. How much of the money was from Mrs. James' private funds? $ ______________.

b. How much did Medicare pay? ______________.

Mathematical computations:

Problem 3: You work for Dr. Coccidioides. He does not accept assignment. He is treating Mr. Robinson for allergies. Mr. Robinson has Medicare Part A. You send in a bill to Medicare for the $135 that Mr. Robinson owes you.

What portion of the bill will Medicare pay? ____

Problem 4: In June, Mr. Fay has an illness that incurs $89 in medical bills. He asks you to bill Medicare, and the physician does not accept assignment. He has paid the deductible at another physician's office.

a. If Medicare allows the entire amount of your fees, the Medicare check to the patient is

$ ______________ (which comes to you).

b. The patient's part of the bill to you is ______________.

Mathematical computations:

Problem 5: Mr. Iba, a Medicare patient with a Medigap insurance policy, is seen for an office visit and the fee is $80. The Medicare-approved amount is $54.44. The patient has met his deductible for the year.

a. The Medicare payment check is $ ________________________.

b. After the claim is submitted to the Medigap insurance, the Medigap payment check is

$ ________________________.

c. To zero out the balance, the Medicare courtesy adjustment is ______________.

Mathematical computations:

Problem 6: Mrs. Smith, a Medicare patient, had surgery, and the participating physician's fee is $1250. This patient is working part-time, and her employer group health plan (primary insurance) allowed $1100, applied $500 to the deductible, and paid 80% of $600.

a. Amount paid by this plan: $ ______________.

b. The spouse's employer group health plan (secondary insurance) is billed for the balance, which is $ ______________. This program also has a $500 deductible. This plan pays 100% of the fee billed, minus the deductible.

c. The spouse's employer group plan makes a payment of ______________.

You send copies of remittance advice from the two group health plans and submit a claim to Medicare (the third insurance) for $1250. The balance at this point is $ ______________.

Mathematical computations:

Problem 7: Beverly James has Medicare Part B coverage. She has $242 in medical bills and has met $100 of the $147 (2013 deductible). Dr. Practon agrees to accept assignment.

Original Bill

a. Medicare allows $200. Medicare payment: ______________________________

b. Beverly James owes Dr. Practon: ______________________________

c. Dr. Practon's courtesy adjustment: ______________________________

Mathematical computations:

Problem 8: Oliver Mills has Medicare Part B coverage. He fell at home and suffered a sprain and Dr. Skeleton treated him. His medical bill totaled $370 and he has met $60 of the $147 (2013 deductible). Dr. Skeleton agrees to accept assignment.

Original Bill

a. Medicare allows $280. Medicare payment: ____________________

b. Oliver Mills owes Dr. Skeleton: ____________________

c. Dr. Skeleton's courtesy adjustment: ____________________

Mathematical computations:

Problem 9: Maria Sanchez has Medicare Part B coverage. She has $565 in medical bills at Dr. Cardi's office and met $45 of the $147 (2013 deductible) at another physician's office. Dr. Cardi agrees to accept assignment.

Original Bill

a. Medicare allows $480. Medicare payment: ____________________

b. Maria Sanchez owes Dr. Cardi: ____________________

c. Dr. Cardi's courtesy adjustment: ____________________

Mathematical computations:

Problem 10: In the late 1980s, Medicare's Resource-Based Relative Value System (RBRVS) became the way payment was determined each year. However, since the early 1990s, annual fee schedules have been supplied by local fiscal intermediaries, and so the RBRVS has become more useful in determining practice cost to convert patients to capitation in negotiations of managed care contracts. Because physicians may request determination of fees for certain procedures to discover actual cost and what compensation ratios should be, it is important to know how Medicare fees are determined. Each year the *Federal Register* publishes geographic practice cost indices by Medicare carrier and locality as well as relative value units and related information. This assignment will give you some mathematical practice in using figures for annual conversion factors to determine fees for given procedures in various regions of the United States. Refer to Figures 12-1 and 12-2, which are pages of the *Federal Register*.

a. HCPCS Code 47600: Removal of gallbladder. The medical practice is located in Phoenix, Arizona.

		Work		*Overhead*		*Malpractice*
RVUs		________		________		________
GPCI	×	________	×	________	×	________

+ ________ + ________ + ________ = Total adjusted RVUs

2013 Conversion factor $34.0230 × Total adjusted RVUs ________ = allowed

amount $ ________.

b. HCPCS Code 47715: Excision of bile duct cyst. The medical practice is located in Arkansas.

		Work		*Overhead*		*Malpractice*
RVUs		________		________		________
GPCI	×	________	×	________	×	________

+ ________ + ________ + ________ = Total adjusted RVUs ________

2013 Conversion factor $34.0230 × Total adjusted RVUs ________ = allowed

amount $ ________.

c. HCPCS Code 48146: Pancreatectomy. The medical practice is located in Fresno, California.

		Work		*Overhead*		*Malpractice*
RVUs		________		________		________
GPCI	×	________	×	________	×	________

+ ________ + ________ + ________ = Total adjusted RVUs ________

2013 Conversion factor $34.0230 × Total adjusted RVUs × = allowed

amount $ ________.

ADDENDUM D.—GEOGRAPHIC PRACTICE COST INDICES BY MEDICARE CARRIER AND LOCALITY					
Carrier number	Locality number	Locality name	Work	Practice expense	Mal-practice
510	5	Birmingham, AL	0.981	0.913	0.824
510	4	Mobile, AL	0.964	0.911	0.824
510	2	North Central AL	0.970	0.867	0.824
510	1	Northwest AL	0.985	0.869	0.824
510	6	Rest of AL	0.975	0.851	0.824
510	3	Southeast AL	0.972	0.869	0.824
1020	1	Alaska	1.106	1.255	1.042
1030	5	Flagstaff (city), AZ	0.983	0.911	1.255
1030	1	Phoenix, AZ	1.003	1.016	1.255
1030	7	Prescott (city), AZ	0.983	0.911	1.255
1030	99	Rest of Arizona	0.987	0.943	1.255
1030	2	Tucson (city), AZ	0.987	0.989	1.255
1030	8	Yuma (city), AZ	0.983	0.911	1.255
520	13	Arkansas	0.960	0.856	0.302
2050	26	Anaheim-Santa Ana, CA	1.046	1.220	1.370
542	14	Bakersfield, CA	1.028	1.050	1.370
542	11	Fresno/Madera, CA	1.006	1.009	1.370
542	13	Kings/Tulare, CA	0.999	1.001	1.370
2050	18	Los Angeles, CA (1st of 8)	1.060	1.196	1.370
2050	19	Los Angeles, CA (2nd of 8)	1.060	1.196	1.370

Figure 12-1

ADDENDUM B.—RELATIVE VALUE UNITS (RVUs) AND RELATED INFORMATION

HCPCS[1]	MOD	Status	Description	Work RVUs	Practice expense RVUs[2]	Mal-practice RVUs	Total	Global period	Update
47399	....	C	Liver surgery procedure	0.00	0.00	0.00	0.00	YYY	S
47400	....	A	Incision of liver duct	19.11	8.62	1.38	29.11	090	S
47420	....	A	Incision of bile duct	15.48	9.59	2.01	27.08	090	S
47425	....	A	Incision of bile duct	14.95	11.84	2.48	29.27	090	S
47440	....	A	Incision of bile duct	18.51	10.61	2.23	31.35	090	S
47460	....	A	Incision of bile duct sphincter	14.57	15.71	1.84	32.12	090	N
47480	....	A	Incision of gallbladder	8.14	7.68	1.61	17.43	090	S
47490	....	A	Incision of gallbladder	6.11	3.61	0.38	10.10	090	N
47500	....	A	Injection for liver x-rays	1.98	1.53	0.14	3.65	000	N
47505	....	A	Injection for liver x-rays	0.77	1.34	0.14	2.25	000	N
47510	....	A	Insert catheter, bile duct	7.47	2.90	0.25	10.62	090	N
47511	....	A	Insert bile duct drain	10.02	2.90	0.25	13.17	090	N
47525	....	A	Change bile duct catheter	5.47	1.61	0.16	7.24	010	N
47530	....	A	Revise, reinsert bile tube	5.47	1.53	0.19	7.19	090	N
47550	....	A	Bile duct endoscopy	3.05	1.58	0.35	4.98	000	S
47552	....	A	Biliary endoscopy, thru skin	6.11	1.38	0.21	7.70	000	S
47553	....	A	Biliary endoscopy, thru skin	6.42	3.84	0.63	10.89	000	N
47554	....	A	Biliary endoscopy, thru skin	9.16	3.97	0.68	13.81	000	S
47555	....	A	Biliary endoscopy, thru skin	7.64	2.66	0.30	10.60	000	N
47556	....	A	Biliary endoscopy, thru skin	8.66	2.66	0.30	11.62	000	N
47600	....	A	Removal of gallbladder	10.80	7.61	1.60	20.01	090	S
47605	....	A	Removal of gallbladder	11.66	8.23	1.77	21.66	090	S
47610	....	A	Removal of gallbladder	14.01	9.47	2.02	25.50	090	S
47612	....	A	Removal of gallbladder	14.91	14.39	3.08	32.38	090	S
47620	....	A	Removal of gallbladder	15.97	11.35	2.39	29.71	090	S
47630	....	A	Removal of bile duct stone	8.40	3.79	0.40	12.59	090	N
47700	....	A	Exploration of bile ducts	13.90	7.71	1.60	23.21	090	S
47701	....	A	Bile duct revision	26.87	8.30	1.92	37.09	090	S
47710	....	A	Excision of bile duct tumor	18.64	12.19	2.49	33.32	090	S
47715	....	A	Excision of bile duct cyst	14.66	8.31	1.73	24.70	090	S
47716	....	A	Fusion of bile duct cyst	12.67	6.63	1.55	20.85	090	S
47720	....	A	Fuse gallbladder and bowel	12.03	9.26	1.95	23.34	090	S
47721	....	A	Fuse upper gi structures	14.57	11.55	2.50	28.62	090	S
47740	....	A	Fuse gallbladder and bowel	14.08	10.32	2.16	26.56	090	S
47760	....	A	Fuse bile ducts and bowel	20.15	11.74	2.56	34.45	090	S
47765	....	A	Fuse liver ducts and bowel	19.25	14.77	3.00	37.02	090	S
47780	....	A	Fuse bile ducts and bowel	20.63	13.22	2.76	36.61	090	S
47800	....	A	Reconstruction of bile ducts	17.91	13.37	2.46	33.74	090	S
47801	....	A	Placement, bile duct support	11.41	5.54	0.82	17.77	090	S
47802	....	A	Fuse liver duct and intestine	16.19	10.38	1.77	28.34	090	S
47999	....	C	Bile tract surgery procedure	0.00	0.00	0.00	0.00	YYY	S
48000	....	A	Drainage of abdomen	13.25	7.13	1.42	21.80	090	S
48001	....	A	Placement of drain, pancreas	15.71	8.22	1.91	25.84	090	S
48005	....	A	Resect/debride pancreas	17.77	9.29	2.16	29.22	090	S
48020	....	A	Removal of pancreatic stone	13.12	6.86	1.59	21.57	090	S
48100	....	A	Biopsy of pancreas	10.30	4.26	0.80	15.36	090	S
48102	....	A	Needle biopsy, pancreas	4.48	2.44	0.25	7.17	010	N
48120	....	A	Removal of pancreas lesion	12.93	9.83	2.09	24.85	090	S
48140	....	A	Partial removal of pancreas	18.47	13.44	2.86	34.77	090	S
48145	....	A	Partial removal of pancreas	19.30	15.88	3.20	38.38	090	S
48146	....	A	Pancreatectomy	21.97	16.67	1.94	40.58	090	S
48148	....	A	Removal of pancrearic duct	14.57	8.32	1.70	24.59	090	S
48150	....	A	Partial removal of pancreas	34.55	22.79	4.80	62.14	090	S
48151	....	D	Partial removal of pancreas	0.00	0.00	0.00	0.00	090	0
48152	....	A	Pancreatectomy	31.33	22.79	4.80	58.92	090	S
48153	....	A	Pancreatectomy	34.55	22.79	4.80	62.14	090	S
48154	....	A	Pancreatectomy	31.33	22.79	4.80	58.92	090	S
48155	....	A	Removal of pancreas	19.65	20.63	4.31	44.59	090	S
48160	....	N	Pancreas removal, transplant	0.00	0.00	0.00	0.00	XXX	0
48180	....	A	Fuse pancreas and bowel	21.11	12.74	2.66	36.51	090	S
48400	....	A	Injection, intraoperative	1.97	1.04	0.24	3.25	ZZZ	S
48500	....	A	Surgery of pancreas cyst	12.17	8.62	1.68	22.47	090	S
48510	....	A	Drain pancreatic pseudocyst	11.34	7.62	1.46	20.42	090	S
48520	....	A	Fuse pancreas cyst and bowel	13.11	11.43	2.46	27.00	090	S
48540	....	A	Fuse pancreas cyst and bowel	15.95	12.80	2.68	31.43	090	S
48545	....	A	Pancreatorrhaphy	14.81	7.75	1.81	24.37	090	S
48547	....	A	Duodenal exclusion	21.42	11.20	2.61	35.23	090	S

[1] All numeric CPT HCPCS Copyright 1993 American Medical Association.
[2] *Indicates reduction of Practice Expense RVUs as a result of OBRA 1993.

Figure 12-2

ASSIGNMENT 12-3 LOCATE HCPCS ALPHANUMERIC CODES

Performance Objective

Task: Insert the correct HCPCS codes for problems presented.

Conditions: Use a pen or pencil, the HCPCS code book or Appendix B in this *Workbook*.

Standards: Time: ______________ minutes

Accuracy: ______________

(Note: The time element and accuracy criteria may be given by your instructor.)

Directions: As you have learned from the *Handbook*, it is necessary to use three levels of codes (CPT, HCPCS, and regional codes) when submitting Medicare claims. Refer to Appendix B in this *Workbook* to complete this HCPCS coding exercise for Medicare claims.

1. Cellular therapy ______________
2. Injection amygdalin, laetrile, vitamin B_{17} ______________
3. Fentanyl citrate injection for local anesthetic ______________
4. Splint, wrist ______________
5. Crutches ______________
6. Cervical head harness ______________
7. 1 mL gamma globulin ______________
8. Injection, vitamin B_{12} ______________
9. Contraceptives (unclassified drugs) ______________
10. Surgical tray ______________
11. Penicillin, procaine, aqueous, injection ______________

ASSIGNMENT 12-4 LOCATE CPT CODES AND HCPCS ALPHANUMERIC MODIFIERS

Performance Objective

Task: Insert the correct CPT codes and HCPCS modifiers for problems presented.

Conditions: Use a pen or pencil, the CPT code book, and a HCPCS code book or Appendix B in this *Workbook*.

Standards: Time: ______________ minutes

Accuracy: ______________

(Note: The time element and accuracy criteria may be given by your instructor.)

Directions: Now get some practice in selecting CPT codes with HCPCS modifiers. For this assignment, in addition to referring to a CPT code book and Appendix A in this *Workbook*, you will need to refer to either a HCPCS code book or Appendix B in this *Workbook* to complete these Medicare problems.

1. Second surgical opinion ordered by a professional review organization, detailed history and examination, low-complexity decision making ______________
2. Chiropractic manipulation of spine, one region, acute treatment ______________
3. Office visit by a locum tenens physician of established patient, problem-focused history and examination with straightforward decision-making ______________
4. Strapping of thumb of left hand ______________

Insurance Claim Assignments

Assignments presented in this section are to give you hands-on experience in completing a variety of Medicare insurance cases by using the CMS-1500 (02-12) claim form. Periodically, newsletters are issued by Medicare fiscal intermediaries relaying new federal policies and guidelines. This may change block requirements on the claim form, codes (procedural and diagnostic) that are covered in the Medicare program, or mean lower reimbursement or denial of reimbursement for a particular code number. Cases shown do not reflect payment policies for a particular procedure or service; this depends on federal guidelines and local medical review policies (LMRPs) at the time of claim submission.

The cases presented in this section are:

Assignment 12-5	Medicare
Assignment 12-6	Medicare/Medicaid (Medi-Medi)
Assignment 12-7	Medicare Secondary Payer (MSP) [advanced]
Assignment 12-8	Medicare/Medigap
Assignment 12-9	Medicare Railroad, Retiree with Advance Beneficiary Notice of Noncoverage [advanced]
Assignment 12-10	Medicare/Medicaid (Medi-Medi)

Additional cases presented on the Student Software Challenge (located on Evolve) are:

Computer Case 8	Medicare
Computer Case 9	Medicare/Medigap
Computer Case 10	Medicare/Medicaid

ASSIGNMENT 12-5 COMPLETE A CLAIM FORM FOR A MEDICARE CASE

Performance Objective

Task: Complete a CMS-1500 (02-12) claim form for a Medicare case, post transactions to the financial accounting record, and define patient record abbreviations.

Conditions: Use the patient's medical record (Figure 12-3) and financial statement (Figure 12-4), one health insurance claim form (print from Evolve website), a computer, procedural and diagnostic code books, and Appendixes A and B in this *Workbook*.

Standards: Claim Productivity Measurement

Time: ______________ minutes

Accuracy: ______________

(Note: The time element and accuracy criteria may be given by your instructor.)

Directions:

1. Complete the CMS-1500 (02-12) claim form, using NUCC guidelines for a Medicare case. If your instructor wants you to direct it to your local fiscal intermediary, obtain the name and address by going to the Evolve website listed in Internet Resources at the end of Chapter 12 in the *Handbook*. Refer to Elsa M. Mooney's patient record for information. Refer to Appendix A in this *Workbook* to locate the fees to be recorded on the claim and posted to the financial statement. Date the claim December 21. Dr. Cardi is a participating physician who is accepting assignment, and Mrs. Mooney has already met her deductible for the year owing to previous medical expenses with another physician. Use the participating provider Medicare fee.

2. Refer to Chapter 7 (Figure 7-6) of the *Handbook* for instructions on how to complete this claim form and a Medicare template.

3. Use your CPT code book or Appendix A in this *Workbook* to determine the correct five-digit code number and modifiers for each professional service rendered. Use your HCPCS Level II code book or refer to Appendix B in this *Workbook* for HCPCS procedure codes and modifiers. If your instructor tells you to also find the ICD-10-CM codes, a draft version may be downloaded from the following website: http://www.cdc.gov/nchs/icd/icd10cm.htm.

4. Record all transactions on the financial accounting record and indicate when you have billed Medicare.

5. On January 12, Medicare sent check No. 115620 and paid 80% of the approved amount for services rendered on December 15, 20xx. Note: For this case, the approved amount will be the participating amount. Post this amount to the patient's financial account and indicate the balance due from the patient.

6. A Performance Evaluation Checklist may be reproduced from the "Instruction Guide to the Workbook" chapter if your instructor wishes you to submit it to assist with scoring and comments.

After the instructor has returned your work to you, either make the necessary corrections and place your work in a three-ring notebook for future reference or, if you received a high score, place it in your portfolio for reference when applying for a job.

Abbreviations pertinent to this record:

Pt	________	LC	________
N	________	MDM	________
EKG	________	adv	________
STAT	________	rtn	________
CPK	________	ofc	________
Dx	________	echo	________
ASCVD	________	RTO	________

Additional Coding and Fee Calculations

1. Refer to Mrs. Mooney's medical record, abstract information, and code procedures that would be billed by outside providers.

Site	*Description of Service*	*Code*
a. College Hospital Laboratory	________	________
b. College Hospital Physiology	________	________
c. College Hospital Radiology	________	________

2. Refer to the Mock Fee Schedule shown in Appendix A in this *Workbook* and complete the following questions:

A. If Dr. Cardi is not participating in the Medicare program, what is the maximum (limiting charge) he can bill for the professional services rendered?

Office visit $ ________ ECG $ ________

B. In the case of a nonparticipating physician, how much will Medicare pay for these services? Note: Use the nonparticipating fees as the allowed amount.

Office visit $ ________ ECG $ ________

C. How much is the patient's responsibility for these services?

Office visit $ ________ ECG $ ________

D. How much will the courtesy adjustment be on the patient's financial record?

Office visit $ ________ ECG $ ________

PATIENT RECORD NO. 12-5

Mooney	Elsa	M.	02-06-30	F	555-452-4968
LAST NAME	FIRST NAME	MIDDLE NAME	BIRTH DATE	SEX	HOME PHONE

5750 Canyon Road	Woodland Hills	XY	12345
ADDRESS	CITY	STATE	ZIP CODE

555-806-3244			Mooney@wb.net
CELL PHONE	PAGER NO.	FAX NO.	E-MAIL ADDRESS

321-XX-2653	R9865549
PATIENT'S SOC. SEC. NO.	DRIVER'S LICENSE

retired secretary	
PATIENT'S OCCUPATION	NAME OF COMPANY

ADDRESS OF EMPLOYER	PHONE

husband deceased	
SPOUSE OR PARENT	OCCUPATION

EMPLOYER	ADDRESS	PHONE

Medicare	self
NAME OF INSURANCE	INSURED OR SUBSCRIBER

321-XX-2653A	
POLICY/CERTIFICATE NO.	GROUP NO.

REFERRED BY: George Gentle, MD, 1000 N. Main Street, Woodland Hills, XY 12345 NPI# 40213102XX

DATE	PROGRESS NOTES
12-15-xx	New pt referred by Dr. Gentle comes in complaining of chest pain and shortness of
	breath; a detailed history was taken. A detailed examination was essentially N. EKG done
	to rule out myocardial infarction; normal sinus rhythm, no abnormalities noted. Pt sent to
	College Hospital for STAT cardiac enzymes (CPK), 2D echocardiogram
	(transthoracic/real-time with Doppler), and complete chest x-ray.
	Working Dx: angina—ASCVD (LC MDM). Pt adv to rtn to ofc this afternoon for test results.
	PC/llf Perry Cardi, MD

Figure 12-3

Acct No. 12-5

STATEMENT
Financial Account
COLLEGE CLINIC
4567 Broad Avenue
Woodland Hills, XY 12345-0001
Tel. 555-486-9002
Fax No. 555-487-8976

Mrs. Elsa M. Mooney
5750 Canyon Road
Woodland Hills, XY 12345-0001

Phone No. (H) (555) 452-4968 (W) ______ Birthdate 02-06-30

Primary Insurance Co. Medicare Policy/Group No. 321-XX-2653A

	REFERENCE	DESCRIPTION	CHARGES	CREDITS PYMNTS.	CREDITS ADJ.	BALANCE
			BALANCE FORWARD →			
12-15-xx		Init OV, D hx/exam, LC decision making				
12-15-xx		EKG with interpret & report				

PLEASE PAY LAST AMOUNT IN BALANCE COLUMN

THIS IS A COPY OF YOUR FINANCIAL ACCOUNT AS IT APPEARS ON OUR RECORDS

Figure 12-4

ASSIGNMENT 12-6 COMPLETE A CLAIM FORM FOR A MEDICARE/MEDICAID CASE

Performance Objective

Task: Complete a CMS-1500 (02-12) claim form for a Medicare/Medicaid case, post transactions to the financial accounting record, and define patient record abbreviations.

Conditions: Use the patient's medical record (Figure 12-5) and financial statement (Figure 12-6), one health insurance claim form (print from Evolve website), a computer, procedural and diagnostic code books, and Appendixes A and B in this *Workbook*.

Standards: Claim Productivity Measurement

Time: ______________ minutes

Accuracy: ______________

(Note: The time element and accuracy criteria may be given by your instructor.)

Directions:

1. Complete the CMS-1500 (02-12) claim form, using NUCC guidelines for a Medicare/Medicaid case. If your instructor wants you to direct it to your local Medicare fiscal intermediary, obtain the name and address by going to the Evolve website listed in Internet Resources at the end of Chapter 12 in the *Handbook*. Refer to Mrs. Helen P. Nolan's patient record for information. Note that Helen's husband is deceased and she collects benefits based on her spouse's earnings; thus, the Medicare number ends with a D. Refer to Appendix A in this *Workbook* to locate the fees to be recorded on the claim and posted to the financial statement. Date the claim May 31.

2. Refer to Chapter 7 and Figure 7-7 of the *Handbook* for instructions on how to complete the CMS-1500 (02-12) claim form.

3. Use your CPT code book or Appendix A in this *Workbook* to determine the correct five-digit code number and modifiers for each professional service rendered. Use your HCPCS Level II code book or refer to Appendix B in this *Workbook* for HCPCS procedure codes and modifiers. If your instructor tells you to also find the ICD-10-CM codes, a draft version may be downloaded from the following website: http://www.cdc.gov/nchs/icd/icd10cm.htm.

4. Record all transactions on the financial record and indicate the proper information when you have billed Medicare/Medicaid. On July 1, you receive a check (number 107621) from Medicare for $600, and on July 15 you receive a voucher (number 3571) from Medicaid for $200. Record these payments on the account, and show a courtesy adjustment to zero the account.

5. A Performance Evaluation Checklist may be reproduced from the "Instruction Guide to the Workbook" chapter if your instructor wishes you to submit it to assist with scoring and comments.

After the instructor has returned your work to you, either make the necessary corrections and place your work in a three-ring notebook for future reference or, if you received a high score, place it in your portfolio for reference when applying for a job.

Abbreviations pertinent to this record:

Pt	__________	phys	__________
hx	__________	prep	__________
BP	__________	hosp	__________
ext	__________	EPF	__________
Dx	__________	exam	__________
int	__________	MC	__________
adv	__________	MDM	__________
Pre-op	__________	slt	__________
adm	__________	PF	__________
UA	__________	SF	__________
auto	__________	RTO	__________
FBS	__________	wk	__________
micro	__________	OV	__________
CXR	__________	p.r.n.	__________

Additional Coding and Fee Calculations

1. Refer to Mrs. Nolan's medical record, abstract information, and code procedures that would be billed by outside providers.

Site	*Description of Service*	*Code*
a. College Hospital Laboratory	__________	__________
b. College Hospital Laboratory	__________	__________
c. College Hospital Laboratory	__________	__________
d. College Hospital Radiology	__________	__________

2. Calculate Dr. Cutler's assistant surgeon fee, which is 18.5% of the primary surgeon's fee:

   Hemorrhoidectomy with fistulectomy: $ __________

PATIENT RECORD NO. 12-6

Nolan	Helen	P.	05-10-37	F	555-660-9878
LAST NAME	FIRST NAME	MIDDLE NAME	BIRTH DATE	SEX	HOME PHONE

2588 Cedar Street	Woodland Hills	XY	12345-0001
ADDRESS	CITY	STATE	ZIP CODE

		555-660-9878	Nolan@wb.net
CELL PHONE	PAGER NO.	FAX NO.	E-MAIL ADDRESS

732-XX-1573	J4022876
PATIENT'S SOC. SEC. NO.	DRIVER'S LICENSE

homemaker	
PATIENT'S OCCUPATION	NAME OF COMPANY

ADDRESS OF EMPLOYER	PHONE

James J. Nolan (deceased)		
SPOUSE OR PARENT	OCCUPATION	BIRTH DATE

EMPLOYER	ADDRESS	PHONE

Medicare/Medicaid	
NAME OF INSURANCE	INSURED OR SUBSCRIBER

632-XX-3209D	19-60-2358490-1-XX
MEDICARE NO.	MEDICAID NO.

REFERRED BY: James B. Jeffers, MD, 100 S. Broadway, Woodland Hills, XY 12345-0001 NPI# 12345069XX

DATE	PROGRESS NOTES
5-1-xx	New pt comes in complaining of constipation, rectal bleeding, and rectal pain. Detailed
	hx taken, BP 120/80. A detailed exam revealed ext hemorrhoids. Diagnostic proctoscopy
	done to further evaluate the hemorrhoids and control bleeding using bipolar cautery.
	Dx: int & ext bleeding hemorrhoids and anorectal fistula. Adv hospitalization for removal
	of hemorrhoids and fistula repair.
	RR/llf Rex Rumsey, MD
5-8-xx	Pre-op testing done prior to adm to College Hospital (UA auto/with micro., hemogram
	auto, FBS quantitative, CXR single frontal view). Admit, phys exam & prep of hospital
	records. Hemorrhoidectomy with fistulectomy performed (authorization no. 7699220012).
	Dr. Clarence Cutler assisted.
	RR/llf Rex Rumsey, MD
5-9-xx	Hosp visit (EPF hx/exam MC MDM). Pt comfortable, slt pain.
	RR/llf Rex Rumsey, MD
5-10-xx	Hosp visit (PF hx/exam SF MDM). No pain.
	RR/llf Rex Rumsey, MD
5-11-xx	Discharged pt to home. RTO in 1 wk.
	RR/llf Rex Rumsey, MD
5-17-xx	OV (PF hx/exam SF MDM). Pt doing well, surgical site healed. Return p.r.n.
	RR/llf Rex Rumsey, MD

Figure 12-5

Acct. No. 12-6

STATEMENT
Financial Account
COLLEGE CLINIC
4567 Broad Avenue
Woodland Hills, XY 12345-0001
Tel. 555-486-9002
Fax No. 555-487-8976

Helen P. Nolan
2588 Cedar Street
Woodland Hills, XY 12345

Phone No. (H) (555) 660-9878 (W) ____ Birthdate 05-10-37

Primary Insurance Co. Medicare/Medicaid Policy/Group No. 632-XX-3209D

	REFERENCE	DESCRIPTION	CHARGES	CREDITS PYMNTS.	CREDITS ADJ.	BALANCE
20XX			BALANCE FORWARD →			
05-01-xx		NP OV				
05-01-xx		Proctoscopy				
05-08-xx		Hemorrhoidectomy with fistulectomy				
05-09-xx		HV				
05-10-xx		HV				
05-11-xx		Discharge				
05-17-xx		OV				

PLEASE PAY LAST AMOUNT IN BALANCE COLUMN

THIS IS A COPY OF YOUR FINANCIAL ACCOUNT AS IT APPEARS ON OUR RECORDS

Figure 12-6

ASSIGNMENT 12-7 COMPLETE A CLAIM FORM FOR A MEDICARE/SECONDARY PAYER CASE

Performance Objective

Task: Complete a CMS-1500 (02-12) claim form for an MSP case, post transactions to the financial accounting record, and define patient record abbreviations.

Conditions: Use the patient's medical record (Figure 12-7) and financial statement (Figure 12-8), one health insurance claim form (print from Evolve website), a computer, procedural and diagnostic code books, and Appendixes A and B in this *Workbook*.

Standards: Claim Productivity Measurement

Time: ______________ minutes

Accuracy: ______________

(Note: The time element and accuracy criteria may be given by your instructor.)

Directions:

1. Complete the CMS-1500 (02-12) claim form, using NUCC guidelines for an MSP case, and direct it to the primary insurance carrier. This assignment requires two claim forms, so make a photocopy of the CMS-1500 (02-12) claim form for the second claim. Refer to Peter F. Donlon's patient record for information. Refer to Appendix A in this *Workbook* to locate the fees to be recorded on the claim and posted to the financial statement. Date the claim May 14. Dr. Antrum is not accepting assignment in this case. For a nonparticipating physician, use the limiting charge column of the Mock Fee Schedule. This should also be considered the allowed amount.

2. See Chapter 7 (Figure 7-9) of the *Handbook* for help in completing these forms.

3. Use your CPT code book or Appendix A in this *Workbook* to determine the correct five-digit code number and modifiers for each professional service rendered. Refer to your HCPCS Level II code book or Appendix B in this *Workbook* for HCPCS procedure codes and modifiers. If your instructor tells you to also find the ICD-10-CM codes, a draft version may be downloaded from the following website: http://www.cdc.gov/nchs/icd/icd10cm.htm.

4. Record all transactions on the financial record and indicate when you have billed the primary insurance carrier.

5. On June 5, Coastal Health Insurance Company paid $800 (check number 45632) on this claim. Post this payment to the patient's financial account and indicate the balance that will be billed to Medicare the following day. Note: The explanation of benefits from Coastal Health would be sent to Medicare with a completed CMS-1500 (02-12) claim form.

6. A Performance Evaluation Checklist may be reproduced from the "Instruction Guide to the Workbook" chapter if your instructor wishes you to submit it to assist with scoring and comments.

After the instructor has returned your work to you, either make the necessary corrections and place your work in a three-ring notebook for future reference or, if you received a high score, place it in your portfolio for reference when applying for a job.

Abbreviations pertinent to this record:

ER	________	adm	________
p.m.	________	MC	________
EPF	________	imp	________
hx	________	PF	________
exam	________	SF	________
LC	________	hosp	________
MDM	________	RTO	________
est	________	OV	________
pts	________	surg	________
cm	________	sched	________
consult	________	ofc	________
c̄	________	post-op	________
MRI	________	wk	________
px	________		

Additional Coding and Fee Calculations

1. Refer to Mr. Donlon's medical record, abstract information, and code procedures that would be billed by outside providers.

Site	*Description of Service*	*Code*
a. Emergency room (ER) physician	________	________
b. ER consult	________	________
c. College Hospital Radiology	________	________
d. College Hospital Radiology	________	________

2. Use your diagnostic code book and code the symptoms that the patient presented with in the ER.

Symptom	*ICD-9-CM Code*	*ICD-10-CM Code*
a. ______________	______________	______________
b. ______________	______________	______________
c. ______________	______________	______________

3. On the septoplasty surgery (May 10, 20xx), assume that Coastal Health Insurance Company paid $459.74.

   a. What would the Medicare payment be? ______________________________

   b. What would the patient responsibility be? __________________________

   c. What would the courtesy adjustment be? ___________________________

PATIENT RECORD NO. 12-7

LAST NAME	FIRST NAME	MIDDLE NAME	BIRTH DATE	SEX	HOME PHONE
Donlon	Peter	F	08-09-38	M	555-762-3580

ADDRESS	CITY	STATE	ZIP CODE
1840 East Chevy Chase Drive	Woodland Hills	XY	12345

CELL PHONE	PAGER NO.	FAX NO.	E-MAIL ADDRESS

PATIENT'S SOC. SEC. NO.	DRIVER'S LICENSE
987-XX-4321	Y2100968

PATIENT'S OCCUPATION	NAME OF COMPANY
chef	Harbor Town Eatery

ADDRESS OF EMPLOYER	PHONE
1116 Harbor Way, Woodland Hills, XY 12345	555-762-0050

SPOUSE OR PARENT	OCCUPATION
wife deceased	

NAME OF PRIMARY INSURANCE	ADDRESS	PHONE
Coastal Health Insurance Co.	10 N. Main Street, Woodland Hills, XY 12345	555-369-4401

NAME OF INSURANCE	INSURED OR SUBSCRIBER

POLICY/CERTIFICATE NO.	GROUP NO.
34276	45A

NAME OF SECONDARY INSURANCE	MEDICARE NO.
Medicare	987-XX-4321A

REFERRED BY:

DATE	PROGRESS NOTES
5-1-xx	Called to ER on Sunday, 11 p.m. ER physician, Dr. Rene Whitney (NPI # 77 536222XX) performed an EPF hx/exam with LC MDM on one of my est pts who was injured at home while walking across lawn pushing garbage can; tripped and hit his head on curb. Pt complains of acute headache, nausea, and nasal pain caused by impact and skin laceration. I sutured a 2.0 cm simple laceration of nose. Pt vomited twice in ER. Requested ER consult c̄ neurologist, Dr. Parkinson (C hx/exam M MDM), who ordered MRI of brain (without contrast) and complete skull series. I performed a C hx and px & adm pt to College Hospital; MDM MC. Imp: Concussion without skull fracture, no loss of consciousness; nasal laceration; deviated septum which may need reconstruction. Disability from work from 5-1 to 5-17.
	CA/llf — *Concha Antrum, MD*
5-2-xx	Hospital visit (PF hx/exam LC MDM).
	CA/llf — *Concha Antrum, MD*
5-3-xx	Hospital visit (PF hx/exam SF MDM).
	CA/llf — *Concha Antrum, MD*
5-4-xx	Discharge from hospital. See hosp records for daily notes. RTO in 2 day for suture removal.
	CA/llf — *Concha Antrum, MD*
5-6-xx	OV. Sutures removed; wound healed. Discussed deviated septum and recommended septoplasty. Surg sched for 5/10/xx at College Hospital.
	CA/llf — *Concha Antrum, MD*
5-10-xx	Adm to College Hospital (D hx/exam LC MDM). Performed septoplasty. Pt doing well; moved to recovery room.
	CA/llf — *Concha Antrum, MD*
5-11-xx	Pt doing well, no hemorrhage, discharged home.
	CA/llf — *Concha Antrum, MD*
5-12-xx	Pt comes into ofc with postop anterior nasal hemorrhage. Cauterized rt side. RTO in 1 wk.
	CA/llf — *Concha Antrum, MD*

Figure 12-7

Acct. No. 12-7

STATEMENT
Financial Account

COLLEGE CLINIC
4567 Broad Avenue
Woodland Hills, XY 12345-0001
Tel. 555-486-9002
Fax No. 555-487-8976

Peter F. Donlon
1840 East Chevy Chase Drive
Woodland Hills, XY 12345

Phone No. (H) (555) 762-3580 (W) (555)762-0050 Birthdate 08-09-38

Insurance Co. Coastal Health Insurance Co./Medicare Policy/Group No. 34276 Grp. 45A
Medicare No. 987-XX-4321A

	REFERENCE	DESCRIPTION	CHARGES	CREDITS PYMNTS.	CREDITS ADJ.	BALANCE
20XX		BALANCE FORWARD →				
05-01-xx		Initial hospital care				
05-01-xx		Skin repair				
05-02-xx		HV				
05-03-xx		HV				
05-04-xx		Discharge				
05-06-xx		Suture removal				
05-10-xx		Admit-Septoplasty				
05-11-xx		Discharge				
05-12-xx		Postop OV				

PLEASE PAY LAST AMOUNT IN BALANCE COLUMN

THIS IS A COPY OF YOUR FINANCIAL ACCOUNT AS IT APPEARS ON OUR RECORDS

Figure 12-8

ASSIGNMENT 12-8 COMPLETE A CLAIM FOR A MEDICARE/MEDIGAP CASE

Performance Objective

Task: Complete a CMS-1500 (02-12) claim form for a Medicare/Medigap case, post transactions to the financial accounting record, and define patient record abbreviations.

Conditions: Use the patient's medical record (Figure 12-9) and financial statement (Figure 12-10), one health insurance claim form (print from Evolve website), a computer, procedural and diagnostic code books, and Appendixes A and B in this *Workbook*.

Standards: Claim Productivity Measurement

Time: ______________ minutes

Accuracy: ______________

(Note: The time element and accuracy criteria may be given by your instructor.)

Directions:

1. Complete the CMS-1500 (02-12) claim form, using Medicare/Medigap NUCC guidelines. If your instructor wants you to direct it to your local fiscal intermediary, obtain the name and address by going to the Evolve website listed in Internet Resources at the end of Chapter 12 in the *Handbook*. This case involves a patient who has a Medigap supplemental policy that is a secondary payer. Refer to Jeremiah W. Diffenderffer's patient record and financial statement for information. See Medicare participating provider fees in Appendix A in this *Workbook* to locate the fees to be recorded on the claim and posted to the financial statement. Fees in the participating column are also the approved amounts. Date the claim June 13. Dr. Coccidioides is accepting assignment in this case. Mr. Diffenderffer has met his deductible for the year, owing to previous care by Dr. Coccidioides.

2. Refer to Chapter 7 and Figure 7-8 of the *Handbook* for instructions on how to complete the CMS-1500 (02-12) claim form.

3. Use your CPT code book or Appendix A in this *Workbook* to determine the correct five-digit code number and modifiers for each professional service rendered. Refer to your HCPCS Level II code book or Appendix B in this *Workbook* for HCPCS procedure codes and modifiers. If your instructor tells you to also find the ICD-10-CM codes, a draft version may be downloaded from the following website: http://www.cdc.gov/nchs/icd/icd10cm.htm.

4. Record all transactions on the financial record, and indicate the proper information when you have billed Medicare and Medigap.

5. On August 3, Medicare check number 654821 was received in the amount of $270.05, paying 80% of the approved amount for all services except the medication charge, of which they allowed $10. Post this payment to the patient's financial account, and calculate and post the courtesy adjustment. On August 15, United American Insurance Company check number 3254 was received in the amount of $67.51, paying 20% of the approved amount for all services, including the $10 allowed amount determined by Medicare for the medication. Post this payment to the patient's financial statement, and indicate the balance due from the patient.

6. A Performance Evaluation Checklist may be reproduced from the "Instruction Guide to the Workbook" chapter if your instructor wishes to submit it to assist with scoring and comments.

After the instructor has returned your work to you, either make the necessary corrections and place your work in a three-ring notebook for future reference or, if you received a high score, place it in your portfolio for reference when applying for a job.

Abbreviations pertinent to this record:

Est	______	hx	______
oft	______	exam	______
p.m.	______	HC	______
SOB	______	MDM	______
adv	______	imp	______
AP	______	RTO	______
lat	______	wk	______
tech	______	c/o	______
CXR	______	HCN	______
ABG	______	PF	______
PFT	______	SF	______
a.m.	______	IV	______
RTO	______	ml	______
CPX	______	appt	______
C	______		

Additional Coding

1. Refer to Mr. Diffenderffer's medical record, abstract information, and code procedures that would be billed by outside providers.

Site	*Description of Service*	*Code*
a. College Hospital Laboratory	______	______
b. College Hospital Respiratory Department	______	______

PATIENT RECORD NO. 12-8

Diffenderffer	Jeremiah	W	08-24-31	M	555-471 9930
LAST NAME	FIRST NAME	MIDDLE NAME	BIRTH DATE	SEX	HOME PHONE

120 Elm Street	Woodland Hills	XY	12345
ADDRESS	CITY	STATE	ZIP CODE

555-218-0087		555-471-9930	Diffenderffer@wb.net
CELL PHONE	PAGER NO.	FAX NO.	E-MAIL ADDRESS

731-XX-7401	none
PATIENT'S SOC. SEC. NO.	DRIVER'S LICENSE

retired painter	
PATIENT'S OCCUPATION	NAME OF COMPANY

ADDRESS OF EMPLOYER	PHONE

deceased	
SPOUSE OR PARENT	OCCUPATION

Medicare	731-XX-7401T
NAME OF INSURANCE	MEDICARE NO

United American Insurance Company,	P.O. Box 810, Dallas, TX 75221	555-328-2841
NAME OF OTHER INSURANCE	ADDRESS	PHONE

007559715	UNITXY003
POLICY/CERTIFICATE NO.	PAYERID NO.

REFERRED BY: John M. Diffenderffer (brother)

DATE	PROGRESS NOTES
6-1-xx	Est pt telephoned ofc this p.m. stating he has been involved in a long painting project in
	his home and when he breathed paint fumes in his kitchen today he experienced
	SOB & coughing. Dr. Coccidioides is out of the ofc this p.m. and was paged. Physician
	adv pt to come into ofc for AP & lat chest x-ray and bilateral bronchogram this afternoon.
	Chest x-ray and bronchogram taken by x-ray tech.
	RH/llf Rene Holmes, CMA
6-2-xx	CXR and bronchogram showed pulmonary emphysema. Adv pt by phone to have ABG for
	direct O_2 saturation and PFT (spirometry) at College Hospital this a.m. and RTO for CPX
	this afternoon.
	BC/llf Brady Coccidioides, MD
6-2-xx	Pt returns for C hx/exam HC MDM. Imp: emphysema, bronchitis and pneumonitis due to
	inhalation of fumes and vapors. Adv no more painting; bed rest. RTO 1 wk.
	BC/llf Brady Coccidioides, MD
6-5-xx	Pt calls as ofc is closing c/o difficulty breathing; he has been ambulating and climbing
	stairs. HCN PF hx/exam SF MDM. Administered Coramine (nikethamide) medication IV
	(unclassified drug, 1.5 ml two ampules @ 12.50 each). Imp: recurrent bronchitis and pneumonitis,
	exertional dyspnea. Adv complete bed rest. RTO for appt on 6-9-xx.
	BC/llf Brady Coccidioides, MD

Figure 12-9

STATEMENT
Financial Account

Acct. No. 12-8

COLLEGE CLINIC
4567 Broad Avenue
Woodland Hills, XY 12345-0001
Tel. 555-486-9002
Fax No. 555-487-8976

Jeremiah W. Diffenderffer
120 Elm Street
Woodland Hills, XY 12345

Phone No. (H) (555) 471-9930 (W) ____________ Birthdate 08-24-31

Insurance Co. Medicare/United American Insurance Co. Policy/Group No. 007559715

Medicare No. 731-XX-7401T

	REFERENCE	DESCRIPTION	CHARGES		CREDITS PYMNTS.		CREDITS ADJ.		BALANCE	
20XX							**BALANCE FORWARD** →		20	00
06-01-xx		Chest x-ray								
06-01-xx		Bronchogram								
06-02-xx		OV								
06-05-xx		HC								
06-05-xx		IV administration								
06-05-xx		Medication								

PLEASE PAY LAST AMOUNT IN BALANCE COLUMN

THIS IS A COPY OF YOUR FINANCIAL ACCOUNT AS IT APPEARS ON OUR RECORDS

Figure 12-10

ASSIGNMENT 12-9 COMPLETE A CLAIM FORM FOR A MEDICARE CASE WITH AN ADVANCE BENEFICIARY NOTICE OF NONCOVERAGE

Performance Objective

Task: Complete a CMS-1500 (02-12) claim form for a Medicare case and an advance beneficiary notice of noncoverage, post transactions to the financial accounting record, and define patient record abbreviations.

Conditions: Use the patient's record (Figure 12-11) and financial statement (Figure 12-12), an advance beneficiary notice of noncoverage form (Figure 12-13), two health insurance claim forms (print from Evolve website), a computer, procedural and diagnostic code books, and Appendixes A and B in this *Workbook*.

Standards: Claim Productivity Measurement

Time: ______________ minutes

Accuracy: ______________

(Note: The time element and accuracy criteria may be given by your instructor.)

Directions:

1. Complete a CMS-1500 (02-12) claim form for a Medicare case, using NUCC guidelines. If your instructor wants you to direct it to your local Medicare Railroad fiscal intermediary, obtain the name and address by going to the Evolve website listed in Internet Resources at the end of Chapter 12 in the *Handbook*. This assignment requires two claim forms, so make a photocopy for the second claim. Refer to Raymond D. Fay's patient record for information. Refer to Appendix A in this *Workbook* to locate the fees to be recorded on the claim and posted to the financial statement. Date the claim December 31. Dr. Antrum is a participating physician and is accepting assignment in this case.

2. Refer to Figure 7-6 in the *Handbook* for instructions on how to complete the CMS-1500 (02-12) claim form.

3. The nystagmus service is disallowed by Medicare, and an advance beneficiary notice of noncoverage needs to be completed. Refer to Figure 12-9 in the *Handbook* for a completed example of this form. Note: When a noncovered service is provided, a fee will not be listed in the Medicare fee schedule; therefore, list the regular (mock) fee.

4. Use your CPT code book or Appendix A in this *Workbook* to determine the correct five-digit code number and modifiers for each professional service rendered. Use your HCPCS Level II code book or refer to Appendix B in this *Workbook* for HCPCS procedure codes and modifiers. The patient has met $71 of the $147 deductible. If your instructor tells you to also find the ICD-10-CM codes, a draft version may be downloaded from the following website: http://www.cdc.gov/nchs/icd/icd10cm.htm.

5. Record all transactions on the financial accounting record, and indicate the proper information when you have billed Medicare.

6. A Performance Evaluation Checklist may be reproduced from the "Instruction Guide to the Workbook" chapter if your instructor wishes you to submit it to assist with scoring and comments.

After the instructor has returned your work to you, either make the necessary corrections and place your work in a three-ring notebook for future reference or, if you received a high score, place it in your portfolio for reference when applying for a job.

Abbreviations pertinent to this record:

Pt	______	RTO	______
D	______	rtn	______
hx	______	OV	______
exam	______	appt(s)	______
retn	______	wk	______
R/O	______	inj.	______
LC	______	Dx	______
MDM	______	PF	______
N	______	SF	______
X	______	sx	______
incl	______	disc	______

Additional Fee Calculations

1. Medicare sent payment on this claim, allowing 80% of the approved amount after the partial deductible was met, which was subtracted from the amount of this claim. Note: For this case, the approved amount will be the limiting charge. Medicare denied payment on code 92531 as a noncovered service.

   a. What is the amount of the Medicare check? ______

   b. What is the amount of the patient responsibility? ______

   c. Is there a courtesy adjustment? ______

PATIENT RECORD NO. 12-9

LAST NAME	FIRST NAME	MIDDLE NAME	BIRTH DATE	SEX	HOME PHONE
Fay	Raymond		02-03-32	M	555-788-9090

ADDRESS	CITY	STATE	ZIP CODE
33 North Pencil Avenue	Woodland Hills	XY	12345

CELL PHONE	PAGER NO.	FAX NO.	E-MAIL ADDRESS
	555-250-4890	555-788-9090	fay@wb.net

PATIENT'S SOC. SEC. NO.	DRIVER'S LICENSE
887-66-1235	R8966543

PATIENT'S OCCUPATION	NAME OF COMPANY
retired railroad engineer	

ADDRESS OF EMPLOYER	PHONE

SPOUSE OR PARENT	OCCUPATION
Marilyn B. Fay	homemaker

EMPLOYER	ADDRESS	PHONE

NAME OF INSURANCE	INSURED OR SUB SCRIBER
Medicare Railroad	self

MEDICARE NO.
A 887-XX-1235A

REFERRED BY: George Gentle, MD, 1000 N. Main St., Woodland Hills, XY 12345 NPI# 402131102XX

DATE	PROGRESS NOTES
10-31-xx	New pt presents, a D hx was taken. Pt complains of skin rash and dizziness for 3 days.
	A detailed exam reveals rash on chest and arms. Retn in 4 days for tests to R/O eye/ear
	causes for dizziness and food allergies (LC MDM).
	CA/llf Concha Antrum, MD
11-4-xx	Comprehensive audiometric threshold evaluation (with speech)—N. 10 intradermal
	allergy tests; delayed reaction. Bilateral mastoid X (complete)—N. Spontaneous nystagmus
	test, incl. gaze—N. RTO in 3 days for skin test results.
	CA/llf Concha Antrum, MD
11-7-xx	Rtn OV for allergy skin test results—positive for 3 substances. Pt to purchase allergen
	extract and make sequential appts next wk for daily immunotherapy inj. Dx: food allergies.
	CA/llf Concha Antrum, MD
11-14-xx thru	Immunotherapy; 3 inj. per/day
11-18-xx	CA/llf Concha Antrum, MD
11-21-xx thru	Immunotherapy; 3 inj. per/day
11-25-xx	CA/llf Concha Antrum, MD
11-28-xx thru	Immunotherapy; 3 inj. per/day
12-2-xx	CA/llf Concha Antrum, MD
12-5-xx thru	Immunotherapy; 3 inj. per/day
12-8-xx	CA/llf Concha Antrum, MD
12-9-xx	OV (PF hx/exam SF MDM) Pt. sx improved. Received final inj and evaluated for disch.
	CA/llf Concha Antrum, MD

Figure 12-11

Acct No. 12-9

STATEMENT
Financial Account

COLLEGE CLINIC
4567 Broad Avenue
Woodland Hills, XY 12345-0001
Tel. 555-486-9002
Fax No. 555-487-8976

Raymond Fay
33 North Pencil Avenue
Woodland Hills, XY 12345

Phone No. (H) (555) 788-9090 (W) ______ Birthdate 02-03-32

Primary Insurance Co. Medicare Railroad Policy/Group No. A 887-XX 1235A

Secondary Insurance Co. N/A Policy/Group No. ______

DATE	REFERENCE	DESCRIPTION	CHARGES	CREDITS PYMNTS.	CREDITS ADJ.	BALANCE
20xx		BALANCE FORWARD →				
10-31-xx		OV				
11-4-xx		Audiometry evaluation				
11-4-xx		Intradermal allergy tests				
11-4-xx		Bilateral mastoid x-rays				
11-4-xx		Spontaneous nystagmus test				
11-7-xx		Allergy test results				
11-14 to 11-18-xx		Immunotherapy inj. (3/day X 5)				
11-21 to 11-25-xx		Immunotherapy inj. (3/day X 5)				
11-28 to 12-2-xx		Immunotherapy inj. (3/day X 5)				
12-5 to 12-9-xx		Immunotherapy inj. (3/day X 5)				
12-9-xx		OV				

PLEASE PAY LAST AMOUNT IN BALANCE COLUMN

THIS IS A COPY OF YOUR FINANCIAL ACCOUNT AS IT APPEARS ON OUR RECORDS

Figure 12-12

A. Notifier:

B. Patient Name: **C. Identification Number:**

Advance Beneficiary Notice of Noncoverage (ABN)

NOTE: If Medicare doesn't pay for **D.** ____________ below, you may have to pay.

Medicare does not pay for everything, even some care that you or your health care provider have good reason to think you need. We expect Medicare may not pay for the **D.** ____________ below.

D.	E. Reason Medicare May Not Pay:	F. Estimated Cost

WHAT YOU NEED TO DO NOW:

- Read this notice, so you can make an informed decision about your care.
- Ask us any questions that you may have after you finish reading.
- Choose an option below about whether to receive the **D.** ____________ listed above.

Note: If you choose Option 1 or 2, we may help you to use any other insurance that you might have, but Medicare cannot require us to do this.

G. OPTIONS: **Check only one box. We cannot choose a box for you.**

☐ **OPTION 1.** I want the **D.** ____________ listed above. You may ask to be paid now, but I also want Medicare billed for an official decision on payment, which is sent to me on a Medicare Summary Notice (MSN). I understand that if Medicare doesn't pay, I am responsible for payment, but **I can appeal to Medicare** by following the directions on the MSN. If Medicare does pay, you will refund any payments I made to you, less co-pays or deductibles.

☐ **OPTION 2.** I want the **D.** ____________ listed above, but do not bill Medicare. You may ask to be paid now as I am responsible for payment. **I cannot appeal if Medicare is not billed.**

☐ **OPTION 3.** I don't want the **D.** ____________ listed above. I understand with this choice I am **not** responsible for payment, and **I cannot appeal to see if Medicare would pay.**

H. Additional Information:

This notice gives our opinion, not an official Medicare decision. If you have other questions on this notice or Medicare billing, call **1-800-MEDICARE** (1-800-633-4227/**TTY:** 1-877-486-2048).

Signing below means that you have received and understand this notice. You also receive a copy.

I. Signature:	J. Date:

According to the Paperwork Reduction Act of 1995, no persons are required to respond to a collection of information unless it displays a valid OMB control number. The valid OMB control number for this information collection is 0938-0566. The time required to complete this information collection is estimated to average 7 minutes per response, including the time to review instructions, search existing data resources, gather the data needed, and complete and review the information collection. If you have comments concerning the accuracy of the time estimate or suggestions for improving this form, please write to: CMS, 7500 Security Boulevard, Attn: PRA Reports Clearance Officer, Baltimore, Maryland 21244-1850.

Form CMS-R-131 (03/11) Form Approved OMB No. 0938-0566

Figure 12-13

ASSIGNMENT 12-10 COMPLETE A CLAIM FORM FOR A MEDICARE/MEDICAID CASE

Performance Objective

Task: Complete a CMS-1500 (02-12) claim form for a Medicare/Medicaid case, post transactions to the financial accounting record, and define patient record abbreviations.

Conditions: Use the patient's medical record (Figure 12-14) and financial statement (Figure 12-15), one health insurance claim form (print from Evolve website), a computer, procedural and diagnostic code books, and Appendixes A and B in this *Workbook*.

Standards: Claim Productivity Measurement

Time: ______________ minutes

Accuracy: ______________

(Note: The time element and accuracy criteria may be given by your instructor.)

Directions:

1. Complete the CMS-1500 (02-12) claim form, using NUCC guidelines for a Medicare/Medicaid case. If your instructor wants you to direct it to your local Medicare fiscal intermediary, obtain the name and address by going to the Evolve website listed in Internet Resources at the end of Chapter 12 in the *Handbook*. Refer to Mr. Harris Fremont's patient record for information. Refer to Appendix A in this *Workbook* to locate the fees to be recorded on the claim and posted to the financial statement. Date the claim October 31.
2. Refer to Chapter 7 and Figure 7-7 of the *Handbook* for instructions on how to complete the CMS-1500 (02-12) claim form.
3. Use your CPT code book or Appendix A in this *Workbook* to determine the correct five-digit code number and modifiers for each professional service rendered. Use your HCPCS Level II code book or refer to Appendix B in this *Workbook* for HCPCS procedure codes and modifiers. If your instructor tells you to also find the ICD-10-CM codes, a draft version may be downloaded from the following website: http://www.cdc.gov/nchs/icd/icd10cm.htm.
4. Record all transactions on the financial account and indicate the proper information when you have billed Medicare/Medicaid.
5. On December 12, Medicare paid $125 (check number 281362) on this claim. Post this payment to the patient's financial account. On December 29, you receive a voucher number 7234 from Medicaid for $45. Post this payment to the patient's financial account and show the courtesy adjustment.
6. A Performance Evaluation Checklist may be reproduced from the "Instruction Guide to the Workbook" chapter if your instructor wishes you to submit it to assist with scoring and comments.

After the instructor has returned your work to you, either make the necessary corrections and place your work in a three-ring notebook for future reference or, if you received a high score, place it in your portfolio for reference when applying for a job.

Abbreviations pertinent to this record:

NP	________________	pt	________________
c/o	________________	lab	________________
hx	________________	CBC	________________
R	________________	auto	________________
L	________________	diff	________________
N	________________	ESR	________________
Rx	________________	R/O	________________
adv	________________	PF	________________
rtn	________________	SF	________________
LC	________________	prn	________________
MDM	________________	imp	________________

Additional Coding

1. Refer to Mr. Fremont's medical record, abstract information, and code procedures that would be billed by outside providers.

Site	*Description of Service*	*Code*
a. ABC Laboratory	____________	____________
b. ABC Laboratory	____________	____________
c. ABC Laboratory	____________	____________
d. ABC Laboratory	____________	____________

2. Use your diagnostic code book and code the symptoms of which the patient complained.

Symptom	*ICD-9-CM Code*	*ICD-10-CM Code*
a. ____________	____________	____________
b. ____________	____________	____________

PATIENT RECORD NO. 12-10

LAST NAME	FIRST NAME	MIDDLE NAME	BIRTH DATE	SEX	HOME PHONE
Fremont	Harris		07-10-23	M	555-899-0109

ADDRESS	CITY	STATE	ZIP CODE
735 North Center Street	Woodland Hills,	XY	12345

CELL PHONE	PAGER NO.	FAX NO.	E-MAIL ADDRESS

PATIENT'S SOC. SEC. NO.	DRIVER'S LICENSE
454-XX-9569	none

PATIENT'S OCCUPATION	NAME OF COMPANY
retired baseball coach	

ADDRESS OF EMPLOYER	PHONE

SPOUSE OR PARENT	OCCUPATION
Emily B. Fremont	homemaker

EMPLOYER	ADDRESS	PHONE

NAME OF INSURANCE	INSURED OR SUBSCRIBER
Medicare/Medicaid	

MEDICARE NO.	MEDICAID NO.
454-XX-9569A	56-10-0020205-0-XX

REFERRED BY: Raymond Skeleton, MD

DATE	PROGRESS NOTES
10-2-xx	NP referred by Dr. Skeleton. He comes in c/o discomfort around toes of both feet and
	has difficulty walking. Pt states he dropped shelf on feet about a month ago. A detailed
	hx reveals gout and mycotic nails. X-ray R and L feet (2 views) N. Detailed exam reveals
	bilateral mycotic nails & ingrown nail on great R toe. Rx: Electrically débride and trimmed
	overgrowth of all nails and adv to rtn if pain continues in great R toe (LC MDM). Gave pt
	order to have lab work done at ABC Laboratory (CBC w/auto diff., ESR (automated), uric acid level)
	R/O gout. Imp: Mycotic nails; difficulty walking.
	NP/llf Nick Pedro, DPM
10-18-xx	Pt returns c/o ingrown nail on R great toe (PF hx/exam SF MDM). Lab work done on
	10/2/xx showed no signs of gout. Performed wedge excision of skin/nail fold.
	Rtn prn. Imp: Ingrown nail – great R toe; toe pain.
	NP/llf Nick Pedro, DPM

Figure 12-14

Acct No. 12-10

STATEMENT
Financial Account

COLLEGE CLINIC
4567 Broad Avenue
Woodland Hills, XY 12345-0001
Tel. 555-486-9002
Fax No. 555-487-8976

Harris Fremont
735 North Center Street
Woodland Hills, XY 12345

Phone No. (H) 555-899-0109 (W) ______ Birthdate 7/10/23

Primary Insurance Co. Medicare Policy/Group No. 454XX9569A

Secondary Insurance Co. Medicaid Policy/Group No. 561000202050XX

DATE	REF-ERENCE	DESCRIPTION	CHARGES	CREDITS PYMNTS.	CREDITS ADJ.	BALANCE
20xx		BALANCE FORWARD →				
10-2-xx		NP OV				
10-2-xx		X-rays R/L feet				
10-2-xx		Débridement nails				
10-18-xx		OV				
10-18-xx		Wedge excision R. great toe				

PLEASE PAY LAST AMOUNT IN BALANCE COLUMN

THIS IS A COPY OF YOUR FINANCIAL ACCOUNT AS IT APPEARS ON OUR RECORDS

Figure 12-15

STUDENT SOFTWARE CHALLENGE

ASSIGNMENT 12-11 ASSIGNMENTS FOR MEDICARE CASES 8 THROUGH 10 ONSCREEN COMPLETION OF CMS-1500 (02-12) INSURANCE CLAIM FORMS

Performance Objective

Task: Enter transactions from patients' onscreen encounter forms (superbills) and complete block-by-block onscreen health insurance claim forms.

Conditions: Onscreen encounter forms (superbills) and computer.

Standards: Time: ______________ minutes

Accuracy: ______________

(Note: The time element and accuracy criteria may be given by your instructor.)

Directions: Log on to your Evolve account at http://evolve.elsevier.com and access the student resources for Fordney: *Insurance Handbook for the Medical Office,* 13th edition. Then choose Student Software Challenge.

1. For these assignments, follow the instructions for entering data into the onscreen CMS-1500 (02-12) health insurance claim form, completing blocks 1 through 33 for cases 8 through 10.
2. Use your CPT code book or Appendix A in this *Workbook* to determine the correct five-digit code number and modifiers for each professional service rendered. If your instructor tells you to also find the ICD-10-CM codes, a draft version may be downloaded from the following website: http://www.cdc.gov/nchs/icd/icd10cm.htm.
3. A Performance Evaluation Checklist may be reproduced from the "Instruction Guide to the Workbook" chapter if your instructor wishes you to submit it to assist with scoring and comments.
4. Print a hard copy of the completed health insurance claim form for each case.
5. After the instructor has returned your work to you, either make the necessary corrections and place your work in a three-ring notebook for future reference or, if you received a high score, place it in your portfolio for reference when applying for a job.

13 Medicaid and Other State Programs

Marilyn T. Fordney

KEY TERMS

Your instructor may wish to select some words pertinent to this chapter for a test. For definitions of the terms, further study, and/or reference, the words, phrases, and abbreviations may be found in the glossary at the end of the Handbook. *Key terms for this chapter follow.*

categorically needy
coinsurance
copayment
covered services
Early and Periodic Screening, Diagnosis, and Treatment
fiscal agent
Maternal and Child Health Program
Medicaid
Medi-Cal
medically needy
prior approval
recipient
share of cost
State Children's Health Insurance Program
Supplemental Security Income

KEY ABBREVIATIONS

See how many abbreviations and acronyms you can translate and then use this as a handy reference list. Definitions for the key abbreviations are located near the back of the Handbook *in the glossary.*

DEFRA ______________________

EPSDT ______________________

FPL ______________________

MCHP ______________________

MN ______________________

MQMB ______________________

OBRA ______________________

OOY claims ______________________

POS machine ______________________

QI program ______________________

QMB ______________________

RA ______________________

SCHIP ______________________

SLMB ______________________

SSI ______________________

TANF ______________________

TEFRA ______________________

PERFORMANCE OBJECTIVES

The student will be able to:

- Define and spell the key terms and key abbreviations for this chapter, given the information from the Handbook glossary, within a reasonable time period and with enough accuracy to obtain a satisfactory evaluation.
- After reading the chapter, answer the fill-in-the-blank, multiple choice, and true/false review questions with enough accuracy to obtain a satisfactory evaluation.
- Fill in the correct meaning of each abbreviation, given a list of common medical abbreviations and symbols that appear in chart notes, within a reasonable time period and with enough accuracy to obtain a satisfactory evaluation.
- Given the patient's medical chart notes, ledger cards, and blank insurance claim forms, complete each CMS-1500 (02-12) Health Insurance Claim Form for billing within a reasonable time period and with enough accuracy to obtain a satisfactory evaluation.
- Correctly post payments, adjustments, and balances on the patient's ledger cards, using the Mock Fee Schedule in Appendix A in this *Workbook*, within a reasonable time period and with enough accuracy to obtain a satisfactory evaluation.

STUDY OUTLINE

History
Medicaid Programs
- Maternal and Child Health Program
- Low-Income Medicare Recipients

Medicaid Eligibility
- Verifying Eligibility
- Categorically Needy
- Medically Needy
- Maternal and Child Health Program Eligibility
- Spousal Impoverishment Protection Law
- New Freedom Initiative
- Accepting Medicaid Patients
  - Program Participation
  - Identification Card
  - Point-of-Service Machine
  - Retroactive Eligibility

Medicaid Benefits
- Covered Services
- Disallowed Services

Medicaid Managed Care
Claim Procedures
- Copayment
- Prior Approval
- Time Limit
- Reciprocity
- Claim Form

After Claim Submission
- Remittance Advice
- Appeals

ASSIGNMENT 13-1 REVIEW QUESTIONS

Part I Fill in the Blank

Review the objectives, key terms, glossary definitions of key terms, chapter information, and figures before completing the following review questions.

1. Medicaid is administered by ________________ with partial ________________ funding.

2. Medicaid is not an insurance program. It is a/an ________________ program.

3. In all other states, the program is known as Medicaid, but in California the program is called ________________.

4. Because the federal government sets minimum requirements, states are free to enhance the Medicaid program. Name two ways in which Medicaid programs vary from state to state.

   a. ________________

   b. ________________

5. SCHIP means ________________ and MCHP means ________________ and covers children of what age group?

   ____

6. Name the three aid programs for low-income Medicare patients.

   a. ________________

   b. ________________

   c. ________________

7. Name two broad classifications of people eligible for Medicaid assistance.

   a. ________________

   b. ________________

8. The name of the program for the prevention, early detection, and treatment of conditions of children receiving welfare is known as ________________. It is abbreviated as ________________.

9. Your Medicaid patient seen today needs long-term hemodialysis services. You telephone for authorization to get verbal approval. Four important items to obtain are:

   a. ________________

   b. ________________

   c. ________________

   d. ________________

10. The time limit for submitting a Medicaid claim varies from ______________________

to ______________________
from the date the service is rendered. In your state, the time limit is

______________________.

11. The insurance claim form for submitting Medicaid claims in all states is

______________________.

12. Your Medicaid patient also has TRICARE. What billing procedure do you follow? Be exact in your steps for a dependent of an active military person.

a. ______________________

b. ______________________

13. Five categories of adjudicated claims that may appear on a Medicaid remittance advice document are:

a. ______________________

b. ______________________

c. ______________________

d. ______________________

e. ______________________

14. Name three levels of Medicaid appeals.

a. ______________________

b. ______________________

c. ______________________

Part II Multiple Choice

Choose the best answer.

15. When professional services are rendered, the Medicaid identification card or electronic verification must show eligibility for
    a. day of service.
    b. year of service.
    c. month of service.
    d. week of service.

16. When a Medicaid patient is injured in an automobile accident and the car has liability insurance, this involves a third-party payer so the insurance claim is sent to the
    a. patient.
    b. automobile insurance carrier.
    c. Medicaid fiscal agent.
    d. none of the above.

17. The only state without a Medicaid program that is similar to those existing in other states that has an alternative prepaid medical assistance program is
    a. Arizona.
    b. California.
    c. Colorado.
    d. New Mexico.

18. A patient's Medicaid eligibility may be verified by
    a. touch-tone telephone.
    b. modem.
    c. special Medicaid terminal equipment.
    d. all of the above.

19. When a Medicaid patient requires a piece of durable medical equipment, the physician must
    a. write a prescription.
    b. obtain prior authorization, preferably written.
    c. instruct the patient on how to use the equipment.
    d. give name and address of where to purchase the equipment.

20. Medicare beneficiaries who are disabled but have annual incomes below the federal poverty level may be eligible for
    a. Medicaid Qualified Medicare Beneficiary Program.
    b. Qualifying Individuals Program.
    c. Specified Low-Income Medicare Beneficiary Program.
    d. all of the above.

Part III True/False

Write "T" or "F" in the blank to indicate whether you think the statement is true or false.

________ 21. Cerebral palsy is a condition that qualifies a child for benefits under the Maternal and Child Health Program.

________ 22. There is only one type of copayment requirement in the Medicaid program.

________ 23. When filing a claim for a Medicaid managed care patient, transmit the claim to the managed care organization and not the Medicaid fiscal agent.

________ 24. Providers must enroll for participation in the Medicaid program with the fiscal agent for their region.

________ 25. A state agency that investigates complaints of mistreatment in long-term care facilities is the Medicaid Fraud Control Unit (MFCU).

ASSIGNMENT 13-2 CRITICAL THINKING

Performance Objective

Task: After reading the scenario, answer the following questions, using critical thinking skills.

Conditions: Use a pen or pencil.

Standards: Time: ______________ minutes

Accuracy: ______________

(Note: The time element and accuracy criteria may be given by your instructor.)

Directions: After reading the scenario, answer questions, using your critical thinking skills. Record your answers on the blank lines.

Scenario: Mrs. Ho suddenly experiences a pain in her right lower abdominal area and rushes to a local hospital for emergency care. Laboratory work verifies that she has a ruptured appendix, and immediate surgery is recommended. Is prior authorization required in a bona fide emergency situation like this?

1. ______________________________

   Reason: ______________________________

   In referring to the instructions for completing a CMS-1500 (02-12) claim form for a Medicaid case, which two blocks on the CMS-1500 (02-12) claim form need to be completed for emergency services?

2. Block ______________________________

   What data should be inserted? ______________________________

3. Block ______________________________

   What data should be inserted and/or document attached?

   ____

ASSIGNMENT 13-3 COMPLETE A CLAIM FORM FOR A MEDICAID CASE

Performance Objective

Task: Complete a CMS-1500 (02-12) claim form, post transactions to the financial accounting record, and define patient record abbreviations.

Conditions: Use the patient's record (Figure 13-1) and financial statement (Figure 13-2), one health insurance claim form (print from Evolve website), a computer, procedural and diagnostic code books, and Appendixes A and B in this *Workbook*.

Standards: Claim Productivity Measurement

Time: ______________ minutes

Accuracy: ______________

(Note: The time element and accuracy criteria may be given by your instructor.)

Directions:

1. Using NUCC guidelines, complete the Health Insurance Claim Form and direct it to Medicaid for Rose Clarkson by referring to her patient record. Date the claim September 6. Refer to Appendix A in this *Workbook* to locate the fees to record on the claim and post them to the financial statement. If your instructor wants you to insert the name and address of your Medicaid fiscal agent on the claim, obtain the address by going to the Evolve website listed in Internet Resources at the end of Chapter 13 in the *Handbook*.

2. Refer to Chapter 7 (Figure 7-4) in the *Handbook* for instructions on how to complete this claim form and a Medicaid template.

3. Use your *Current Procedural Terminology* (CPT) code book or Appendix A in this *Workbook* to determine the correct five-digit code number and modifiers for each professional service rendered. Use your Healthcare Common Procedure Coding System (HCPCS) Level II code book or refer to Appendix B in this *Workbook* for HCPCS procedure codes and modifiers.

If your instructor tells you to also find the ICD-10-CM codes, a draft version may be downloaded from the following website: http://www.cdc.gov/nchs/icd/icd10cm.htm.

4. Record all transactions on the financial account, and indicate the date when you have billed Medicaid.

5. Refer to Appendix A in this *Workbook* for the clinic and hospital provider numbers that are needed for completing Medicaid forms.

6. A Performance Evaluation Checklist may be reproduced from the "Instruction Guide to the Workbook" chapter if your instructor wishes you to submit it to assist with scoring and comments.

After the instructor has returned your work to you, either make the necessary corrections and place your work in a three-ring notebook for future reference or, if you received a high score, place it in your portfolio for reference when applying for a job.

PATIENT RECORD NO. 13-3

LAST NAME	FIRST NAME	MIDDLE NAME	BIRTH DATE	SEX	HOME PHONE
Clarkson	Rose		03-09-54	F	555-487-2209

ADDRESS	CITY	STATE	ZIP CODE
3408 Jackson Street	Hempstead	XY	11551-0300

CELL PHONE	PAGER NO.	FAX NO.	E-MAIL ADDRESS
	555-340-2200		

PATIENT'S SOC. SEC. NO.	DRIVER'S LICENSE
030-XX-9543	R3207897

PATIENT'S OCCUPATION	NAME OF COMPANY
unemployed	

ADDRESS OF EMPLOYER	PHONE

SPOUSE OR PARENT	OCCUPATION

EMPLOYER	ADDRESS	PHONE

NAME OF INSURANCE	INSURED OR SUBSCRIBER
Medicaid	self

MEDICAID NO.	GROUP NO.
CC99756329346X	

REFERRED BY: James Jackson, MD, 100 North Main Street, Hempstead, XY 11551 NPI# 72011337XX

DATE	PROGRESS NOTES
9-4-xx	New pt presents complaining of cough & SOB. A detailed hx was taken which revealed
	mitral valve prolapse. A D exam was done indicating elevated cardiac and respiratory rates,
	diminished breath sounds, distended neck veins, and edema of both ankles. 12 lead ECG
	performed; normal sinus rhythm and elevated heart rate. Echocardiogram done
	(2D, complete with pulsed wave Doppler) to evaluate mitral valve, cardiac chamber size, and ventricular
	function; presence of mitral valve regurgitation. Single view chest x-ray indicated presence
	of fluid in lungs. Primary diagnosis: congestive heart disease and mitral valve prolapse
	(LC MDM). Pt given Rx for diuretic, digitalis, and vasodilator. Restrict fluid and sodium
	intake. Retn in 2 wks.
	PC/llf Perry Cardi, MD

Figure 13-1

Acct No. 13-3

STATEMENT
Financial Account

COLLEGE CLINIC
4567 Broad Avenue
Woodland Hills, XY 12345-0001
Tel. 555-486-9002
Fax No. 555-487-8976

Rose Clarkson
3408 Jackson Street
Hempstead, XY 11551-0300

Phone No. (H) (555) 487-2209 (W) ______ Birthdate 3-9-54

Primary Insurance Co. Medicaid Policy/Group No. C99756E

Secondary Insurance Co. None Policy/Group No. ______

DATE	REFERENCE	DESCRIPTION	CHARGES	CREDITS		BALANCE
				PYMNTS.	ADJ.	
20xx			BALANCE FORWARD →			
9-4-xx		OV NP				
9-4-xx		12 lead ECG				
9-4-xx		Echocardiogram c̄ Doppler				
9-4-xx		Chest x-ray				

PLEASE PAY LAST AMOUNT IN BALANCE COLUMN

THIS IS A COPY OF YOUR FINANCIAL ACCOUNT AS IT APPEARS ON OUR RECORDS

Figure 13-2

Abbreviations pertinent to this record:

Pt	____________	LC	____________
SOB	____________	MDM	____________
hx	____________	Rx	____________
D	____________	retn	____________
ECG	____________	wks	____________

ASSIGNMENT 13-4 COMPLETE A CLAIM FORM FOR A MEDICAID CASE

Performance Objective

Task: Complete a CMS-1500 (02-12) claim form for a Medicaid case, post transactions to the financial accounting record, and define patient record abbreviations.

Conditions: Use the patient's record (Figure 13-3) and financial statement (Figure 13-4), one health insurance claim form (print from Evolve website), a computer, procedural and diagnostic code books, and Appendixes A and B in this *Workbook*.

Standards: Claim Productivity Measurement

Time: ______________ minutes

Accuracy: ______________

(Note: The time element and accuracy criteria may be given by your instructor.)

Directions:

1. Using NUCC guidelines, complete the Health Insurance Claim Form and direct it to Medicaid for Stephen M. Drake by referring to his patient record. Refer to Appendix A in this *Workbook* to locate the fees to record on the claim, and post them to the financial statement. On May 1, the fee for the injection of Bicillin is $10. As learned in Chapter 6, injectable drugs and medications may be billed separately for Medicaid patients. Date the claim May 26. If your instructor wants you to insert the name and address of your Medicaid fiscal agent on the claim, obtain it by going to the Evolve website listed in Internet Resources at the end of Chapter 13 in the *Handbook*. Do not list services not charged for (NC) on the claim form; however, do list postoperative follow-up visits during the global period on the financial statement. Locate the correct code number in the CPT Medicine section.

   Remember that the physician must always sign all forms on Medicaid cases; stamped signatures are not allowed.

2. Refer to Chapter 7 (Figure 7-4) in the *Handbook* for instructions on how to complete this claim form and a Medicaid template.

3. Use your CPT code book or Appendix A in this *Workbook* to determine the correct five-digit code number and modifiers for each professional service rendered. Use your HCPCS Level II code book or refer to Appendix B in this *Workbook* for HCPCS procedure codes and modifiers. If your instructor tells you to also find the ICD-10-CM codes, a draft version may be downloaded from the following website: http://www.cdc.gov/nchs/icd/icd10cm.htm.

4. Record all transactions of the financial account and indicate the date when you have billed Medicaid.

5. Refer to Appendix A in this *Workbook* for the clinic and hospital provider numbers that are needed for completing Medicaid forms.

6. On July 1, Medicaid paid $200 on this claim. Post this payment (warrant number 766504) to the patient's financial account and adjust the balance, using the same line.

7. A Performance Evaluation Checklist may be reproduced from the "Instruction Guide to the Workbook" chapter if your instructor wishes you to submit it to assist with scoring and comments.

PATIENT RECORD NO. 13-4

LAST NAME	FIRST NAME	MIDDLE NAME	BIRTH DATE	SEX	HOME PHONE
Drake	Stephen	M	04-03-91	M	555-277-5831

ADDRESS	CITY	STATE	ZIP CODE
2317 Charnwood Avenue	Woodland Hills	XY	12345

CELL PHONE	PAGER NO.	FAX NO.	E-MAIL ADDRESS

PATIENT'S SOC. SEC. NO.	DRIVER'S LICENSE
566-XX-0081	

PATIENT'S OCCUPATION	NAME OF COMPANY
full time student	

ADDRESS OF EMPLOYER	PHONE

SPOUSE OR PARENT	OCCUPATION
Mrs. Virginia B. Drake (mother)	none—family on welfare

EMPLOYER	ADDRESS	PHONE

NAME OF INSURANCE	INSURED OR SUBSCRIBER
Medicaid	

POLICY/CERTIFICATE NO.	GROUP NO.
Child's identification number	19-37-1524033-16X

REFERRED BY: James B. Jeffers, MD, 100 S. Broadway, Woodland Hills, XY 12345 Provider No. 12345069XX

DATE	PROGRESS NOTES
5-1-xx	NP comes in complaining of severe sore throat since April 4. A detailed hx was taken.
	Mother states Stephen has had many bouts of adenoid symptoms and tonsillitis since age 4. He has missed
	school on three occasions this year due to throat infections. Did complete phys exam (D)
	which showed enlargement & inflam of tonsils and adenoids. Temp 101.2. Strep culture done
	(screening) with a preliminary report; positive for strep. Administered penicillin G (Bicillin)
	1.2 million units IM and wrote Rx to start AB and continue x 10 d. Imp: Acute tonsillitis
	(LC MDM). RTO 1 week.
	GP/llf Gerald Practon, MD
5-8-xx	Pt returns; sore throat improved but still swollen. Tonsils are 4+ hypertrophic. Received
	medical records from past primary physician which indicated hx of 5 bouts of strep over
	last 3 yrs. Adv. tonsillectomy and adenoidectomy. Phoned for prior authorization 3 p.m.,
	Auth. No. 45042, given by Mrs. Jane Michaels. Pt to be admitted tomorrow for one day
	surgery (PF HX/PX SF MDM).
	GP/llf Gerald Practon, MD
5-9-xx	Admit to College Hospital. Tonsillectomy and adenoidectomy performed. Pt doing well,
	discharged 4:00 P.M. RTC 1 week.
	GP/llf Gerald Practon, MD
5-17-xx	PO visit. No complaints. Temp 98.1. Retn if necessary (PF HX/PX SF MDM).
	GP/llf Gerald Practon, MD

Figure 13-3

Acct No. 13-4

STATEMENT
Financial Account
COLLEGE CLINIC
4567 Broad Avenue
Woodland Hills, XY 12345-0001
Tel. 555-486-9002
Fax No. 555-487-8976

Stephen M. Drake
c/o Virginia B. Drake
2317 Charnwood Avenue
Woodland Hills, XY 12345

Phone No. (H) (555) 277-5831 (W) ____ Birthdate 4-3-91

Primary Insurance Co. Medicaid Policy/Group No. 19-37-1524033-16X

Secondary Insurance Co. N/A Policy/Group No. ____

DATE	REFERENCE	DESCRIPTION	CHARGES	CREDITS PYMNTS.	CREDITS ADJ.	BALANCE
20xx		BALANCE FORWARD →				
5-1-xx		NP OV				
5-1-xx		Strep culture				
5-1-xx		Injection AB				
5-1-xx		Bicillin				
5-8-xx		OV				
5-9-xx		T & A				
5-17-xx		PO OV				

PLEASE PAY LAST AMOUNT IN BALANCE COLUMN

THIS IS A COPY OF YOUR FINANCIAL ACCOUNT AS IT APPEARS ON OUR RECORDS

Figure 13-4

After the instructor has returned your work to you, either make the necessary corrections and place your work in a three-ring notebook for future reference or, if you received a high score, place it in your portfolio for reference when applying for a job.

Abbreviations pertinent to this record:

NP	______________	imp	______________
hx	______________	LC	______________
D	______________	MDM	______________
phys	______________	RTO	______________
inflam	______________	yrs	______________
temp	______________	adv	______________
strep	______________	PF	______________
IM	______________	SF	______________
Rx	______________	RTC	______________
AB	______________	PO	______________
X	______________	retn	______________
d	______________		

Additional Coding

1. Using your diagnostic code book, code the symptoms that the patient presented with on May 1, 20xx.

	Symptom	*ICD-9-CM Code*	*ICD-10-CM Code*
a.	______________	______________	______________
b.	______________	______________	______________
c.	______________	______________	______________

ASSIGNMENT 13-5 COMPLETE A CLAIM FORM FOR A MEDICAID CASE

Performance Objective

Task: Complete a CMS-1500 (02-12) claim form for a Medicaid case, post transactions to the financial accounting record, and define patient record abbreviations.

Conditions: Use the patient's record (Figure 13-5) and financial statement (Figure 13-6), one health insurance claim form (print from Evolve website), a computer, procedural and diagnostic code books, and Appendixes A and B in this *Workbook.*

Standards: Claim Productivity Measurement

Time: ______________ minutes

Accuracy: ______________

(Note: The time element and accuracy criteria may be given by your instructor.)

Directions:

1. Using NUCC guidelines, complete the Health Insurance Claim Form and direct it to Medicaid for Barry L. Brooke by referring to his patient record. Refer to Appendix A in this *Workbook* to locate the fees to record on the claim, and post them to the financial statement. The financial statement should be sent in care of (c/o) the patient's parents because he is a minor. Date the claim June 10. If your instructor wants you to insert the name and address of your Medicaid fiscal agent on the claim, obtain it by going to the Evolve website listed in Internet Resources at the end of Chapter 13 in the *Handbook*.

2. Refer to Chapter 7 (Figure 7-4) in the *Handbook* for instructions on how to complete this claim form and a Medicaid template.

3. Use your CPT code book or Appendix A in this *Workbook* to determine the diagnostic codes and the correct five-digit code number and modifiers for each professional service rendered. Use your HCPCS Level II code book or refer to Appendix B in this *Workbook* for HCPCS procedure codes and modifiers.

   If your instructor tells you to also find the ICD-10-CM codes, a draft version may be downloaded from the following website: http://www.cdc.gov/nchs/icd/icd10cm.htm.

4. Record all transactions on the financial account and indicate the date when you have billed Medicaid.

5. Refer to Appendix A in this *Workbook* for the clinic and hospital provider numbers that are needed for completing Medicaid forms.

6. On July 1, Medicaid paid $75 (warrant number 329670) on this claim. Post this payment to the patient's financial statement and adjust the balance.

7. A Performance Evaluation Checklist may be reproduced from the "Instruction Guide to the Workbook" chapter if your instructor wishes you to submit it to assist with scoring and comments.

PATIENT RECORD NO. 13-5

Brooke	Barry	L	02-03-90	M	555-487-9770
LAST NAME	FIRST NAME	MIDDLE NAME	BIRTH DATE	SEX	HOME PHONE

3821 Ocean Drive	Woodland Hills	XY	12345
ADDRESS	CITY	STATE	ZIP CODE

			brooke@wb.net
CELL PHONE	PAGER NO.	FAX NO.	E-MAIL ADDRESS

776-XX-1931	
PATIENT'S SOC. SEC. NO.	DRIVER'S LICENSE

child—full time student	
PATIENT'S OCCUPATION	NAME OF COMPANY

ADDRESS OF EMPLOYER	PHONE

Robert D. Brooke (father)	none—family on welfare (father totally disabled)
SPOUSE OR PARENT	OCCUPATION

EMPLOYER	ADDRESS	PHONE

Medicaid	Barry
NAME OF INSURANCE	INSURED OR SUBSCRIBER

54-32-7681533-10X
MEDICAID NO.

REFERRED BY: Virginia B. Drake (friend)

DATE	PROGRESS NOTES
5-28-xx	Sunday evening, new pt seen in ER at College Hospital. Pt twisted L knee while playing
	baseball at Grove Park. X-rays (3 views of L knee) were ordered –N for fx. Imp: effusion
	and ligament strain lt knee. Tx: aspirated lt knee and removed 5 cc bloody fluid.
	Discussion is held with mother and son; bracing versus casting. Mother insists on a cast
	because she states he is noncompliant and thinks he will remove the brace and injure his
	leg further. Barry agrees to have cast. Applied long leg fiberglass walking cast. Pt to be
	seen in office in 2 wks (D HX/PX M MDM).
	RS/llf Raymond Skeleton, MD
6-10-xx	Pt returns c/o continued knee pain and wants cast removed. He is in tears and says he
	has been miserable. Mother agrees to have cast removed; leg examined. Fitted pt with
	orthotic device for his knee (straight-leg canvas immobilizer, longitudinal, prefabricated $85).
	Ordered MRI without contrast of L knee to be done at College Hospital Radiology. Pt given directions and
	precautions regarding ambulation with brace (EPF HX/PX LC MDM). RTO 2 wks.
	RS/llf Raymond Skeleton, MD

Figure 13-5

Acct No. 13-5

STATEMENT

Financial Account

COLLEGE CLINIC
4567 Broad Avenue
Woodland Hills, XY 12345-0001
Tel. 555-486-9002
Fax No. 555-487-8976

Barry L Brooke
c/o Robert D. Brooke
3821 Ocean Drive
Woodland Hills, XY 12345

Phone No. (H) (555) 487-9770 (W) ______ Birthdate 2-3-90

Primary Insurance Co. Medicaid Policy/Group No. 5432768153310X

Secondary Insurance Co. ______ Policy/Group No. ______

DATE	REFERENCE	DESCRIPTION	CHARGES	CREDITS PYMNTS.	CREDITS ADJ.	BALANCE
20xx		BALANCE FORWARD →				
5-28-xx		ER				
5-28-xx		Aspiration L knee				
5-28-xx		Cast application				
6-10-xx		OV				
6-10-xx		L Knee immobilizer				

PLEASE PAY LAST AMOUNT IN BALANCE COLUMN

THIS IS A COPY OF YOUR FINANCIAL ACCOUNT AS IT APPEARS ON OUR RECORDS

Figure 13-6

After the instructor has returned your work to you, either make the necessary corrections and place your work in a three-ring notebook for future reference or, if you received a high score, place it in your portfolio for reference when applying for a job.

Abbreviations pertinent to this record:

Pt	____________	lt	____________
ER	____________	tx	____________
L	____________	cc	____________
N	____________	MRI	____________
fx	____________	RTO	____________
imp	____________	wks	____________

Additional Coding

1. Refer to Barry Brooke's medical record, abstract information, and code procedures that would be billed by outside providers.

Site	*Description of Service*	*Code*
a. College Hospital Radiology	____________	____________
b. College Hospital Central Supply	____________	____________
c. College Hospital Radiology	____________	____________

14 TRICARE and Veterans' Health Care

Marilyn T. Fordney

KEY TERMS

Your instructor may wish to select some words pertinent to this chapter for a test. For definitions of the terms, further study, and/or reference, the words, phrases, and abbreviations may be found in the glossary at the end of the Handbook. *Key terms for this chapter follow.*

active duty service member
allowable charge
authorized provider
beneficiary
catastrophic cap
catchment area
cooperative care
coordination of benefits
cost share
Defense Enrollment Eligibility Reporting System
Department of Veterans Affairs
emergency
health benefits advisor
health care finder
medically (or psychologically) necessary
Military Treatment Facility
nonparticipating physician or provider
other health insurance
participating physician or provider
partnership program
point-of-service option
preauthorization
primary care manager
quality assurance program
regional contractor
service benefit program
service-connected injury
service retiree (military retiree)
sponsor
summary payment voucher
total, permanent, service-connected disability
TRICARE Extra
TRICARE for Life
TRICARE Prime
TRICARE service center
urgent care
veteran
Veterans Health Administration

KEY ABBREVIATIONS

See how many abbreviations and acronyms you can translate and then use this as a handy reference list. Definitions for the key abbreviations are located near the back of the Handbook *in the glossary.*

ADSM ____________________

CHAMPVA ____________________

DEERS ____________________

FTM ____________________

HAC ____________________

HBA ____________________

HCF ____________________

MHS ____________________

MTF ____________________

NAS ____________________

nonpar ____________________

OHI ____________________

par ____________________

PCM ____________________

POS option ____________________

SHCP ____________________

TFL ____________________

TMA ____________________

TPR ______________________________

TPRADFM ______________________________

TSC ______________________________

USFHP ______________________________

VA ______________________________

PERFORMANCE OBJECTIVES

The student will be able to:

- Define and spell the key terms and key abbreviations for this chapter, given the information from the *Handbook* glossary, within a reasonable time period and with enough accuracy to obtain a satisfactory evaluation.
- After reading the chapter, answer the fill-in-the-blank, multiple choice, and true/false review questions with enough accuracy to obtain a satisfactory evaluation.
- Fill in the correct meaning of each abbreviation, given a list of common medical abbreviations and symbols that appear in chart notes, within a reasonable time period and with enough accuracy to obtain a satisfactory evaluation.
- Given the patient's medical chart notes, ledger cards, and blank insurance claim forms, complete each CMS-1500 (02-12) Health Insurance Claim Form for billing within a reasonable time period and with enough accuracy to obtain a satisfactory evaluation.
- Using the Mock Fee Schedule in Appendix A in this *Workbook*, correctly post payments, adjustments, and balances on the patients' ledger cards within a reasonable time period and with enough accuracy to obtain a satisfactory evaluation.
- Compute mathematical calculations, given TRICARE problem situations, within a reasonable time period and with enough accuracy to obtain a satisfactory evaluation.

STUDY OUTLINE

History of TRICARE
TRICARE Programs
- Eligibility
- Nonavailability Statement

TRICARE Standard
- Enrollment
- Identification Card
- Benefits
- Fiscal Year
- Authorized Providers of Health Care
- Preauthorization
- Payment

TRICARE Extra
- Enrollment
- Identification Card
- Benefits
- Network Provider
- Preauthorization
- Payments

TRICARE Prime
- Enrollment
- Identification Card
- Benefits
- Primary Care Manager
- Preauthorization
- Payments

TRICARE Reserve Select
TRICARE Retired Reserve
TRICARE Young Adult
TRICARE for Life
- Enrollment
- Identification Card
- Benefits
- Referral and Preauthorization
- Payment

TRICARE Plus
- Enrollment
- Identification Card
- Benefits
- Payment

TRICARE Prime Remote Program
- Enrollment
- Identification Card
- Benefits
- Referral and Preauthorization
- Payments

Supplemental Health Care Program
- Enrollment
- Identification Card
- Benefits
- Referral and Preauthorization
- Payments

ASSIGNMENT 14-1 REVIEW QUESTIONS

Part I Fill in the Blank

Review the objectives, key terms, glossary definitions of key terms, chapter information, and figures before completing the following review questions.

1. CHAMPUS, the acronym for Civilian Health and Medical Program of the Uniformed Services, is now called ________________ and was organized to control escalating medical costs and to standardize benefits for active duty families and military retirees.

2. An active duty service member is known as a/an ________________; once retired, this former member is called a/an ________________________________.

3. An individual who qualifies for TRICARE is known as a/an ________________________________.

4. A system for verifying an individual's TRICARE eligibility is called ____.

5. Mrs. Hancock, a TRICARE beneficiary, lives 2 miles from a Uniformed Services Medical Treatment Facility but needs to be hospitalized for mental health care services at Orlando Medical Center, a civilian hospital. What type of authorization does she require?
____

6. TRICARE Standard and Veterans Health Administration (CHAMPVA) beneficiary identification cards are issued to ________________ and ________________. Information must be obtained from ________________ and ________________ of the card and placed on the health insurance claim form.

7. Programs that allow TRICARE Standard beneficiaries to receive treatment, services, or supplies from civilian providers are called ________________ and ________________.

8. For patients whose sponsor is a rank of E4 and below, the TRICARE Standard deductible for outpatient care is how much per patient?________________________________
Per family? ________________________________

9. For patients whose sponsor is a rank of E5 and above, the TRICARE Standard deductible for outpatient care is how much per patient? ________________________________
Per family? ________________________________

10. For TRICARE Standard, dependents of active duty members pay what percentage for outpatient services after the deductible has been met? ________________________________
What percentage does TRICARE pay? ________________________________

11. For retired members or their dependents on TRICARE Standard, what is their deductible responsibility for outpatient services? Per person? ________________________________
Per family? ________________________________

12. For TRICARE Standard, retired members or their dependents pay what percentage for outpatient services after the deductible has been met? ______________________
What percentage does TRICARE pay? ______________________

13. A voluntary TRICARE health maintenance organization type of option is known as ______________________.

14. CHAMPVA is the acronym for ______________________, now known as the ______________________.

15. Those individuals who serve in the United States Armed Forces, finish their service, and are honorably discharged are known as ______________________.

16. Veterans Health Administration (CHAMPVA) is not an insurance program but is considered as a/an ______________________ program.

17. Which individuals are entitled to Veterans Health Administration (CHAMPVA) medical benefits?
a. ______________________
b. ______________________
c. ______________________

18. The public law establishing a person's right to review and contest inaccuracies in personal medical records is known as the ______________________.

19. An organization that contracts with the government to process TRICARE and Veterans Health Administration (CHAMPVA) health insurance claims is known as a/an ______________________.

20. The time limit for submitting a TRICARE Standard or CHAMPVA claim for outpatient service is ______________________;
for inpatient service, it is ______________________.

Part II Multiple Choice

Choose the best answer.

21. The TRICARE fiscal year
    a. begins January 1 and ends December 31.
    b. begins April 1 and ends March 30.
    c. begins June 1 and ends May 30.
    d. begins October 1 and ends September 30.

22. A health care professional who helps a patient who is under the TRICARE Standard program obtain preauthorization for care is called a/an
    a. primary care physician (PCP).
    b. health care finder (HCF).
    c. health benefits advisor (HBA).
    d. participating provider.

23. TRICARE standard beneficiaries pay a certain amount each year for the cost share and annual deductible, which is known as
    a. catastrophic cap.
    b. limiting charge.
    c. coinsurance.
    d. payment limitation.

24. To qualify for TRICARE for Life (TFL), a beneficiary must be
    a. a TRICARE beneficiary.
    b. eligible for Medicare Part A.
    c. enrolled in Medicare Part B.
    d. all of the above.

25. The time limit for filing a TRICARE Standard claim is
    a. the end of the calendar year after the fiscal year in which services were furnished.
    b. within 1 year from the date a service is provided.
    c. within 1 year from the month of service.
    d. within 2 years from when service is provided.

Part III True/False

Write "T" or "F" in the blank to indicate whether you think the statement is true or false.

________ 26. Medically necessary treatment needed for immediate illness or injury that would not result in further disability or death if not treated immediately is known as urgent care.

________ 27. TRICARE beneficiaries who use nonauthorized providers and receive medical services may be responsible for their entire bill.

________ 28. When an individual on TRICARE Prime shows you their identification card, it guarantees TRICARE eligibility.

________ 29. TRICARE Prime Remote (TPR) is a program designed for military retirees and their families.

________ 30. Beneficiaries of the Veterans Health Administration (CHAMPVA) program have complete freedom of choice in selecting their civilian health care providers.

ASSIGNMENT 14-2 CRITICAL THINKING

Performance Objective

Task: After reading the scenarios, answer the following questions, using critical thinking skills.

Conditions: Use a pen or pencil.

Standards: Time: ______________ minutes

Accuracy: ______________

(Note: The time element and accuracy criteria may be given by your instructor.)

Directions: After reading the scenarios, answer the following questions, using your critical thinking skills. Record your answers on the blank lines.

1. If Bertha Evans is seen for an office visit and has other insurance besides TRICARE, and she is the dependent of an active military person, whom do you bill first?

   ____

   Reason: ____

2. If Jason Williams, a TRICARE beneficiary who became disabled at age 10 years and who is also receiving Medicare Part A and Medicare Part B benefits, is seen for a consultation, whom do you bill first?

   ____

   Reason: ____

3. If Tanner Vine, a Veterans Health Administration (CHAMPVA) and Medicaid beneficiary, is seen on an emergency basis in the office, whom do you bill first?

   ____

   Reason: ____

ASSIGNMENT 14-3 CALCULATE MATHEMATICAL PROBLEMS

Performance Objective

Task: Calculate and insert the correct amounts for three TRICARE scenarios.

Conditions: Use a pen or pencil, the description of the problem, and calculation formulas.

Standards: Time: ____________ minutes

Accuracy: ____________

(Note: The time element and accuracy criteria may be given by your instructor.)

Directions: Calculate and insert the correct amounts for the following scenarios using these formulas.

Basic calculation formulas

TRICARE

$	TRICARE allowed amount
– ________	Minus deductible
$	Balance on which pmt calculated
× ______ %	Multiply TRICARE plan %
$	TRICARE payment

PATIENT

$	Allowed amount after deductible
× ______ %	Multiply TRICARE plan %
$	
+ ________	Add any deductible amt owed
$	Amount patient pays

ADJUSTED AMOUNT

$	Billed amount
– ________	Minus allowable amount
$	Adjusted amount

Problem 1: On October 1, in consultation, Dr. Caesar sees the wife of a Navy man who is stationed at Port Hueneme. Dr. Caesar orders her to the hospital because of a suspected ectopic pregnancy. She undergoes a laparotomy and salpingectomy. Her husband is a rank of E5. Here are her bills. Indicate what TRICARE Standard will pay.

Outpatient Services:	*TRICARE Standard*		
	Bill/Allowable	**TRICARE Payment**	**Patient Owes**
Consultation	$75	$ ________	$ ________
Inpatient services:			
Salpingectomy	$600		
Assistant surgeon	$120		
Anesthesiologist	$400		
3-day stay (drugs, laboratory tests, operating room)	$2500		
Total	$ ________		$ ________

Mathematical computations:

Problem 2: This is the same situation as in Problem 1, except that the patient is the wife of a retired military man and has TRICARE Standard.

Outpatient Services:	*TRICARE Standard*		
	Bill/Allowable	**TRICARE Payment**	**Patient Owes**
Consultation	$75	$ ________	$ ________
Inpatient services with separately billed professional charges			
	Bill/Allowable	**TRICARE Payment**	**Patient Owes**
Salpingectomy	$600	$ ________	$ ________
Assistant surgeon	$120	$ ________	$ ________
Anesthesiologist	$400	$ ________	$ ________
Inpatient services billed by hospital			
3-day stay (drugs, laboratory tests, operating room)	$2500	$ ________	
Total payment owed by patient to Dr. Caesar			$ ________

Mathematical computations:

Problem 3: A TRICARE patient whose sponsor is a rank of E5 asks Dr. Caesar to accept assignment on her medical care, and Dr. Caesar agrees. She has not met her deductible. She is the wife of an active duty man. She has TRICARE Extra.

Dr. Caesar's bill:

Consultation	$50	Allowable:	$50
Complete blood cell count	20		20
Urinalysis	5		5
Blood serology and complement fixation	25		25
Posteroanterior and lateral chest radiograph	40		40
Electrocardiogram	35		30
Spirometry	40		40
Total	$215		$210

How much is Dr. Caesar's check from TRICARE Extra? $ ______________. The patient owes the doctor $ ______________. Dr. Caesar's courtesy adjustment is $ ______________.

Mathematical computations:

ASSIGNMENT 14-4 COMPLETE A CLAIM FORM FOR A TRICARE STANDARD CASE

Performance Objective

Task: Complete a CMS-1500 (02-12) claim form for a TRICARE Standard case, post transactions to the financial accounting record, and define patient record abbreviations.

Conditions: Use the patient's record (Figure 14-1) and financial statement (Figure 14-2), one health insurance claim form (print from Evolve website), a computer, procedural and diagnostic code books, and Appendixes A and B in this *Workbook*.

Standards: Claim Productivity Measurement

Time: ______________ minutes

Accuracy: ______________

(Note: The time element and accuracy criteria may be given by your instructor.)

Directions:

1. Using NUCC guidelines, complete the CMS-1500 (02-12) claim form. If your instructor wants you to direct it to your local TRICARE fiscal intermediary, go to the website http://www.tricare.osd.mil. On the map, click on the area where you reside and then choose a state to access claims information for that state. Refer to Miss Rosa M. Sandoval's patient record for information and Appendix A to locate the fees to record on the claim and post to the financial statement. Date the claim May 31. Dr. Atrics is not accepting assignment on this TRICARE Standard case but is completing the claim for the patient's convenience. The family of this patient has not previously met its deductible.

2. Refer to Chapter 7 (Figure 7-9) of the *Handbook* for instructions on how to complete this claim form and to view a TRICARE template.

3. Use your *Current Procedural Terminology* (CPT) code book or Appendix A in this *Workbook* to determine the correct five-digit code number and modifiers for each professional service rendered. Use your Healthcare Common Procedure Coding System (HCPCS) Level II code book or refer to Appendix B in this *Workbook* for HCPCS procedure codes and modifiers. If your instructor tells you to also find the ICD-10-CM codes, a draft version may be downloaded from the following website: http://www.cdc.gov/nchs/icd/icd10cm.htm.

4. On May 8, Miss Sandoval makes a partial payment of $20 by check (No. 4013). Record the proper information on the financial record but not on the claim form, and note the date you have billed TRICARE (May 31).

5. A Performance Evaluation Checklist may be reproduced from the "Instruction Guide to the Workbook" chapter if your instructor wishes you to submit it to assist with scoring and comments.

After the instructor has returned your work to you, either make the necessary corrections and place your work in a three-ring notebook for future reference or, if you received a high score, place it in your portfolio for reference when applying for a job.

Abbreviations pertinent to this record:

pt	________________	ofc	________________
rt	________________	FU	________________
EPF	________________	retn	________________
yr(s)	________________	PO	________________
temp	________________	PF	________________
adv	________________	HX	________________
SF	________________	PX	________________
MDM	________________	wk	________________
$\bar{c}$	________________	T	________________

PATIENT RECORD NO. 14-4

Sandoval	Rosa	M	11-01-91	F	555-456-3322
LAST NAME	FIRST NAME	MIDDLE NAME	BIRTH DATE	SEX	HOME PHONE

209 West Maple Street	Woodland Hills	XY	12345
ADDRESS	CITY	STATE	ZIP CODE

CELL PHONE	PAGER NO.	FAX NO.	E-MAIL ADDRESS

994-XX-1164	
PATIENT'S SOC. SEC. NO.	DRIVER'S LICENSE

Child—full time student (lives with mother)	
PATIENT'S OCCUPATION	NAME OF COMPANY

ADDRESS OF EMPLOYER	PHONE

Hernan J. Sandoval (father)	Staff Sargeant—Grade 9 (active duty)
SPOUSE OR PARENT	OCCUPATION

United States Army	HHC 3rd Batt, 25th Infantry, APO New York, New York, 10030	
EMPLOYER	ADDRESS	PHONE

TRICARE Standard	father (DOB 2/10/70)
NAME OF INSURANCE	INSURED OR SUBSCRIBER

886-XX-0999	
POLICY/CERTIFICATE NO.	GROUP NO.

REFERRED BY: Maria Sandoval (mother)

DATE	PROGRESS NOTES
5-1-xx	New pt comes in complaining of pain in rt ear for 3 days. An EPF history was taken which
	revealed several ear infections (suppurative) over the past 3 yrs. An EPF exam revealed
	fluid and pus in rt ear. Temp 101°. Adv mother a myringotomy was necessary. Scheduled
	outpatient surg at College Hospital this afternoon. Imp: Acute rt suppurative otitis media
	(SF MDM). The prior authorization number is 2076500781.
	PA/llf Pedro Atrics, MD
5-1-xx	Pt admitted to outpatient surgery (College Hospital). Rt myringotomy c̄ aspiration
	performed. Pt did well. To be seen in ofc for FU in 2 days.
	PA/llf Pedro Atrics, MD
5-3-xx	Pt retns PO (PF HX/PX SF MDM). No pain rt ear. Pt progressing well. Retn in 1 wk.
	PA/llf Pedro Atrics, MD
5-8-xx	Pt retns PO (PF HX/PX SF MDM). T 98°, no fluid or pus in rt ear. No pain. Pt discharged,
	retn prn.
	PA/llf Pedro Atrics, MD

Figure 14-1

Acct No. 14-4

STATEMENT
Financial Account

COLLEGE CLINIC
4567 Broad Avenue
Woodland Hills, XY 12345-0001
Tel. 555-486-9002
Fax No. 555-487-8976

Rosa M. Sandoval
c/o Maria Sandoval
209 West Maple Street
Woodland Hills, XY 12345-0001

Phone No. (H) (555) 456-3322 (W) ______ Birthdate 11-9-91

Primary Insurance Co. TRICARE Standard Policy/Group No. 886-XX-0999

Secondary Insurance Co. ______ Policy/Group No. ______

DATE	REFERENCE	DESCRIPTION	CHARGES	CREDITS PYMNTS.	CREDITS ADJ.	BALANCE
20xx		BALANCE FORWARD →				
5-1-xx		NP OV				
5-1-xx		Myringotomy				
5-3-xx		PO OV				
5-8-xx		PO OV				

PLEASE PAY LAST AMOUNT IN BALANCE COLUMN

THIS IS A COPY OF YOUR FINANCIAL ACCOUNT AS IT APPEARS ON OUR RECORDS

Figure 14-2

ASSIGNMENT 14-5 COMPLETE A CLAIM FORM FOR A TRICARE EXTRA CASE

Performance Objective

Task: Complete a CMS-1500 (02-12) claim form for a TRICARE Extra case, post transactions to the financial accounting record, and define patient record abbreviations.

Conditions: Use the patient's record (Figure 14-3) and financial statement (Figure 14-4), one health insurance claim form (print from Evolve website), a computer, procedural and diagnostic code books, and Appendixes A and B in this *Workbook*.

Standards: Claim Productivity Measurement

Time: ______________ minutes

Accuracy: ______________

(Note: The time element and accuracy criteria may be given by your instructor.)

Directions:

1. Using NUCC guidelines, complete the CMS-1500 (02-12) claim form. If your instructor wants you to direct it to your local TRICARE fiscal intermediary, go to the website http://www.tricare.osd.mil. On the map, click on the area where you reside and then choose a state to access claims information for that state. Refer to Mrs. Darlene B. Drew's patient record for information and Appendix A to locate the fees to record on the claim and post to the financial statement. Date the claim February 3. Assume that the Nonavailability Statement (NAS) has been transmitted electronically so that the physician can treat the patient at College Hospital. Dr. Ulibarri is accepting assignment on this TRICARE Extra case. This patient met her deductible last November when seen by a previous physician.

2. Refer to Chapter 7 (Figure 7-9) of the *Handbook* for instructions on how to complete this claim form and to view a TRICARE template.

3. Use your CPT code book or Appendix A in this *Workbook* to determine the correct five-digit code number and modifiers for each professional service rendered. Use your HCPCS Level II code book or refer to Appendix B in this *Workbook* for HCPCS procedure codes and modifiers. If your instructor tells you to also find the ICD-10-CM codes, a draft version may be downloaded from the following website: http://www.cdc.gov/nchs/icd/icd10cm.htm.

4. Record the proper information on the financial record and claim form and note the date when you have billed TRICARE Extra.

5. A Performance Evaluation Checklist may be reproduced from the "Instruction Guide to the Workbook" chapter if your instructor wishes you to submit it to assist with scoring and comments.

After the instructor has returned your work to you, either make the necessary corrections and place your work in a three-ring notebook for future reference, or, if you received a high score, place it in your portfolio for reference when applying for a job.

Abbreviations pertinent to this record:

Pt	________________	LC	________________
D	________________	MDM	________________
HX	________________	PF	________________
PX	________________	rec	________________
UA	________________	SF	________________
WBC	________________	C	________________
RBC	________________	M	________________
cc	________________	surg	________________
lab	________________	ofc	________________
Rx	________________	PO	________________
caps	________________	OV	________________
t.i.d	________________	rtn	________________
Retn	________________	PRN	________________
Dx	________________		

PATIENT RECORD NO. 14-5

LAST NAME	FIRST NAME	MIDDLE NAME	BIRTH DATE	SEX	HOME PHONE
Drew	Darlene	B	12-22-51	F	555-466-1002

ADDRESS	CITY	STATE	ZIP CODE
720 Ganley Street,	Woodland Hills,	XY	12345

CELL PHONE	PAGER NO.	FAX NO.	E-MAIL ADDRESS
555-320-9988	555-210-9400	555-466-1002	drew@wb.net

PATIENT'S SOC. SEC. NO.	DRIVER'S LICENSE
450-XX-3762	H0492188

PATIENT'S OCCUPATION	NAME OF COMPANY
Seamstress	J. B. Talon Company

ADDRESS OF EMPLOYER	PHONE
2111 Ventura Road, Merck, XY 12346	555-733-0156

SPOUSE OR PARENT	OCCUPATION
Harry M. Drew	U.S. Navy Lieutenant Commander (L/C), Active Status

Service #221-XX-0711 Social Security No. 221-XX-0711 Grade12 — BIRTH DATE: 4-15-37

ADDRESS: P.O. Box 2927, A.P.O., New York, New York 09194

NAME OF INSURANCE	TRICARE EXTRA I.D. CARD NO.	EFFECTIVE DATE
TRICARE Extra	67531	01-01-80

REFERRED BY: James B. Jeffers, MD, 100 S. Broadway, Woodland Hills, XY 12345 Tax ID#77621074X

DATE	PROGRESS NOTES
1-13-xx	New pt comes in complaining of large sore in vagina causing extreme pain. Performed a
	D HX/PX. UA (non-automated with microscopy) loaded with WBCs and RBCs. Upon pelvic
	examination, a very tender mass is located in the paraurethral area (Skene's gland).
	I incised and drained the abscess and obtained 10 cc greenish pus; took culture and sent
	to lab. Pt feels much better. Rx Terramycin 30 caps 1 t.i.d. Retn in 5 days. Dx: Paraurethral
	abscess (LC/MDM).
	GU/llf Gene Ulibarri, MD
1-18-xx	Pt returns and a PF HX/PX performed. Abscess is filled with fluid again, opened, and a
	wick of Iodoform gauze placed to help with drainage. Rec daily sitz baths and outpatient
	hospitalization to remove gland. Culture results show pseudomonas organism.
	Arrangements made for surgery on the 24th, admit at 5:30 a.m., surgery at 7:30 a.m.
	(SF MDM).
	GU/llf Gene Ulibarri, MD
1-24-xx	Admit to College Hospital outpatient facility (C HX/PX M MDM). Surg: Excision of Skene's
	gland. To be seen in ofc next week for PO exam. Renewed Rx Terramycin.
	GU/llf Gene Ulibarri, MD
1-27-xx	PO OV (PF HX/PX SF/MDM). Pt doing well. No pain, urethral tissue and perineum looks
	healthy, healing well. Rtn PRN.
	GU/llf Gene Ulibarri, MD

Figure 14-3

Acct No. 14-5

STATEMENT
Financial Account
COLLEGE CLINIC
4567 Broad Avenue
Woodland Hills, XY 12345-0001
Tel. 555-486-9002
Fax No. 555-487-8976

Darlene B. Drew
720 Ganley Street
Woodland Hills, XY 12345

Phone No. (H) 555-466-1002 (W) 555-733-0156 Birthdate 12-22-51

Primary Insurance Co. TRICARE Extra Policy/Group No. 221-XX-0711

Secondary Insurance Co. ______ Policy/Group No. ______

DATE	REFERENCE	DESCRIPTION	CHARGES	CREDITS PYMNTS.	CREDITS ADJ.	BALANCE
20xx		BALANCE FORWARD →				
1-13-xx		NP OV				
1-13-xx		UA				
1-13-xx		Drainage of Skene's gland abscess				
1-13-xx		Handling/Transport culture specimen				
1-18-xx		OV				
1-24-xx		Excision Skene's gland				
1-27-xx		PO OV				

PLEASE PAY LAST AMOUNT IN BALANCE COLUMN

THIS IS A COPY OF YOUR FINANCIAL ACCOUNT AS IT APPEARS ON OUR RECORDS

Figure 14-4

ASSIGNMENT 14-6 COMPLETE THREE CLAIM FORMS FOR A TRICARE STANDARD CASE

Performance Objective

Task: Complete three CMS-1500 (02-12) claim forms for a TRICARE Standard case, post transactions to the financial accounting record, and define patient record abbreviations.

Conditions: Use the patient's record (Figure 14-5) and financial statement (Figure 14-6), health insurance claim forms (print from Evolve website), a computer, procedural and diagnostic code books, and Appendixes A and B in this *Workbook*.

Standards: Claim Productivity Measurement

Time: ______________ minutes

Accuracy: ______________

(Note: The time element and accuracy criteria may be given by your instructor.)

Directions:

1. This case requires three claim forms. Make photocopies of a CMS-1500 (02-12) claim form or print from Evolve website. Using NUCC guidelines, complete the CMS-1500 (02-12) claim forms. If your instructor wants you to direct them to your local TRICARE fiscal intermediary, go to the website http://www.tricare.osd.mil. On the map, click on the area where you reside and then choose a state to access claims information for that state. Refer to Mrs. Mae I. Abbreviate's patient record for information and Appendix A in this *Workbook* to locate the fees to record on the claim, and post them to the financial statement. Date the claims January 31. Dr. Coccidioides is not accepting assignment on this TRICARE Standard case but is completing the claim for the patient's convenience.

2. Refer to Chapter 7 (Figure 7-9) of the *Handbook* for instructions on how to complete these claim forms and to view a TRICARE template.

3. Use your CPT code book or Appendix A in this *Workbook* to determine the correct five-digit code number and modifiers for each professional service rendered. Use your HCPCS Level II code book or refer to Appendix B in this *Workbook* for HCPCS procedure codes and modifiers. If your instructor tells you to also find the ICD-10-CM codes, a draft version may be downloaded from the following website: http://www.cdc.gov/nchs/icd/icd10cm.htm.

4. Record the proper information on the financial record and note the date when you have billed TRICARE.

5. A Performance Evaluation Checklist may be reproduced from the "Instruction Guide to the Workbook" chapter if your instructor wishes you to submit it to assist with scoring and comments.

After the instructor has returned your work to you, either make the necessary corrections and place your work in a three-ring notebook for future reference, or, if you received a high score, place it in your portfolio for reference when applying for a job.

Abbreviations pertinent to this record:

NP	________	F	________
W	________	P	________
PE	________	R	________
CC	________	EENT	________
wk	________	GGE	________
X	________	HC	________
pt	________	MDM	________
PH	________	STAT	________
UCHD	________	CBC	________
T & A	________	diff	________
aet	________	WBC	________
Grav	________	RTO	________
Para1	________	RTW	________
D & C	________	CT	________
DUB	________	dx	________
LMP	________	a.m.	________
surg	________	D	________
OS	________	MC	________
yr	________	cm	________
FH	________	lt	________
CA	________	C & S	________
L & W	________	gm	________
GB	________	mg	________
SH	________	IM	________
PX	________	retn	________
ht	________	ofc	________
wt	________	OV	________
lbs	________	PF	________
BP	________	SF	________
T	________	HC	________

Additional Coding

1. Refer to Mrs. Abbreviate's medical record, abstract information, and code procedures that would be billed by outside providers.

Site	*Description of Service*	*Code*
a. College Hospital Radiology	____________	____________
b. College Hospital Laboratory	____________	____________
c. College Hospital Laboratory	____________	____________
d. College Hospital Radiology	____________	____________
e. College Hospital Microbiology	____________	____________
f. College Hospital Radiology	____________	____________

2. Use your diagnostic code book and code the symptoms that the patient complained of on January 14, 20xx.

Symptom	*ICD-9-CM Code*	*ICD-10-CM Code*
a. ____________	____________	____________
b. ____________	____________	____________
c. ____________	____________	____________
d. ____________	____________	____________

PATIENT RECORD NO. 14-6

LAST NAME	FIRST NAME	MIDDLE NAME	BIRTH DATE	SEX	HOME PHONE
Abbreviate	Mae	I	01-02-52	F	555-986-7667

ADDRESS	CITY	STATE	ZIP CODE
4667 Symbol Road	Woodland Hills	XY	12345

CELL PHONE	PAGER NO.	FAX NO.	E-MAIL ADDRESS
555-740-3300		555-986-7667	abbreviate@wb.net

PATIENT'S SOC. SEC. NO.	DRIVER'S LICENSE
865-XX-2311	E0598247

PATIENT'S OCCUPATION	NAME OF COMPANY
administrative assistant	U. R. Wright Company

ADDRESS OF EMPLOYER	PHONE
6789 Abridge Road, Woodland Hills, XY 12346	555-988-7540

SPOUSE OR PARENT	OCCUPATION
Shorty S. Abbreviate	Staff Sargeant, Grade 12 (Active Duty)

EMPLOYER	ADDRESS	PHONE
United States Army	HHC, 2nd Batt., 27th Infantry, APO New York, New York, 10030	

NAME OF INSURANCE	INSURED OR SUBSCRIBER
TRICARE Standard	husband (DOB 3/25/40)

POLICY/CERTIFICATE NO.	GROUP NO.
023-XX-7866	

REFERRED BY: Jane B. Accurate (friend)

Figure 14-5a

Continued

DATE	PROGRESS NOTES No. 14-6
1-14-xx	NP, 45-year-old W F in for complete PE. CC: Recent onset of flu-like symptoms of
	approximate 2 wk duration, including cough; chest pain X 2 days. Pt states beginning to
	cough up moderate amounts of greenish sputum with blood streaks, fatigue, fever, and chills.
	Comprehensive history includes PH: UCHD, T & A aet 6, Grav 1 Para 1, D & C aet 41 for
	DUB, LMP 12-18-XX, surg on OS after accident last yr. FH: Father expired of kidney CA aet
	63; mother L & W after GB surg in 1999; no siblings. SH: Pt admits to past alcohol abuse,
	denies alcohol use in last 6 months. No smoking, denies drug abuse. Comprehensive PX:
	Ht 5' 7", wt 150 lbs, BP 150/80, T 100.5 F, P 88, R 18; EENT $\overline{o}$ except OS opaque;
	chest, rales scattered bilaterally, pt is dyspneic. Abdomen soft, nontender.
	GGE (HC MDM). Pt would like to avoid hospitalization if at all possible. Sent to College
	Hospital for STAT chest x-ray (2 views) and laboratory tests (electrolyte panel and complete
	CBC, automated with diff WBC. RTO tomorrow morning for test results. Disability from work began Jan. 13
	Completed disability form for work; estimated RTW, 2 weeks.
	BC/llf Brady Coccicioides, MD
1-14-xx	Call received from hospital radiology department: Chest x-rays revealed probable lung
	abscess in left lower lobe; inconclusive. Ordered STAT CT of thorax without contrast for
	more definitive dx. Contacted pt and recommended she have CT done this evening.
	RTO tomorrow a.m.
	BC/llf Brady Coccicioides, MD
1-15-xx	Pt returns to office for test results (D HX/PX MC/MDM). CT reveals lung abscess of
	3.0 cm in lt lower lobe. Pt able to produce sputum for C & S (Gram stain smear), sent to
	College Hospital laboratory, microbiology department. Rocephin (Ceftriaxone sodium)
	1 gm ($5 per 250 mg and 1000 mg = 1 gm) given IM in office, instructed pt to retn to ofc daily
	for Rocephin injections; reevaluate on Friday.
	BC/llf Brady Coccicioides, MD
1-16-xx	Rocephin 1 gm IM ordered by Dr. Coccicioides; administered by medical assistant in left
	gluteus maximus.
	BC/llf Ali Marie Hobkins, CMA
1-17-xx	Rocephin 1 gm IM ordered by Dr. Coccicioides; administered by medical assistant in right
	gluteus maximus.
	BC/llf Ali Marie Hobkins, CMA
1-18-xx	Pt returns for reevaluation (OV PF HX/PX SF MDM). Culture revealed streptococcal
	pneumoniae. Administered Rocephin 1 gm IM. Will continue daily injections.
	Arrangements made for house call over weekend.
	BC/llf Brady Coccicioides, MD
1-19-xx	HC Saturday (PF HX/PX SF MDM). Rocephin 1 gm IM. Pt states she is feeling much
	better, fatigue gone, cough decreased, afebrile. Ordered repeat chest x-ray (2 views) at
	College Hospital Monday. RTO Monday afternoon.
	BC/llf Brady Coccicioides, MD
1-21-xx	OV (PF HX/PX SF MDM). Repeat chest x-ray negative except few residual shadows.
	No injection today, start oral antibiotics. Pt to return in 1 wk for f/u or call sooner if
	symptoms reappear. Estimated RTW, 1/28/XX.
	BC/llf Brady Coccicioides, MD

Figure 14-5b, cont'd

Acct No. 14-6

STATEMENT
Financial Account
COLLEGE CLINIC
4567 Broad Avenue
Woodland Hills, XY 12345-0001
Tel. 555-486-9002
Fax No. 555-487-8976

Mae I. Abbreviate
4667 Symbol Road
Woodland Hills, XY 12345

Phone No. (H) 555-986-7667 (W) 555-988-7540 Birthdate 01/02/52

Primary Insurance Co. TRICARE Standard Policy/Group No. 023-XX-7866

Secondary Insurance Co. ________ Policy/Group No. ________

DATE	REFERENCE	DESCRIPTION	CHARGES	CREDITS		BALANCE
				PYMNTS.	ADJ.	
20xx		BALANCE FORWARD →				
1-14-xx		NP OV				
1-15-xx		OV				
1-15-xx		Injection AB				
1-15-xx		Rocefin 1 gm				
1-16-xx		Injection AB				
1-16-xx		Rocefin 1 gm				
1-17-xx		Injection AB				
1-17-xx		Rocefin 1 gm				
1-18-xx		OV				
1-18-xx		Injection AB				
1-18-xx		Rocefin 1 gm				
1-19-xx		HC				
1-19-xx		Injection AB				
1-19-xx		Rocefin 1 gm				
1-21-xx		OV				

PLEASE PAY LAST AMOUNT IN BALANCE COLUMN

THIS IS A COPY OF YOUR FINANCIAL ACCOUNT AS IT APPEARS ON OUR RECORDS

Figure 14-6

STUDENT SOFTWARE CHALLENGE

ASSIGNMENT 14-7 FOR TRICARE CASE 7 ONSCREEN COMPLETION OF CMS-1500 (02-12) INSURANCE CLAIM FORM

Performance Objective

Task: Enter transactions from patient's onscreen encounter form (superbill) and complete block-by-block onscreen health insurance claim form.

Conditions: Onscreen encounter form (superbill) and computer

Standards: Time: ______________ minutes

Accuracy: ______________

(Note: The time element and accuracy criteria may be given by your instructor.)

Directions: Log on to your Evolve account at http://evolve.elsevier.com and access the student resources for Fordney: *Insurance Handbook for the Medical Office,* 13th edition. Then choose Student Software Challenge.

1. For this assignment, follow the instructions for entering data into the onscreen CMS-1500 (02-12) health insurance claim form, completing blocks 1 through 33 for Case 7.
2. Use your CPT code book or Appendix A in this *Workbook* to determine the correct five-digit code number and modifiers for each professional service rendered. If your instructor tells you to also find the ICD-10-CM codes, a draft version may be downloaded from the following website: http://www.cdc.gov/nchs/icd/icd10cm.htm.
3. A Performance Evaluation Checklist may be reproduced from the "Instruction Guide to the Workbook" chapter if your instructor wishes you to submit it to assist with scoring and comments.
4. Print a hard copy of the completed health insurance claim form.
5. After the instructor has returned your work to you, either make the necessary corrections and place your work in a three-ring notebook for future reference, or, if you received a high score, place it in your portfolio for reference when applying for a job.

15 Workers' Compensation

Marilyn T. Fordney

KEY TERMS

Your instructor may wish to select some words pertinent to this chapter for a test. For definitions of the terms, further study, and/or reference, the words, phrases, and abbreviations may be found in the glossary at the end of the Handbook. *Key terms for this chapter follow.*

accident
adjudication
by report
claims examiner
compromise and release
deposition
ergonomic
extraterritorial
Federal Employees' Compensation Act
fee schedule
injury
insurance adjuster
lien
medical service order
nondisability claim
occupational illness or disease
Occupational Safety and Health Administration
permanent and stationary
permanent disability
petition
second-injury fund
sequelae
sub rosa films
subsequent-injury fund
temporary disability
third-party liability
third-party subrogation
waiting period
work hardening
Workers' Compensation Appeals Board
workers' compensation insurance

KEY ABBREVIATIONS

See how many abbreviations and acronyms you can translate and then use this as a handy reference list. Definitions for the key abbreviations are located near the back of the Handbook *in the glossary.*

AME ______________________

BR ______________________

C&R ______________________

ERISA ______________________

FECA ______________________

IAIABC ______________________

IME ______________________

LHWCA ______________________

MSDS ______________________

ND claim ______________________

OSHA ______________________

P&S ______________________

PD ______________________

QME ______________________

ROM ______________________

SIF ______________________

TD ______________________

WCAB ______________________

WP ______________________

PERFORMANCE OBJECTIVES

The student will be able to:

- Define and spell the key terms and key abbreviations for this chapter, given the information from the *Handbook* glossary, within a reasonable time period and with enough accuracy to obtain a satisfactory evaluation.
- After reading the chapter, answer the fill-in-the-blank, multiple choice, and true/false review questions with enough accuracy to obtain a satisfactory evaluation.
- Given a list of common medical abbreviations and symbols that appear in chart notes, fill in the correct meaning of each abbreviation within a reasonable time period and with enough accuracy to obtain a satisfactory evaluation.
- Given the patients' medical chart notes, ledger cards, and blank insurance forms, complete each workers' compensation form for billing, within a reasonable time period and with enough accuracy to obtain a satisfactory evaluation.
- Given the patients' medical chart notes, ledger cards, and blank insurance claim forms, complete each CMS-1500 (02-12) Health Insurance Claim Form for submission to a workers' compensation insurance company within a reasonable time period and with enough accuracy to obtain a satisfactory evaluation.
- Using the Mock Fee Schedule in Appendix A in this *Workbook*, correctly post payments, adjustments, and balances on the patients' ledger cards within a reasonable time period and with enough accuracy to obtain a satisfactory evaluation.

STUDY OUTLINE

History
- Workers' Compensation Statutes
- Workers' Compensation Reform

Workers' Compensation Laws and Insurance
- Purposes of Workers' Compensation Laws
- Self-Insurance
- Managed Care

Eligibility
- Industrial Accident
- Occupational Illness

Coverage
- Federal Laws
- State Laws
- State Disability and Workers' Compensation

Benefits

Types of State Claims
- Nondisability Claim
- Temporary Disability Claim
- Permanent Disability Claim

Fraud and Abuse

Occupational Safety and Health Administration Act of 1970
- Background
- Coverage
- Regulations
- Filing a Complaint
- Inspection
- Record Keeping and Reporting

Legal Situations
- Medical Evaluator
- Depositions
- Medical Testimony
- Liens
- Third-Party Subrogation

Medical Reports
- Health Information Record Keeping
- Terminology

Reporting Requirements
- Employer's Report
- Medical Service Order
- Physician's First Report
- Progress or Supplemental Report
- Final Report

Claim Submission
- Financial Responsibility
- Fee Schedules
- Helpful Billing Tips
- Billing Claims
- Out-of-State Claims
- Delinquent or Slow Pay Claims

Procedure 15-1: Completing the Doctor's First Report of Occupational Injury or Illness

ASSIGNMENT 15-1 REVIEW QUESTIONS

Part I Fill in the Blank

Review the objectives, key terms, glossary definitions of key terms, chapter information, and figures before completing the following review questions.

1. Name two kinds of statutes under workers' compensation.

   a. ______________________________

   b. ______________________________

2. An unexpected, unintended event that occurs at a particular time and place, causing injury to an individual not of his or her own making, is called a/an

   ______________________________.

3. Maria Cardoza works in a plastics manufacturing company and inhales some fumes that cause bronchitis. Because this condition is associated with her employment, it is called a/an

   ______________________________.

4. Name the federal workers' compensation acts that cover workers.

   a. ______________________________

   b. ______________________________

   c. ______________________________

   d. ______________________________

5. State compensation laws that require each employer to accept its provisions and provide for specialized benefits for employees who are injured at work are called

   ______________________________.

6. State compensation laws that may be accepted or rejected by the employer are

   known as ______________________________.

7. State five methods used for funding workers' compensation.

   a. ______________________________

   b. ______________________________

   c. ______________________________

   d. ______________________________

   e. ______________________________

8. Who pays the workers' compensation insurance premiums?

   ____

9. What is the time limit in your state for submitting the employers' and/or physicians' report on an industrial accident?

   ____

10. When an employee with a preexisting condition is injured at work and the injury produces a disability greater than what would have been caused by the second injury alone, the benefits are derived from a/an

____.

11. Name jobs that may not be covered by workers' compensation insurance.

a. ____

b. ____

c. ____

d. ____

e. ____

f. ____

12. What is the minimum number of employees per business needed in your state for workers' compensation statutes to become effective? _______________

13. What waiting period must elapse in your state before workers' compensation payments begin? _______________

14. List five types of workers' compensation benefits.

a. ____

b. ____

c. ____

d. ____

e. ____

15. Who can treat an industrial injury?

____

____

16. What are three types of workers' compensation claims and the differences among them?

a. ____

____

b. ____

____

c. ____

____

17. Weekly temporary disability payments are based on

____.

18. After suffering an industrial injury, Mr. Fields is in a treatment program in which he is given real work tasks for building strength and endurance. This form of therapy is called ______________________________.

19. When an industrial case reaches the time for rating the disability, this is accomplished by what state agency? ______________________________

20. May an injured person appeal his or her case if he or she is not satisfied with the rating? ______________________________ If so, to whom does he or she appeal? ______________________________ or ______________________________

21. When fraud or abuse is suspected in a workers' compensation case, the physician should report the situation to ______________________________.

22. Explain third-party subrogation.

____

____

23. When an individual suffers a work-related injury or illness, the employer must complete and send a form called a/an ______________________________ to the insurance company and workers' compensation state offices, and if the employee is sent to a physician's office for medical care, the employer must complete a form called a/an ______________________________, which authorizes the physician to treat the employee.

Part II Multiple Choice

Choose the best answer.

24. Employers are required to meet health and safety standards for their employees under federal and state statutes known as the
    a. Occupational Safety and Health Administration (OSHA) Act of 1970.
    b. Health Insurance Portability and Accountability Act (HIPAA).
    c. Clinical Laboratory Improvement Amendment (CLIA).
    d. Employee Retirement Income Security Act (ERISA).

25. The process of carrying on a lawsuit is called
    a. lien.
    b. litigation.
    c. deposition.
    d. adjudication.

26. A proceeding during which an attorney questions a witness who answers under oath but not in open court is called a/an
    a. subpoena.
    b. subrogation.
    c. petition.
    d. deposition.

27. The legal promise of a patient to satisfy a debt to the physician from proceeds received from a litigated case is termed a/an
    a. medical service order.
    b. subpoena.
    c. lien.
    d. promissory note.

28. When a physician treats an industrial injury, he or she must complete a First Treatment Medical Report or Doctor's First Report of Occupational Injury or Illness and send it to the following:
    a. Insurance carrier
    b. Employer
    c. State workers' compensation office
    d. All of the above

Part III True/False

Write "T" or "F" in the blank to indicate whether you think the statement is true or false.

________ 29. The first thing an employee should do after he or she is injured on the job is to notify his or her employer or immediate supervisor.

________ 30. A roofer takes his girlfriend to a roofing job and she is injured. She is covered under workers' compensation insurance.

________ 31. A stamped physician's signature is acceptable on the Doctor's First Report of Occupational Injury or Illness form.

________ 32. In a workers' compensation case, bills should be submitted monthly or at the time of termination of treatment, and a claim becomes delinquent after a time frame of 45 days.

________ 33. If an individual seeks medical care for a workers' compensation injury from another state, the state's regulations are followed in which the injured person's claim was originally filed.

________ 34. When a patient arrives at a medical office and says he or she was hurt at work, you should verify insurance information with the benefits coordinator for the employer.

ASSIGNMENT 15-2 COMPLETE A DOCTOR'S FIRST REPORT OF OCCUPATIONAL INJURY OR ILLNESS FORM FOR A WORKERS' COMPENSATION CASE

Performance Objective

Task: Complete a Doctor's First Report of Occupational Injury or Illness form and define patient record abbreviations.

Conditions: Use the patient's record (Figure 15-1), a Doctor's First Report of Occupational Injury or Illness form (Figure 15-2), and a computer.

Standards: Claim Productivity Measurement

Time: ______________ minutes

Accuracy: ______________

(Note: The time element and accuracy criteria may be given by your instructor.)

Directions:

1. Complete the Doctor's First Report of Occupational Injury or Illness form (see Figure 15-2) for this nondisability type of claim.

2. Define abbreviations found in the patient's medical record.

After the instructor has returned your work to you, either make the necessary corrections and place your work in a three-ring notebook for future reference or, if you received a high score, place it in your portfolio for reference when applying for a job.

Abbreviations pertinent to this record:

Apt	______________	CT	______________
Lt	______________	Neg	______________
pt	______________	MC	______________
ED	______________	MDM	______________
Hosp	______________	DC	______________
ER	______________	PD	______________
C	______________	FU	______________
HX	______________	Wks	______________
PX	______________	Approx	______________
c/o	______________	RTW	______________
L	______________	WC	______________

PATIENT RECORD NO. 15-2-3

LAST NAME	FIRST NAME	MIDDLE NAME	BIRTH DATE	SEX	HOME PHONE
Hiranuma	Glen	M	12-24-55	M	555-467-3383

ADDRESS	CITY	STATE	ZIP CODE
4372 Hanley Avenue	Woodland Hills	XY	12345

CELL PHONE	PAGER NO.	FAX NO.	E-MAIL ADDRESS
555-908-3433		555-467-3383	hiranuma@wb.net

PATIENT'S SOC. SEC. NO.	DRIVER'S LICENSE
558-XX-9960	U3402189

PATIENT'S OCCUPATION	NAME OF COMPANY
house painter	Pittsburgh Paint Company (commercial painting company)

ADDRESS OF EMPLOYER	PHONE
3725 Bonfeld Avenue, Woodland Hills, XY 12345	555-486-9070

SPOUSE OR PARENT	OCCUPATION
Esme M. Hiranuma	homemaker

EMPLOYER	ADDRESS	PHONE

NAME OF INSURANCE: State Compensation Insurance Fund, 14156 Magnolia Boulevard, Torres, XY 12349

POLICY/CERTIFICATE NO.	GROUP NO.
016-2432-211	

REFERRED BY: Pittsburgh Paint Company

DATE	PROGRESS NOTES
5-22-xx	At 9:30 a.m. this ♂ house painter was painting an apt ceiling (apt located at 3540 W. 87th Street, Woodland Hills, XY 12345, County of Woodland Hills) when he slipped and fell from a tall ladder landing on his head and lt side of body; brief unconsciousness for approximately 15 minutes. Employer was notified by coworker and pt was sent to College Hosp ED. I was called to the hosp at request of employer and saw pt in ER at 5 p.m. (performed a C HX/PX). Pt c/o L shoulder pain and swelling; L leg and hip pain; neck and head pain. X-rays were taken of lt hip (complete), lt femur (2 views), and cervical spine (3 views) as well as CT of brain (without contrast)—all neg. I admitted pt for overnight stay in hosp for concussion. Applied sling for L shoulder sprain. Cleaned and dressed L hip and leg abrasions (MC/MDM). Plan to DC 5/23/xx. No PD expected. Pt to FU in 2 wks. Approx. RTW 6/6 xx. Prepared WC report.
	GP/llf Gerald Practon, MD
5-23-xx	Pt's HA gone. Vital signs normal. Discharged home. RTO 1 wk.
	GP/llf Gerald Practon, MD

Figure 15-1

DOCTOR'S FIRST REPORT OF OCCUPATIONAL INJURY OR ILLNESS

Within 5 days of initial examination, for every occupational injury or illness, send 2 copies of this report to the employers' workers' compensation insurance carrier or the self-insured employer. Failure to file a timely doctor's report may result in assessment of a civil penalty. In the case of diagnosed or suspected pesticide poisoning, send a copy of this report to Division of Labor Statistics and Research.

1. INSURER NAME AND ADDRESS

2. EMPLOYER NAME Policy No.

3. Address No. and Street City Zip

4. Nature of business (e.g., food manufacturing, building construction, retailer of women's clothes)

5. PATIENT NAME (first, middle initial, last name) | 6. Sex ☐Male ☐Female | 7. Date of Birth Mo. Day Yr.

8. Address No. and Street City Zip | 9. Telephone Number

10. Occupation (Specific job title) | 11. Social Security Number

12. Injured at: No. and Street City County

13. Date and hour of injury or onset or illness Mo. Day Yr. Hour _____a.m____p.m | 14. Date last worked Mo. Day Yr.

15. Date and hour of first examination or treatment Mo. Day Yr. Hour _____a.m____p.m | 16. Have you (or your office) previously treated patient? ☐Yes ☐No

Patient please complete this portion, if able to do so. Otherwise, doctor please complete immediately. Inability or failure of a patient to complete this portion shall not affect his/her rights to workers' compensation under the Labor Code.
17. DESCRIBE HOW THE ACCIDENT OR EXPOSURE HAPPENED (Give specific object, machinery or chemical.)

18. SUBJECTIVE COMPLAINTS (Describe fully.)

19. OBJECTIVE FINDINGS

A. Physical examination

B. X-ray and laboratory results (State if none or pending.)

20. DIAGNOSIS (If occupational illness specify etiologic agent and duration of exposure.) Chemical or toxic compound involved? ICD-9 Code ☐Yes ☐No

21. Are your findings and diagnosis consistent with patient's account of injury or onset of illness? ☐Yes ☐No If "no" please explain

22. Is there any other current condition that will impede or delay patient's recovery? ☐ Yes ☐ No If "yes" please explain

23. TREATMENT REQUIRED

24. If further treatment required, specify treatment plan/estimated duration.

25. If hospitalized as inpatient, give hospital name and location Date admitted Mo. Day Yr. Estimated stay

26. WORK STATUS –Is patient able to perfom usual work? ☐ Yes ☐ No
If "no," date when patient can return to: Regular work____/____/
Modified work____/____/ Specify restrictions

Doctor's Signature ________ License Number ________
Doctor's Name and Degree ________ IRS Number ________
Address ________ Telephone Number ________

Figure 15-2

ASSIGNMENT 15-3 COMPLETE A CLAIM FORM FOR A WORKERS' COMPENSATION CASE

Performance Objectives

Task: Complete a CMS-1500 (02-12) claim form for a workers' compensation case and post transactions to the financial accounting record.

Conditions: Use the patient's record (see Figure 15-1) and financial statement (Figure 15-3), a CMS-1500 (02-12) claim form (print from Evolve website), a computer, procedural and diagnostic code books, and Appendix A in this *Workbook*.

Standards: Claim Productivity Measurement

Time: ______________ minutes

Accuracy: ______________

(Note: The time element and accuracy criteria may be given by your instructor.)

Directions:

1. Using NUCC guidelines, complete a CMS-1500 (02-12) claim form and direct it to the proper workers' compensation carrier. Refer to Mr. Glen M. Hiranuma's patient record for information and Appendix A in this *Workbook* to locate the fees to record on the claim, and post them to the financial statement. Date the claim May 24 of the current year.

2. Refer to Chapter 7 (Figure 7-11) of the *Handbook* for instructions on how to complete this claim form and a workers' compensation template.

3. Use your CPT code book or Appendix A in this *Workbook* to determine the correct five-digit code number and modifiers for each professional service rendered. Use your HCPCS Level II code book or refer to Appendix B in this Workbook for HCPCS procedure codes and modifiers. Note: In your state, a workers' compensation fee schedule may be available with this information. If your instructor tells you to also find the ICD-10-CM codes, a draft version may be downloaded from the following website: http://www.cdc.gov/nchs/icd/icd10cm.htm.

4. Record the proper information on the financial record and claim form, and note the date you have billed the workers' compensation carrier.

5. A Performance Evaluation Checklist may be reproduced from the "Instruction Guide to the Workbook" chapter if your instructor wishes you to submit it to assist with scoring and comments.

After the instructor has returned your work to you, either make the necessary corrections and place your work in a three-ring notebook for future reference or, if you received a high score, place it in your portfolio for reference when applying for a job.

Additional Coding

1. Refer to Mr. Glen M. Hiranuma's medical record, abstract information, and code procedures that would be billed by outside providers.

Site	*Description of Service*	*Code*
a. College Hospital Radiology	____________________	_______________
b. College Hospital Radiology	____________________	_______________
c. College Hospital Radiology	____________________	_______________
d. College Hospital Radiology	____________________	_______________

Acct No. 15-2-3

STATEMENT
Financial Account

COLLEGE CLINIC
4567 Broad Avenue
Woodland Hills, XY 12345-0001
Tel. 555-486-9002
Fax No. 555-487-8976

Workers' Compensation

State Compensation Insurance Fund
14156 Magnolia Boulevard
Torres, CY 12349-0218

Patient's Name Glen M. Hiranuma — Social Security No. 558-XX-9960

Date of Injury 5-22-xx — Employer Pittsburgh Paint Company — Policy No. 016-2432-211

Phone No. (H) 555-467-3383 — Phone No. (W) 555-486-9070 — Claim No. unassigned

DATE	REFERENCE	DESCRIPTION	CHARGES	CREDITS PYMNTS.	CREDITS ADJ.	BALANCE
20xx		BALANCE FORWARD →				
5-22-xx		Hospital Admit				
5-22-xx		WC Report				
5-23-xx		Discharge				

PLEASE PAY LAST AMOUNT IN BALANCE COLUMN

THIS IS A COPY OF YOUR FINANCIAL ACCOUNT AS IT APPEARS ON OUR RECORDS

Figure 15-3

ASSIGNMENT 15-4 COMPLETE A DOCTOR'S FIRST REPORT OF OCCUPATIONAL INJURY OR ILLNESS FORM FOR A WORKERS' COMPENSATION CASE

Performance Objective

Task: Complete a Doctor's First Report of Occupational Injury or Illness form and define patient record abbreviations.

Conditions: Use the patient's record (Figure 15-4), a Doctor's First Report of Occupational Injury or Illness form (Figure 15-5), and a computer.

Standards: Claim Productivity Measurement

Time: ______________ minutes

Accuracy: ______________

(Note: The time element and accuracy criteria may be given by your instructor.)

Directions:

1. Complete the Doctor's First Report of Occupational Injury or Illness form for this temporary disability type of claim. Refer to Carlos A. Giovanni's patient record for November 11 through November 15.
2. Define abbreviations found in the patient's medical record.

After the instructor has returned your work to you, either make the necessary corrections and place your work in a three-ring notebook for future reference or, if you received a high score, place it in your portfolio for reference when applying for a job.

Abbreviations pertinent to this record:

pt	______________	H	______________
ER	______________	MDM	______________
C	______________	TD	______________
HX	______________	RTW	______________
PX	______________	approx	______________
CT	______________	HV	______________
R	______________	EPF	______________
tr	______________	M	______________
adm	______________	PO	______________
DC	______________	PF	______________
Hosp	______________	SF	______________
OV	______________	X	______________
LC	______________	adv	______________
HA	______________	trt	______________
BP	______________	reg	______________
RTO	______________	W	______________
Wks	______________	Cons	______________

PATIENT RECORD NO. 15-4-5

Giovanni	Carlos	A	10-24-55	M	555-677-3485
LAST NAME	FIRST NAME	MIDDLE NAME	BIRTH DATE	SEX	HOME PHONE

89 Beaumont Court	Woodland Hills	XY	12345
ADDRESS	CITY	STATE	ZIP CODE

	555-230-7788	555-677-3485	giovannic@wb.net
CELL PHONE	PAGER NO.	FAX NO.	E-MAIL ADDRESS

556-XX-9699	Y0394876
PATIENT'S SOC. SEC. NO.	DRIVER'S LICENSE

TV repairman	Giant Television Co. (TV repair company)
PATIENT'S OCCUPATION	NAME OF COMPANY

8764 Ocean Avenue, Woodland Hills, XY 12345	555-647-8851
ADDRESS OF EMPLOYER	PHONE

Maria B. Giovanni	homemaker
SPOUSE OR PARENT	OCCUPATION

EMPLOYER	ADDRESS	PHONE

State Compensation Insurance Fund, 600 S. Lafayette Park Place, Ehrlich, XY 12350
NAME OF INSURANCE

57780	
POLICY/CERTIFICATE NO.	GROUP NO.

REFERRED BY: Giant Television Company

Figure 15-4

Patient: Giovanni, Carlos A. Patient Record No. 15-04-05

DATE	PROGRESS NOTES
11-11-xx	Pt referred to College Hospital ER by employer for workers' compensation injury. I was called in as on-call neurosurgeon to evaluate the pt. Pt states that today at 2 p.m. he fell from the roof of a private home while installing an antenna at 2231 Duarte St., Woodland Hills, XY 12345 in Woodland Hills County. He describes the incident as follows: "When I was attaching the base of an antenna, the weight of the antenna shifted and knocked me off the roof." Pt complains of head pain and indicates brief loss of consciousness. I performed a C HX/PX. Complete skull x-rays showed fractured skull. CT of head/brain (without contrast) indicates well-defined R. subdural hematoma. Pt suffering from cerebral concussion; no open wound. Tr plan: Adm pt to College Hospital (5 p.m.) and schedule R infratentorial craniotomy to evacuate hematoma. (H/MDM). Obtained authorization and prepared Dr.'s First Report.
	AP/llf Astro Parkinson, MD
11-12-xx	Performed R infratentorial craniotomy and evacuated subdural hematoma. Pt stable and returned to room; will be seen daily. TD: Estimated RTW 1-15-xx. Possible cranial defect & head disfigurement resulting. Pt to be hospitalized for approx 2 weeks.
	AP/llf Astro Parkinson, MD
11-13-xx	HV (EPF HX/PX M/MDM). Pt improving; recommend consult with Dr. Graff for cranial defect. Authorization obtained from adjuster (Steve Burroughs) at State Comp.
	AP/llf Astro Parkinson, MD
11-14-xx	Pt seen in cons by Dr. Cosmo Graff who stated he does not recommend correcting PO cranial defect. Both Dr. Graff and I explained how the defect resulted from the injury; there may be some improvement over time. Pt states he is grateful to be alive (EPF HX/PX M/MDM).
	AP/llf Astro Parkinson, MD
11-15-xx	Daily HV (EPF HX/PX M/MDM). Pt progressing appropriately; no complications have occurred.
thru	
11-29-xx	AP/llf Astro Parkinson, MD
11-30-xx	DC from hosp. Permanent cranial defect resulting from fracture and surgery. RTO 1 wk.
	AP/llf Astro Parkinson, MD
12-7-xx	OV (EPF HX/PX LC/MDM) Pt doing very well. No HA or visual disturbances, BP 120/80, alert and oriented. He is anxious to return to work. Pt cautioned about maintaining low activity level until released. RTO 2 wks.
	AP/llf Astro Parkinson, MD
12-21-xx	OV (PF HX/PX SF/MDM). Pt continues to improve. Suggested he start a walking program 3 x wk and monitor symptoms. May do light activity and lifting (10 lbs). Adv to call if any symptoms return. RTO 10 days.
	AP/llf Astro Parkinson, MD
12-29-xx	OV (PF HX/PX SF/MDM). Pt did not experience any symptoms with increased activity. No further trt necessary. Pt will increase activity and call if any problems occur. Pt scheduled to resume reg W on 1-15-xx. Final report submitted to workers' compensation carrier.
	AP/llf Astro Parkinson, MD

Figure 15-4, cont'd

DOCTOR'S FIRST REPORT OF OCCUPATIONAL INJURY OR ILLNESS

Within 5 days of initial examination, for every occupational injury or illness, send 2 copies of this report to the employers' workers' compensation insurance carrier or the self-insured employer. Failure to file a timely doctor's report may result in assessment of a civil penalty. In the case of diagnosed or suspected pesticide poisoning, send a copy of this report to Division of Labor Statistics and Research.

1. INSURER NAME AND ADDRESS

2. EMPLOYER NAME

Policy No.

3. Address No. and Street City Zip

4. Nature of business (e.g., food manufacturing, building construction, retailer of woman's clothes)

5. PATIENT NAME (first, middle initial, last name)	6. Sex ☐ Male ☐ Female	7. Date of Birth Mo. Day Yr.
8. Address No. and Street City Zip		9. Telephone Number
10. Occupation (Specific job title)		11. Social Security Number
12. Injured at: No. and Street City		County
13. Date and hour of injury or onset or illness Mo. Day Yr. Hour _____a.m____p.m		14. Date last worked Mo. Day Yr.
15. Date and hour of first examination or treatment Mo. Day Yr. Hour _____a.m____p.m		16. Have you (or your office) previously treated patient? ☐ Yes ☐ No

Patient please complete this portion, if able to do so. Otherwise, doctor please complete immediately. Inability or failure of a patient to complete this portion shall not affect his/her rights to workers' compensation under the Labor Code.

17. DESCRIBE HOW THE ACCIDENT OR EXPOSURE HAPPENED (Give specific object, machinery or chemical.)

18. SUBJECTIVE COMPLAINTS (Describe fully.)

19. OBJECTIVE FINDINGS

A. Physical examination

B. X-ray and laboratory results (State if none or pending.)

20. DIAGNOSIS (if occupational illness specify etiologic agent and duration of exposure.) Chemical or toxic compound involved? ICD-9 Code ☐ Yes ☐ No

21. Are your findings and diagnosis consistent with patient's account of injury or onset of illness? ☐ Yes ☐ No If "no" please explain

22. Is there any other current condition that will impede or delay patient's recovery? ☐ Yes ☐ No If "yes" please explain

23. TREATMENT REQUIRED

24. If further treatment required, specify treatment plan/estimated duration.

25. If hospitalized as inpatient, give hospital name and location Date admitted Mo. Day Yr. Estimated stay

26. WORK STATUS –is patient able to perfom usual work? ☐ Yes ☐ No

If "no," date when patient can return to: Regular work____/____/

Modified work____/____/ Specify restrictions

Doctor's Signature ________________ License Number __________
Doctor's Name and Degree ________________ IRS Number __________
Address ________________ Telephone Number __________

Figure 15-5

ASSIGNMENT 15-5 COMPLETE A CLAIM FORM FOR A WORKERS' COMPENSATION CASE

Performance Objective

Task: Complete a CMS-1500 (02-12) claim form for a workers' compensation case and post transactions to the financial accounting record.

Conditions: Use the patient's record (see Figure 15-4) and financial statement (Figure 15-6), a CMS-1500 (02-12) claim form (print from Evolve website), a computer, procedural and diagnostic code books, and Appendix A in this *Workbook*.

Standards: Claim Productivity Measurement

Time: ______________ minutes

Accuracy: ______________

(Note: The time element and accuracy criteria may be given by your instructor.)

Directions:

1. Using NUCC guidelines, complete a CMS-1500 (02-12) claim form for November dates of service and direct it to the correct workers' compensation carrier for this temporary disability workers' compensation claim. Refer to Mr. Carlos A. Giovanni's patient record for information and Appendix A in this *Workbook* to locate the fees to record on the claim and post to the financial statement. Date the claim November 30 of the current year.

   Note: A progress report is being submitted with this claim; services for December will be billed on a separate claim (see Assignment 15-6).

2. Refer to Chapter 7 (Figure 7-11) of the *Handbook* for instructions on how to complete this claim form and a workers' compensation template.

3. Use your CPT code book or Appendix A in this *Workbook* to determine the correct five-digit code number and modifiers for each professional service rendered. Use your HCPCS Level II code book or refer to Appendix B in this Workbook for HCPCS procedure codes and modifiers. If your instructor tells you to also find the ICD-10-CM codes, a draft version may be downloaded from the following website: http://www.cdc.gov/nchs/icd/icd10cm.htm.

4. Record the proper information on the financial record and claim form, and note the date you have billed the workers' compensation insurance carrier.

5. A Performance Evaluation Checklist may be reproduced from the "Instruction Guide to the Workbook" chapter if your instructor wishes you to submit it to assist with scoring and comments.

After the instructor has returned your work to you, either make the necessary corrections and place your work in a three-ring notebook for future reference or, if you received a high score, place it in your portfolio for reference when applying for a job.

Additional Coding

1. Refer to Mr. Giovanni's medical record, abstract information, and code procedures that would be billed by outside providers.

Site	*Description of Service*	*Code*
a. College Hospital Radiology	________________	____________
b. College Hospital Radiology	________________	____________

Acct No. 15-5

STATEMENT

Financial Account

Workers' Compensation

COLLEGE CLINIC
4567 Broad Avenue
Woodland Hills, XY 12345-0001
Tel. 555-486-9002
Fax No. 555-487-8976

State Compensation Insurance Fund
14156 Magnolia Boulevard
Torres, CY 12349-0218

Patient's Name Carlos A. Giovanni

Social Security No. 556-XX9699

Date of Injury 11-11-20xx Employer Giant Television Company

Policy No. 57780

Phone No. (H) 555-677-3485 Phone No. (W) 555-647-8851

Claim No. unassigned

DATE	REFERENCE	DESCRIPTION	CHARGES	CREDITS		BALANCE
				PYMNTS.	ADJ.	
20xx		BALANCE FORWARD →				
11-11-xx		Hospital admit				
11-11-xx		WC Report				
11-12-xx		Craniotomy				
11-13 to 11-29-xx		HV				
11-30-xx		Discharge				
12-7-xx		OV				
12-21-xx		OV				
12-29-xx		OV				
12-29-xx		Medical Report				

PLEASE PAY LAST AMOUNT IN BALANCE COLUMN

THIS IS A COPY OF YOUR FINANCIAL ACCOUNT AS IT APPEARS ON OUR RECORDS

Figure 15-6

ASSIGNMENT 15-6 COMPLETE A CLAIM FORM FOR A WORKERS' COMPENSATION CASE

Performance Objective

Task: Complete a CMS-1500 (02-12) claim form for a workers' compensation case and post transactions to the financial accounting record.

Conditions: Use the patient's record (see Figure 15-4) and financial statement (see Figure 15-6), a CMS-1500 (02-12) claim form (print from Evolve website), a computer, procedural and diagnostic code books, and Appendix A in this *Workbook*.

Standards: Claim Productivity Measurement

Time: ______________ minutes

Accuracy: ______________

(Note: The time element and accuracy criteria may be given by your instructor.)

Directions:

1. Using NUCC guidelines, complete a CMS-1500 (02-12) claim form for December services and direct it to the correct workers' compensation carrier for this temporary disability workers' compensation claim. Refer to Mr. Carlos A. Giovanni's patient record for information and Appendix A in this *Workbook* to locate the fees to record on the claim, and post them to the financial statement. Date the claim December 29 of the current year.

2. Refer to Chapter 7 (Figure 7-11) of the *Handbook* for instructions on how to complete this claim form and a workers' compensation template.

3. Use your CPT code book or Appendix A in this *Workbook* to determine the correct five-digit code number and modifiers for each professional service rendered. Use your HCPCS Level II code book or refer to Appendix B in this *Workbook* for HCPCS procedure codes and modifiers. If your instructor tells you to also find the ICD-10-CM codes, a draft version may be downloaded from the following website: http://www.cdc.gov/nchs/icd/icd10cm.htm.

4. Record the proper information on the financial record and claim form, and note the date you have billed the workers' compensation insurance carrier.

5. A Performance Evaluation Checklist may be reproduced from the "Instruction Guide to the Workbook" chapter if your instructor wishes you to submit it to assist with scoring and comments.

After the instructor has returned your work to you, either make the necessary corrections and place your work in a three-ring notebook for future reference or, if you received a high score, place it in your portfolio for reference when applying for a job.

6. Ledger lines: Insert date of service (DOS), reference (CPT code number, check number, or dates of service for posting adjustments or when insurance was billed), description of the transaction, charge amounts, payments, adjustments, and running current balance. The posting date is the actual date the transaction is recorded. If the DOS differs from the posting date, list the DOS in the reference or description column.

16 Disability Income Insurance and Disability Benefits Programs

Karen Levein

KEY TERMS

Your instructor may wish to select some words pertinent to this chapter for a test. For definitions of the terms, further study, and/or reference, the words, phrases, and abbreviations may be found in the glossary at the end of the Handbook.

Some of the insurance terms presented in this chapter are shown marked with an asterisk (*) and may seem familiar from previous chapters. However, their meanings may or may not have a slightly different connotation when referring to disability income insurance. Key terms for this chapter follow.

accidental death and dismemberment
Armed Services Disability
benefit period*
Civil Service Retirement System
consultative examiner
cost-of-living adjustment
Disability Determination Services
disability income insurance
double indemnity
exclusions*
Federal Employees Retirement System
future purchase option
guaranteed renewable*
hearing
long-term disability insurance
noncancelable clause*
partial disability*
reconsideration
regional office
residual benefits*
residual disability
short-term disability insurance
Social Security Administration
Social Security Disability Insurance program
State Disability Insurance
supplemental benefits
Supplemental Security Income
temporary disability*
temporary disability insurance
total disability*
unemployment compensation disability
Veterans Affairs disability program
VA outpatient clinic card
voluntary disability insurance
waiting period*
waiver of premium*

KEY ABBREVIATIONS

See how many abbreviations and acronyms you can translate and then use this as a handy reference list. Definitions for the key abbreviations are located near the back of the Handbook *in the glossary.*

AIDS ______________________

CE ______________________

CSRS ______________________

DDS ______________________

FERS ______________________

HIV ______________________

OASDHI ______________________

RO ______________________

SDI ______________________

SSA ______________________

SSDI program ______________________

SSI ______________________

TDI ______________________

UCD ______________________

VA ______________________

PERFORMANCE OBJECTIVES

The student will be able to:

- Define and spell the key terms and key abbreviations for this chapter, given the information from the *Handbook* glossary, within a reasonable time period, and with enough accuracy to obtain a satisfactory evaluation.
- After reading the chapter, answer the fill-in-the-blank, multiple choice, and true/false review questions with enough accuracy to obtain a satisfactory evaluation.
- Fill in the correct meaning of each abbreviation, given a list of common medical abbreviations and symbols that appear in chart notes, within a reasonable time period and with enough accuracy to obtain a satisfactory evaluation.
- Complete each state disability form, given the patients' medical chart notes and blank state disability forms, within a reasonable time period and with enough accuracy to obtain a satisfactory evaluation.

STUDY OUTLINE

Disability Claims
History
Disability Income Insurance
    Individual
    Group
Federal Disability Programs
    Workers' Compensation
    Disability Benefit Programs
State Disability Insurance
    Background
    State Programs
    Funding
    Eligibility
    Benefits
    Time Limits
    Medical Examinations
    Restrictions
Voluntary Disability Insurance
Claims Submission Guidelines
    Disability Income Claims
Conclusion

ASSIGNMENT 16-1 REVIEW QUESTIONS

Part I Fill in the Blank

Review the objectives, key terms, glossary definitions of key terms, chapter information, and figures before completing the following review questions.

1. Health insurance that provides monthly or weekly income when an individual is unable to work because of a nonindustrial illness or injury is called

   ____

2. Some insurance contracts that pay twice the face amount of the policy if accidental death occurs may have a provision titled ______________________________.

3. When an individual who is insured under a disability income insurance policy cannot perform one or more of his or her regular job duties, this is known as

   ____________________ or ____________________ disability.

4. When an individual becomes permanently disabled and cannot pay the insurance premium, a desirable provision in an insurance contract is ______________________________.

5. Ezra Jackson has disability income insurance under a group policy paid for by his employer. Ezra makes no contribution toward the policy premiums. One evening he goes inline skating and suffers a complex fracture of the patella, which necessitates several months off from work. Are his monthly disability benefits taxable?

   ____________________ Why or why not? ____________________

   ____

6. Two federal programs for individuals younger than 65 years of age who have a severe disability are

   a. ____

   b. ____

7. The Social Security Administration may hire a physician to evaluate an applicant's disability. A physician's role may be any one of the following:

   a. ____

   b. ____

   c. ____

8. Jamie Woods, a Navy petty officer, suffers an accident aboard the USS *Denebola* 3 weeks following his honorable discharge. To receive veteran's benefits for this injury, the time limit in which a claim must be filed is

   ____.

9. Name the states and the territory that have nonindustrial state disability programs.

a. ______________________________

b. ______________________________

c. ______________________________

d. ______________________________

e. ______________________________

f. ______________________________

10. Temporary disability insurance claims must be filed within how many days in your state?

____

11. How long can a person continue to draw state disability insurance benefits?

____

12. After a claim begins, when do basic state disability benefits become payable if the patient is confined to his or her home? ______________________________
If the patient is hospitalized?

____

13. Nick Tyson has recovered since a previous illness ended and becomes ill again with the same ailment. Is he entitled to state disability benefits? ______________________________

14. John S. Thatcher stubbed his toe as he was leaving work and going to his car parked on the street. Because the injury was only slightly uncomfortable, he thought no more about it. The next morning he found that his foot was too swollen to fit in his shoe, so he stayed home. When the swelling did not subside after 3 days, John went to the doctor. Radiographs showed a broken toe, which kept John home for 2 weeks. After 1 week he applied for temporary state disability benefits.

Will he be paid? ______________________ Why or why not? ______________________

15. Peggy Jonson has an ectopic pregnancy and is unable to work because of complications of this condition. Can she receive state temporary disability benefits?

____

16. Four states that allow for maternity benefits in normal pregnancy are

a. ______________________________

b. ______________________________

c. ______________________________

d. ______________________________

17. Betty T. Kraft had to stay home from her job because her 10-year-old daughter had measles. She applied for temporary state disability benefits. Will she be paid?

______________________ Why or why not? ______________________

18. Vincent P. Michael was ill with a bad cold for 1 week. Will he receive temporary state disability benefits? ____________________

Why or why not? ____________________

19. Betsy C. Palm works in Hawaii and had an emergency appendectomy. She was hospitalized for 3 days. Will she receive state disability benefits?

____

Why or why not? ____________________

20. Frank E. Thompson is a box boy at a supermarket on Saturdays and Sundays while a full-time student at college. He broke his leg while skiing and cannot work at the market, but he is able to attend classes with his leg in a cast. Can he collect state disability benefits for his part-time job? ____________ Why or why not?

____

21. Jerry L. Slate is out of a job and is receiving unemployment insurance benefits. He is now suffering from severe intestinal flu. The employment office calls him to interview for a job, but he is too ill to go. Can he collect temporary state disability benefits for this illness when he might have been given a job?

____

Why or why not? ____________________

22. While walking the picket line with other employees on strike, Gene J. Berry came down with pneumonia and was ill for 2 weeks. Can he collect temporary state disability benefits? ____________________

Why or why not? ____________________

Gene went back to work for 3 weeks and then developed a slight cold and cough, which again was diagnosed as pneumonia. The doctor told him to stay home from work. Would he be able to collect temporary disability benefits again? ____________________

Why or why not? ____________________

23. A month after he retired, Roger Reagan had a gallbladder operation. Can he receive temporary state disability benefits? ____________________

Why or why not? ____________________

24. Jane M. Lambert fell in the back yard of her home and fractured her left ankle. She had a nonunion fracture and could not work for 28 weeks. For how long will she collect temporary state disability benefits? ____________________

25. Dr. Kay examines Ben Yates and completes a disability income claim form because of a prolonged illness. On receiving the information, the insurance adjuster notices some conflicting data. Name other documents that may be requested to justify payment of benefits.

a. ____________________

b. ____________________

c. ____________________

26. Trent Walters, a permanently disabled individual, applies for federal disability benefits. To establish eligibility for benefits under this program, data allowed must be

    ________________________ year/years old.

27. A Veterans Affairs patient is seen on an emergency basis by Dr. Onion. Name the two methods or options for billing this case.

    a. ____

    b. ____

Part II Multiple Choice

Choose the best answer.

28. Another disability income insurance term for benefits is
    a. indemnity.
    b. supplemental benefits.
    c. guarantee.
    d. compensation.

29. When the purchase of insurance is investigated, the word/words to look for in the insurance contract that mean the premium cannot be increased at renewal time is/are
    a. guaranteed renewable.
    b. conditional provision.
    c. noncancelable clause.
    d. optional provision.

30. Provisions that limit the scope of insurance coverage are known as
    a. clauses.
    b. deductibles.
    c. conditions.
    d. exclusions.

31. A Social Security Administration division that determines an individual's eligibility to be placed under the federal disability program is called
    a. Disability Determination Services.
    b. Social Security Disability.
    c. Supplemental Security Income.
    d. none of the above.

32. The time period from the beginning of disability to receiving the first payment of benefits is called a/an
    a. exclusion period.
    b. waiting period.
    c. insurance period.
    d. elimination phase.

Part III True/False

Write "T" or "F" in the blank to indicate whether you think the statement is true or false.

________ 33. When a person insured under a disability income insurance policy cannot, for a limited period of time, perform all functions of his or her regular job duties, this is known as permanent disability.

________ 34. To be eligible to apply for disability benefits under Social Security, an individual must be unable to perform any type of work for a period of not less than 12 months.

________ 35. Hospital benefits may be paid for nonoccupational illness or injury under state temporary disability benefits.

________ 36. If a woman has an abnormal condition that arises from her pregnancy (e.g., diabetes or varicose veins) and is unable to work because of the condition, she may not receive state disability benefits.

________ 37. When a claim form is submitted for a patient applying for state disability benefits, the most important item required on the form is the claimant's Social Security number.

ASSIGNMENT 16-2 COMPLETE TWO STATE DISABILITY INSURANCE FORMS

Performance Objective

Task: Complete two state disability insurance forms and define patient record abbreviations.

Conditions: Use the patient's record (Figure 16-1), a Claim Statement of Employee form (Figure 16-2), a Doctor's Certificate form (Figure 16-3), and a computer.

Standards: Time: ______________ minutes

Accuracy: ______________

(Note: The time element and accuracy criteria may be given by your instructor.)

Directions:

1. To familiarize you with what information the employee must furnish, this assignment will encompass completing both the Claim Statement of Employee (see Figure 16-2) and the Doctor's Certificate (see Figure 16-3).
2. Mr. Broussard (see Figure 16-1) is applying for state disability benefits, and he does not receive sick leave pay from his employer. The language he prefers is English. He does not want any disclosure of benefit payment information to his employer. During his disability, he was not in the custody of law enforcement authorities for any violation and he has no alcoholic tendencies.
3. Date the Claim Statement of Employee November 5, and date the Doctor's Certificate November 10. Remember that this is not a claim for payment to the physician, and so no financial accounting record (ledger card) has been furnished for this patient.
4. Refer to Chapter 16 and Figures 16-3 and 16-4 of the *Handbook* to assist you in completing this form.

After the instructor has returned your work to you, either make the necessary corrections and place your work in a three-ring notebook for future reference or, if you received a high score, place it in your portfolio for reference when applying for a job.

Abbreviations pertinent to this record:

NP	______________	c/o	______________
LBP	______________	pt	______________
lt	______________	wk	______________
reg	______________	exam	______________
SLR	______________	rt	______________
WNL	______________	STAT	______________
MRI	______________	RTO	______________
imp	______________	retn	______________

PATIENT RECORD NO. 16-2

Broussard	Jeff	L	03-09-52	M	555-466-2490
LAST NAME	FIRST NAME	MIDDLE NAME	BIRTH DATE	SEX	HOME PHONE

3577 Plain Street	Woodland Hills	XY	12345
ADDRESS	CITY	STATE	ZIP CODE

555-667-7654	555-399-5903	555-466-2490	broussard@wb.net
CELL PHONE	PAGER NO.	FAX NO.	E-MAIL ADDRESS

566-XX-0090	F0394588
PATIENT'S SOC. SEC. NO.	DRIVER'S LICENSE

carpenter Payroll #2156	Ace Construction Company
PATIENT'S OCCUPATION	NAME OF COMPANY

4556 West Eighth Street, Dorland, XY 12347	555-447-8900
ADDRESS OF EMPLOYER	PHONE

Harriet M. Broussard	secretary
SPOUSE OR PARENT	OCCUPATION

Merit Accounting Company, 6743 Main Street, Woodland Hills, XY 12345	555-478-0980
EMPLOYER ADDRESS	PHONE

Blue Cross	Jeff L. Broussard
NAME OF INSURANCE	INSURED OR SUBSCRIBER

466-XX-9979	6131
POLICY/CERTIFICATE NO.	GROUP NO.

REFERRED BY: Harold B. Hartburn (friend)

DATE	PROGRESS NOTES
09-12-xx	8:30 a.m. NP seen c/o ongoing LBP. On 8-15-XX after swinging a golf club, pt had sudden onset of severe
	pain in low back with radiation to lt side. Pt unable to work 8-16 but resumed wk on 8-17 and has been working
	full time but doing no lifting while working. Pain is exacerbating affecting his work and reg duties. Exam
	showed SLR strongly positive on lt, on rt causes pain into lt side. Neurological exam WNL. Ordered STAT
	MRI. Off work. RTO.
	RS/mtf Raymond Skeleton, MD
09-13-xx	Pt returns for test results. MRI showed huge defect of L4-5. Imp: acute herniated disc L4-5 with spinal stenosis.
	Recommended laminotomy, foraminotomy, and diskectomy L4-5.
	RS/mtf Raymond Skeleton, MD
09-14-xx	Admit to College Hospital. Operation: Lumbar laminotomy with exploration and decompression of spinal
	cord with diskectomy L4-5; lumbar anteriorarthrodesis.
	RS/mtf Raymond Skeleton, MD
11-5-xx	Pt seen daily in hosp. At 3 p.m. pt discharged to home. Will retn to wk 12-15-XX.
	RS/mtf Raymond Skeleton, MD

Figure 16-1

Your disability claim can also be filed online at www.edd.ca.gov/

PLEASE PRINT WITH BLACK INK.

250104122

PART A - CLAIMANT'S STATEMENT

A1. YOUR SOCIAL SECURITY NUMBER

A2. IF YOU HAVE PREVIOUSLY BEEN ASSIGNED AN EDD CUSTOMER ACCOUNT NUMBER, ENTER THAT NUMBER HERE

A3. CALIFORNIA DRIVER LICENSE OR ID NUMBER

A4. GENDER MALE FEMALE

A5. IF YOU EVER USED OTHER SOCIAL SECURITY NUMBERS, ENTER THOSE NUMBERS BELOW

A6. STATE GOVERNMENT EMPLOYEE (IF "YES" INDICATE BARGAINING UNIT#) YES NO UNIT#

A7. YOUR DATE OF BIRTH M M D D Y Y Y Y

A8. YOUR LEGAL NAME (FIRST) (MI) (LAST) SUFFIX

A9. OTHER NAMES, IF ANY, UNDER WHICH YOU HAVE WORKED

(FIRST) (MI) (LAST) SUFFIX

(FIRST) (MI) (LAST) SUFFIX

A10. YOUR HOME AREA CODE AND TELEPHONE NUMBER

A11. YOUR CELL AREA CODE AND TELEPHONE NUMBER

A12. LANGUAGE YOU PREFER TO USE

ENGLISH SPANISH CANTONESE VIETNAMESE ARMENIAN PUNJABI TAGALOG OTHER

A13. YOUR MAILING ADDRESS, PO BOX OR NUMBER/STREET/APARTMENT, SUITE, SPACE#, OR PMB# (PRIVATE MAIL BOX)

CITY STATE ZIP OR POSTAL CODE COUNTRY (IF NOT U.S.A.)

A14. YOUR RESIDENCE ADDRESS, REQUIRED IF DIFFERENT FROM YOUR MAILING ADDRESS NUMBER/STREET/APARTMENT OR SPACE#

CITY STATE ZIP OR POSTAL CODE COUNTRY (IF NOT U.S.A.)

A15. YOUR LAST OR CURRENT EMPLOYER - IF YOUR LAST OR CURRENT EMPLOYMENT WAS SELF-EMPLOYMENT, ENTER "SELF" AND FILL-IN THIS OPTION. ☐ SELF

NAME OF YOUR EMPLOYER [STATE GOVERNMENT EMPLOYEES: PROVIDE THE AGENCY NAME (FOR EXAMPLE: CALTRANS)]

NUMBER/STREET/SUITE# (STATE GOVERNMENT EMPLOYEES: PLEASE PROVIDE THE ADDRESS OF YOUR PERSONNEL OFFICE)

CITY STATE ZIP OR POSTAL CODE COUNTRY (IF NOT U.S.A.)

EMPLOYER'S TELEPHONE NUMBER

A16. AT ANY TIME DURING YOUR DISABILITY, WERE YOU IN THE CUSTODY OF LAW ENFORCEMENT AUTHORITIES BECAUSE YOU WERE CONVICTED OF VIOLATING A LAW OR ORDINANCE? YES NO

A17. BEFORE YOUR DISABILITY BEGAN, WHAT WAS THE LAST DAY YOU WORKED? M M D D Y Y Y Y

A18. WHEN DID YOUR DISABILITY BEGIN? M M D D Y Y Y Y

A19. DATE YOU WANT YOUR CLAIM TO BEGIN IF DIFFERENT THAN THE DATE ENTERED IN A18 M M D D Y Y Y Y

A20. SINCE YOUR DISABILITY BEGAN, HAVE YOU WORKED OR ARE YOU WORKING ANY FULL OR PARTIAL DAYS? YES NO

A21 A. IF YOU RECOVERED, ENTER DATE: M M D D Y Y Y Y

A21 B. IF YOU RETURNED TO WORK, ENTER DATE: M M D D Y Y Y Y

DE 2501 Rev. 78 (4-12)

Figure 16-2

250104123

PART A - CLAIMANT'S STATEMENT - CONTINUED

A22. PLEASE RE-ENTER YOUR SOCIAL SECURITY NUMBER

A23. WHAT IS YOUR REGULAR OR CUSTOMARY OCCUPATION?

A24. WHY DID YOU STOP WORKING? (SELECT ONLY ONE BOX)
- ☐ ILLNESS, INJURY, OR PREGNANCY
- ☐ LAYOFF
- ☐ UNPAID LEAVE OF ABSENCE
- ☐ VOLUNTARILY QUIT OR RETIRED
- ☐ TERMINATED
- ☐ OTHER REASON

A25. HOW WOULD YOU DESCRIBE OR CLASSIFY YOUR JOB?
- ☐ Mostly sit; occasionally stand or walk; occasionally lift, carry, push, pull, or otherwise move objects that weigh 10 lbs. or less.
- ☐ Mostly walk/stand; occasionally lift, carry, push, pull, or otherwise move objects that weigh up to 20 lbs.
- ☐ Constantly lift, carry, push, pull, or otherwise move objects that weigh up to 10 lbs.; frequently up to 20 lbs.; occasionally up to 50 lbs.
- ☐ Constantly lift, carry, push, pull, or otherwise move objects that weigh up to 20 lbs.; frequently up to 50 lbs.; occasionally up to 100 lbs.
- ☐ Constantly lift, carry, push, pull, or otherwise move objects that weigh over 20 lbs.; frequently over 50 lbs.; occasionally over 100 lbs.

A26. IF YOUR EMPLOYER(S) CONTINUED OR WILL CONTINUE TO PAY YOU DURING YOUR DISABILITY, INDICATE TYPE OF PAY:
SICK ☐ VACATION ☐ Paid Time Off (PTO) ☐ ANNUAL ☐ OTHER (EXPLAIN)

A27. MAY WE DISCLOSE BENEFIT PAYMENT INFORMATION TO YOUR EMPLOYER(S)?
YES ☐ NO ☐

A28. SECOND EMPLOYER NAME (IF YOU HAVE MORE THAN ONE EMPLOYER)

NUMBER/STREET/SUITE#

CITY | STATE | ZIP OR POSTAL CODE | COUNTRY (IF NOT U.S.A.)

BEFORE YOUR DISABILITY BEGAN, WHAT WAS THE LAST DAY YOU WORKED FOR THIS EMPLOYER? M M D D Y Y Y Y

EMPLOYER'S TELEPHONE NUMBER

A29. IF YOU HAVE MORE THAN 2 EMPLOYERS CHECK HERE. ☐

A30. IF YOU ARE A RESIDENT OF AN ALCOHOLIC RECOVERY HOME OR A DRUG-FREE RESIDENTIAL FACILITY, PROVIDE THE FOLLOWING:
NAME OF FACILITY

NUMBER/STREET/SUITE#

CITY | STATE | ZIP OR POSTAL CODE | AREA CODE AND TELEPHONE NUMBER

A31. HAVE YOU FILED OR DO YOU INTEND TO FILE FOR WORKERS' COMPENSATION BENEFITS?
- ☐ YES - COMPLETE ITEMS A32 THROUGH A38
- ☐ NO - SKIP ITEMS A33 THROUGH A38

A32. WAS THIS DISABILITY CAUSED BY YOUR JOB?
☐ YES ☐ NO

A33. DATE(S) OF INJURY SHOWN ON YOUR WORKERS' COMPENSATION CLAIM
M M D D Y Y Y Y | M M D D Y Y Y Y | M M D D Y Y Y Y | M M D D Y Y Y Y

A34. WORKERS' COMPENSATION INSURANCE COMPANY NAME | AREA CODE AND TELEPHONE NUMBER | EXTENSION (IF ANY)

NUMBER/STREET/SUITE#

CITY | STATE | ZIP CODE | WORKERS' COMPENSATION CLAIM NUMBER

DE 2501 Rev. 78 (4-12)

Figure 16-2, cont'd

Continued

250104124

PART A - CLAIMANT'S STATEMENT - CONTINUED

A35. PLEASE RE-ENTER YOUR SOCIAL SECURITY NUMBER

A36. WORKERS' COMPENSATION ADJUSTER'S NAME | AREA CODE AND TELEPHONE NUMBER | EXTENSION (IF ANY)

A37. EMPLOYER'S NAME SHOWN ON YOUR WORKERS' COMPENSATION CLAIM | AREA CODE AND TELEPHONE NUMBER | EXTENSION (IF ANY)

A38. YOUR ATTORNEY'S NAME (IF ANY) FOR YOUR WORKERS' COMPENSATION CASE | AREA CODE AND TELEPHONE NUMBER | EXTENSION (IF ANY)

ATTORNEY'S ADDRESS NUMBER/STREET/SUITE#

CITY | STATE | ZIP CODE | WORKERS' COMPENSATION APPEALS BOARD/ADJ CASE NUMBER

PLEASE REVIEW, SIGN, AND DATE ITEM A39, AND IF APPLICABLE, ITEMS A40 AND A41

A39. Declaration and Signature. By my signature on this claim statement, I claim benefits and certify that for the period covered by this claim I was unemployed and disabled. I understand that willfully making a false statement or concealing a material fact in order to obtain payment of benefits is a violation of California law and that such violation is punishable by imprisonment or fine or both. I declare under penalty of perjury that the foregoing statement, including any accompanying statements, is to the best of my knowledge and belief true, correct, and complete. By my signature on this claim statement, I authorize the California Department of Industrial Relations and my employer to furnish and disclose to State Disability Insurance all facts concerning my disability, wages or earnings, and benefit payments that are within their knowledge. By my signature on this claim statement, I authorize release and use of information as stated in the "Information Collection and Access" portion of this form (see Informational Instructions, page D). I agree that photocopies of this authorization shall be as valid as the original, and I understand that authorizations contained in this claim statement are granted for a period of fifteen years from the date of my signature or the effective date of the claim, whichever is later.

CLAIMANT'S SIGNATURE (DO NOT PRINT) OR SIGNATURE MADE BY MARK (X) | DATE SIGNED M M D D Y Y Y Y

A40. IF YOUR SIGNATURE IS MADE BY MARK (X), CHECK THE BOX AND IT MUST BE ATTESTED BY TWO WITNESSES WITH THEIR ADDRESSES. ☐

1st WITNESS SIGNATURE (PRINT AND SIGN) | DATE SIGNED M M D D Y Y Y Y

NUMBER/STREET/APARTMENT OR SPACE#, PO BOX OR PRIVATE MAIL BOX ADDRESSES NOT ACCEPTABLE.

CITY | STATE | ZIP CODE

2nd WITNESS SIGNATURE (PRINT AND SIGN) | DATE SIGNED M M D D Y Y Y Y

NUMBER/STREET/APARTMENT OR SPACE#, PO BOX OR PRIVATE MAIL BOX ADDRESSES NOT ACCEPTABLE.

CITY | STATE | ZIP CODE

A41. ☐ CHECK THIS BOX IF YOU ARE THE PERSONAL REPRESENTATIVE SIGNING ON BEHALF OF CLAIMANT AND COMPLETE THE FOLLOWING:

I, (FIRST) (MI) (LAST), REPRESENT THE CLAIMANT IN THIS MATTER AS AUTHORIZED BY ☐ DECLARATION OF INDIVIDUAL CLAIMING DISABILITY INSURANCE BENEFITS DUE AN INCAPACITATED OR DECEASED CLAIMANT, DE 2522 (SEE INSTRUCTION & INFORMATION A, UNDER HOW TO APPLY #4) ☐ POWER OF ATTORNEY (ATTACH COPY)

PERSONAL REPRESENTATIVE'S SIGNATURE (DO NOT PRINT) | DATE SIGNED M M D D Y Y Y Y

DE 2501 Rev. 78 (4-12)

Figure 16-2, cont'd

Claim for Disability Insurance (DI) Benefits - Physician/Practitioner's Certificate
PLEASE PRINT WITH BLACK INK.

250104125

PART B - PHYSICIAN/PRACTITIONER'S CERTIFICATE

B1. PATIENT'S SOCIAL SECURITY NUMBER

B2. PATIENT'S FILE NUMBER

B3. IF YOU KNOW THE PATIENT'S ELECTRONIC RECEIPT NUMBER, ENTER IT HERE:
R

B4. PATIENT'S DATE OF BIRTH
M M D D Y Y Y Y

B5. PATIENT'S NAME (FIRST) (MI) (LAST)

B6. PHYSICIAN/PRACTITIONER'S LICENSE NUMBER

B7. STATE **OR** COUNTRY (IF NOT U.S.A.) THAT ISSUED LICENSE NUMBER ENTERED IN B6
STATE COUNTRY

B8. PHYSICIAN/PRACTITIONER LICENSE TYPE

B9. SPECIALTY (IF ANY)

B10. PHYSICIAN/PRACTITIONER'S NAME AS SHOWN ON LICENSE
(FIRST) (MI) (LAST) SUFFIX

B11. PHYSICIAN/PRACTITIONER'S ADDRESS
MAILING ADDRESS, PO BOX OR NUMBER/STREET/SUITE#
CITY STATE ZIP OR POSTAL CODE COUNTRY (IF NOT U.S.A.)

COUNTY HOSPITAL/GOVERNMENT FACILITY ADDRESS
FACILITY NAME (IF APPLICABLE)
FACILITY ADDRESS, NUMBER/STREET/SUITE#
CITY STATE ZIP OR POSTAL CODE COUNTRY (IF NOT U.S.A.)

B12. THIS PATIENT HAS BEEN UNDER MY CARE AND TREATMENT FOR THIS MEDICAL PROBLEM
FROM M M D D Y Y Y Y TO M M D D Y Y Y Y ☐ CHECK HERE TO INDICATE YOU ARE STILL TREATING THE PATIENT
AT INTERVALS OF: ☐ DAILY ☐ WEEKLY ☐ MONTHLY ☐ AS NEEDED ☐ OTHER

B13. AT ANY TIME DURING YOUR ATTENDANCE FOR THIS MEDICAL PROBLEM, HAS THE PATIENT BEEN INCAPABLE OF PERFORMING HIS/HER REGULAR OR CUSTOMARY WORK?
☐ YES - ENTER DATE DISABILITY BEGAN M M D D Y Y Y Y ☐ NO - SKIP TO B33
WAS THE DISABILITY CAUSED BY AN ACCIDENT OR TRAUMA? ☐ YES ☐ NO
M M D D Y Y Y Y IF YES, INDICATE THE DATE THE ACCIDENT OR TRAUMA OCCURRED.

B14. DATE YOU RELEASED OR ANTICIPATE RELEASING PATIENT TO RETURN TO HIS/HER REGULAR OR CUSTOMARY WORK
("UNKNOWN", "INDEFINITE", ETC., NOT ACCEPTABLE.) M M D D Y Y Y Y
☐ CHECK HERE TO INDICATE PATIENT'S DISABILITY IS PERMANENT AND YOU NEVER ANTICIPATE RELEASING PATIENT TO RETURN TO HIS/HER REGULAR OR CUSTOMARY WORK

B15. IF PATIENT IS NOW PREGNANT OR HAS BEEN PREGNANT, PLEASE CHECK THE APPROPRIATE BOX AND ENTER THE FOLLOWING:
☐ ESTIMATED DELIVERY DATE: M M D D Y Y Y Y ☐ DATE PREGNANCY ENDED: M M D D Y Y Y Y
TYPE OF DELIVERY, IF PATIENT HAS DELIVERED: ☐ VAGINAL ☐ CESAREAN

DE 2501 Rev. 78 (4-12)

Figure 16-3

Continued

250104126

PART B - PHYSICIAN/PRACTITIONER'S CERTIFICATE - CONTINUED

B16. PLEASE RE-ENTER PATIENT'S SOCIAL SECURITY NUMBER

B17. IF THE PATIENT HAS NOT DELIVERED AND YOU DO NOT ANTICIPATE RELEASING THE PATIENT TO RETURN TO REGULAR OR CUSTOMARY WORK PRIOR TO THE ESTIMATED DELIVERY DATE, ENTER THE **NUMBER OF DAYS** THAT THE PATIENT WILL BE DISABLED POSTPARTUM, FOR EACH DELIVERY TYPE:

VAGINAL DELIVERY ☐☐ CESAREAN DELIVERY ☐☐

B18. IN CASE OF AN ABNORMAL PREGNANCY AND/OR DELIVERY, STATE THE COMPLICATION(S) CAUSING MATERNAL DISABILITY

B19. ICD DIAGNOSIS CODE(S) FOR DISABLING CONDITION THAT PREVENT THE PATIENT FROM PERFORMING HIS/HER REGULAR OR CUSTOMARY WORK (REQUIRED)

EXAMPLE OF HOW TO COMPLETE ICD CODES

ICD-9 3 2 0 ▪ 1

ICD-10 G 0 0 ▪ 1

(Check only one box)

☐ **ICD-9**

☐ **ICD-10**

PRIMARY

SECONDARY

SECONDARY

SECONDARY

B20. DIAGNOSIS (REQUIRED) - IF NO DIAGNOSIS HAS BEEN DETERMINED, ENTER A DETAILED STATEMENT OF SYMPTOMS

B21. FINDINGS - STATE NATURE, SEVERITY, AND EXTENT OF THE INCAPACITATING DISEASE OR INJURY, INCLUDE ANY OTHER DISABLING CONDITIONS

B22. TYPE OF TREATMENT/MEDICATION RENDERED TO PATIENT

B23. IF PATIENT WAS HOSPITALIZED, PROVIDE DATES OF ENTRY AND DISCHARGE M M D D Y Y Y Y TO M M D D Y Y Y Y

☐ CHECK HERE TO INDICATE THE PATIENT IS STILL HOSPITALIZED

B24. ☐ CHECK HERE IF PATIENT IS DECEASED, PLEASE PROVIDE DATE OF DEATH M M D D Y Y Y Y

CITY COUNTY STATE

DE 2501 Rev. 78 (4-12)

Figure 16-3, cont'd

250104127

PART B - PHYSICIAN/PRACTITIONER'S CERTIFICATE - CONTINUED

B25. PLEASE RE-ENTER PATIENT'S SOCIAL SECURITY NUMBER

B26. WAS THE PATIENT SEEN PREVIOUSLY BY ANOTHER PHYSICIAN/PRACTITIONER OR MEDICAL FACILITY FOR THE CURRENT DISABILITY/ILLNESS/INJURY?

☐ YES ☐ NO ☐ UNKNOWN IF YES, WHAT WAS THE DATE OF FIRST TREATMENT? M M D D Y Y Y Y

B27. DATE AND TYPE OF SURGERY/PROCEDURE MOST RECENTLY PERFORMED OR TO BE PERFORMED

M M D D Y Y Y Y

WAS THE PATIENT UNABLE TO WORK IMMEDIATELY PRIOR TO THE SURGERY OR PROCEDURE? ☐ YES ☐ NO

M M D D Y Y Y Y IF YES, PLEASE PROVIDE THE FIRST DATE THE PATIENT WAS UNABLE TO WORK BEFORE THE SURGERY OR PROCEDURE

B28. ICD PROCEDURE CODE(S) ☐ ICD-9 ☐ ICD-10

CPT CODE(S) (DO NOT INCLUDE MODIFIERS)

B29. WAS THIS DISABLING CONDITION CAUSED AND/OR AGGRAVATED BY THE PATIENT'S REGULAR OR CUSTOMARY WORK? ☐ YES ☐ NO

B30. ARE YOU COMPLETING THIS FORM FOR THE SOLE PURPOSE OF REFERRAL/RECOMMENDATION TO AN ALCOHOLIC RECOVERY HOME OR DRUG-FREE RESIDENTIAL FACILITY AS INDICATED BY THE PATIENT IN QUESTION A30? ☐ YES ☐ NO

B31. DATE YOUR PATIENT BECAME A RESIDENT OF A DRUG OR ALCOHOL FACILITY (IF KNOWN) M M D D Y Y Y Y

B32. WOULD DISCLOSURE OF THE INFORMATION ON THIS FORM BE MEDICALLY OR PSYCHOLOGICALLY DETRIMENTAL TO YOUR PATIENT? ☐ YES ☐ NO

B33. **ALL PERSONS AUTHORIZED TO CERTIFY (REQUIRED) (CHECK ONE)**

☐ **ALL PHYSICIANS** (MEDICAL OR OSTEOPATHIC PHYSICIAN, SURGEON, CHIROPRACTOR, DENTIST, PODIATRIST, OPTOMETRIST OR PSYCHOLOGIST)

I CERTIFY UNDER PENALTY OF PERJURY THAT THE PATIENT IS UNABLE TO PERFORM HIS/HER REGULAR OR CUSTOMARY WORK BECAUSE OF THE DISABLING CONDITION(S) LISTED ABOVE AND I HAVE TREATED THE PATIENT WITHIN MY SCOPE OF PRACTICE.

☐ **NURSE PRACTITIONER**

I CERTIFY UNDER PENALTY OF PERJURY THAT THE PATIENT IS UNABLE TO PERFORM HIS/HER REGULAR OR CUSTOMARY WORK BECAUSE OF THE DISABLING CONDITION(S) LISTED ABOVE AND I HAVE TREATED THE PATIENT WITHIN MY SCOPE OF PRACTICE. IF FOR A CONDITION OTHER THAN A NORMAL PREGNANCY OR DELIVERY, I CERTIFY THAT I HAVE PERFORMED A PHYSICAL EXAMINATION AND HAVE COLLABORATED WITH A PHYSICIAN OR SURGEON.

☐ **REGISTRAR OF A COUNTY HOSPITAL IN CALIFORNIA OR MEDICAL OFFICER OF A US GOVERNMENT MEDICAL FACILITY**

I CERTIFY UNDER PENALTY OF PERJURY THAT THE PATIENT IS UNABLE TO PERFORM HIS/HER REGULAR OR CUSTOMARY WORK BECAUSE OF THE DISABLING CONDITION(S) LISTED ABOVE AND THESE CONDITIONS ARE SHOWN BY THE PATIENT'S HOSPITAL CHART.

☐ **OTHER:** TITLE OF PERSON IF NOT COVERED ABOVE: (MUST BE ABLE TO LEGALLY CERTIFY TO A DISABILITY)

PHYSICIAN/PRACTITIONER'S ORIGINAL SIGNATURE - **RUBBER STAMP IS NOT ACCEPTABLE**	DATE SIGNED	AREA CODE/PHONE NUMBER
	M M D D Y Y Y Y	

UNDER SECTIONS 2116 AND 2122 OF THE CALIFORNIA UNEMPLOYMENT INSURANCE CODE, IT IS A VIOLATION FOR ANY INDIVIDUAL WHO, WITH INTENT TO DEFRAUD, FALSELY CERTIFIES THE MEDICAL CONDITION OF ANY PERSON IN ORDER TO OBTAIN DISABILITY INSURANCE BENEFITS, WHETHER FOR THE MAKER OR FOR ANY OTHER PERSON, AND IS PUNISHABLE BY IMPRISONMENT AND/OR A FINE NOT EXCEEDING $20,000. SECTION 1143 REQUIRES ADDITIONAL ADMINISTRATIVE PENALTIES.

DE 2501 Rev. 78 (4-12)

OSP 12 127141

Figure 16-3, cont'd

ASSIGNMENT 16-3 COMPLETE TWO STATE DISABILITY INSURANCE FORMS

Performance Objective

Task: Complete two state disability insurance forms and define patient record abbreviations.

Conditions: Use the patient's record (Figure 16-4), a Doctor's Certificate form (Figure 16-5), a Physician's Supplementary Certificate form (Figure 16-6), and a computer.

Standards: Time: ____________ minutes

Accuracy: ____________

(Note: The time element and accuracy criteria may be given by your instructor.)

Directions:

1. Assume that the Claim Statement of Employee has been completed satisfactorily by Mr. Fred E. Thorndike (see Figure 16-4). Complete the Doctor's Certificate form (see Figure 16-5) and date it December 2. In completing this portion of the assignment, look at the first entry made by Dr. Practon on November 25 only.

2. Mr. Thorndike returns to see Dr. Practon on December 7, at which time his disability leave needs to be extended. Complete the Physician's Supplementary Certificate form (see Figure 16-6) by referring to the entry made during the second visit, and date the certificate December 7. Remember that this is not a claim for payment to the physician, and so no ledger card has been furnished for this patient.

3. Refer to Chapter 16 and Figures 16-4 and 16-5 of the *Handbook* to assist you in completing these forms.

After the instructor has returned your work to you, either make the necessary corrections and place your work in a three-ring notebook for future reference or, if you received a high score, place it in your portfolio for reference when applying for a job.

Abbreviations pertinent to this record:

pt	____________	SDI	____________
PE	____________	wks	____________
dx	____________	Cont	____________
RTO	____________	wk	____________
est	____________	FU	____________
$\bar{c}$	____________	CXR	____________
reg	____________		

PATIENT RECORD NO. 16-3

Thorndike	Fred	E	02-17-54	M	555-465-7820
LAST NAME	FIRST NAME	MIDDLE NAME	BIRTH DATE	SEX	HOME PHONE

5784 Helen Street	Woodland Hills	XY	12345
ADDRESS	CITY	STATE	ZIP CODE

555-432-7744	555-320-5500	555-466-7820	thorndike@wb.net
CELL PHONE	PAGER NO.	FAX NO.	E-MAIL ADDRESS

549-XX-8721	M00430548
PATIENT'S SOC. SEC. NO.	DRIVER'S LICENSE

salesman Payoll No. 6852	Easy on Paint Company
PATIENT'S OCCUPATION	NAME OF COMPANY

4586 West 20th Street, Woodland Hills, XY 12345	555-467-8898
ADDRESS OF EMPLOYER	PHONE

Jennifer B. Thorndike	homemaker
SPOUSE OR PARENT	OCCUPATION

EMPLOYER	ADDRESS	PHONE

Pacific Mutual Insurance Company,120 South Main Street, Merck, XY 12346
NAME OF INSURANCE

	6709	Fred E. Thorndike
POLICY/CERTIFICATE NO.	GROUP NO.	INSURED OR SUBSCRIBER

REFERRED BY: John Diehl (Friend)

DATE	PROGRESS NOTES
11-25-xx	On or about 11-3-xx, pt began to have chest pain and much coughing. On 11-24-xx, pt too ill to work and
	decided to file for SDI benefits. Pt states illness is not work connected and he does not receive sick pay.
	PE: Pt examined and complained of productive cough of 3 wks duration and chest pain. Chest x-rays
	confirmed dx-mucopurulent chronic bronchitis. Cont home rest and prescribed antibiotic medication. RTO
	12-7-xx. Pt will be capable of returning to wk 12-8-xx.
	GP/mtf Gerald Practon, MD
12-07-xx	Est pt returns for F/U c bronchitis. Chest pain improved. Still running low grade temp c̄ productive cough.
	F/U CXR shows clearing. Recommended bed rest x 7d. Will extend disability to 12-15-xx at which time pt
	can resume reg work. No complications anticipated.
	GP/mtf Gerald Practon, MD

Figure 16-4

Claim for Disability Insurance (DI) Benefits - Physician/Practitioner's Certificate
PLEASE PRINT WITH BLACK INK.

250104125

PART B - PHYSICIAN/PRACTITIONER'S CERTIFICATE

B1. PATIENT'S SOCIAL SECURITY NUMBER

B2. PATIENT'S FILE NUMBER

B3. IF YOU KNOW THE PATIENT'S ELECTRONIC RECEIPT NUMBER, ENTER IT HERE:

R

B4. PATIENT'S DATE OF BIRTH

M M D D Y Y Y Y

B5. PATIENT'S NAME (FIRST) (MI) (LAST)

B6. PHYSICIAN/PRACTITIONER'S LICENSE NUMBER

B7. STATE **OR** COUNTRY (IF NOT U.S.A.) THAT ISSUED LICENSE NUMBER ENTERED IN B6

STATE COUNTRY

B8. PHYSICIAN/PRACTITIONER LICENSE TYPE

B9. SPECIALTY (IF ANY)

B10. PHYSICIAN/PRACTITIONER'S NAME AS SHOWN ON LICENSE
(FIRST) (MI) (LAST) SUFFIX

B11. PHYSICIAN/PRACTITIONER'S ADDRESS

MAILING ADDRESS, PO BOX OR NUMBER/STREET/SUITE#

CITY STATE ZIP OR POSTAL CODE COUNTRY (IF NOT U.S.A.)

COUNTY HOSPITAL/GOVERNMENT FACILITY ADDRESS

FACILITY NAME (IF APPLICABLE)

FACILITY ADDRESS, NUMBER/STREET/SUITE#

CITY STATE ZIP OR POSTAL CODE COUNTRY (IF NOT U.S.A.)

B12. THIS PATIENT HAS BEEN UNDER MY CARE AND TREATMENT FOR THIS MEDICAL PROBLEM

FROM M M D D Y Y Y Y TO M M D D Y Y Y Y ☐ CHECK HERE TO INDICATE YOU ARE STILL TREATING THE PATIENT

AT INTERVALS OF: ☐ DAILY ☐ WEEKLY ☐ MONTHLY ☐ AS NEEDED ☐ OTHER

B13. AT ANY TIME DURING YOUR ATTENDANCE FOR THIS MEDICAL PROBLEM, HAS THE PATIENT BEEN INCAPABLE OF PERFORMING HIS/HER REGULAR OR CUSTOMARY WORK?

☐ YES - ENTER DATE DISABILITY BEGAN M M D D Y Y Y Y ☐ NO - SKIP TO B33

WAS THE DISABILITY CAUSED BY AN ACCIDENT OR TRAUMA? ☐ YES ☐ NO

M M D D Y Y Y Y IF YES, INDICATE THE DATE THE ACCIDENT OR TRAUMA OCCURRED.

B14. DATE YOU RELEASED OR ANTICIPATE RELEASING PATIENT TO RETURN TO HIS/HER REGULAR OR CUSTOMARY WORK
("UNKNOWN", "INDEFINITE", ETC., NOT ACCEPTABLE.) M M D D Y Y Y Y

☐ CHECK HERE TO INDICATE PATIENT'S DISABILITY IS PERMANENT AND YOU NEVER ANTICIPATE RELEASING PATIENT TO RETURN TO HIS/HER REGULAR OR CUSTOMARY WORK

B15. IF PATIENT IS NOW PREGNANT OR HAS BEEN PREGNANT, PLEASE CHECK THE APPROPRIATE BOX AND ENTER THE FOLLOWING:

☐ ESTIMATED DELIVERY DATE: M M D D Y Y Y Y ☐ DATE PREGNANCY ENDED: M M D D Y Y Y Y

TYPE OF DELIVERY, IF PATIENT HAS DELIVERED: ☐ VAGINAL ☐ CESAREAN

DE 2501 Rev. 78 (4-12)

Figure 16-5

Continued

250104126

PART B - PHYSICIAN/PRACTITIONER'S CERTIFICATE - CONTINUED

B16. PLEASE RE-ENTER PATIENT'S SOCIAL SECURITY NUMBER

B17. IF THE PATIENT HAS NOT DELIVERED AND YOU DO NOT ANTICIPATE RELEASING THE PATIENT TO RETURN TO REGULAR OR CUSTOMARY WORK PRIOR TO THE ESTIMATED DELIVERY DATE, ENTER THE **NUMBER OF DAYS** THAT THE PATIENT WILL BE DISABLED POSTPARTUM, FOR EACH DELIVERY TYPE:

VAGINAL DELIVERY ☐☐ CESAREAN DELIVERY ☐☐

B18. IN CASE OF AN ABNORMAL PREGNANCY AND/OR DELIVERY, STATE THE COMPLICATION(S) CAUSING MATERNAL DISABILITY

B19. ICD DIAGNOSIS CODE(S) FOR DISABLING CONDITION THAT PREVENT THE PATIENT FROM PERFORMING HIS/HER REGULAR OR CUSTOMARY WORK (REQUIRED)

EXAMPLE OF HOW TO COMPLETE ICD CODES

ICD-9 3 2 0 ▪ 1

ICD-10 G 0 0 ▪ 1

(Check only one box)

☐ ICD-9

☐ ICD-10

PRIMARY ☐☐☐▪☐☐☐☐

SECONDARY ☐☐☐▪☐☐☐☐

SECONDARY ☐☐☐▪☐☐☐☐

SECONDARY ☐☐☐▪☐☐☐☐

B20. DIAGNOSIS (REQUIRED) - IF NO DIAGNOSIS HAS BEEN DETERMINED, ENTER A DETAILED STATEMENT OF SYMPTOMS

B21. FINDINGS - STATE NATURE, SEVERITY, AND EXTENT OF THE INCAPACITATING DISEASE OR INJURY, INCLUDE ANY OTHER DISABLING CONDITIONS

B22. TYPE OF TREATMENT/MEDICATION RENDERED TO PATIENT

B23. IF PATIENT WAS HOSPITALIZED, PROVIDE DATES OF ENTRY AND DISCHARGE M M D D Y Y Y Y TO M M D D Y Y Y Y

☐ CHECK HERE TO INDICATE THE PATIENT IS STILL HOSPITALIZED

B24. ☐ CHECK HERE IF PATIENT IS DECEASED, PLEASE PROVIDE DATE OF DEATH M M D D Y Y Y Y

CITY COUNTY STATE

DE 2501 Rev. 78 (4-12)

Figure 16-5, cont'd

250104127

PART B - PHYSICIAN/PRACTITIONER'S CERTIFICATE - CONTINUED

B25. PLEASE RE-ENTER PATIENT'S SOCIAL SECURITY NUMBER

B26. WAS THE PATIENT SEEN PREVIOUSLY BY ANOTHER PHYSICIAN/PRACTITIONER OR MEDICAL FACILITY FOR THE CURRENT DISABILITY/ILLNESS/INJURY?

☐ YES ☐ NO ☐ UNKNOWN IF YES, WHAT WAS THE DATE OF FIRST TREATMENT? M M D D Y Y Y Y

B27. DATE AND TYPE OF SURGERY/PROCEDURE MOST RECENTLY PERFORMED OR TO BE PERFORMED

M M D D Y Y Y Y

WAS THE PATIENT UNABLE TO WORK IMMEDIATELY PRIOR TO THE SURGERY OR PROCEDURE? ☐ YES ☐ NO

M M D D Y Y Y Y IF YES, PLEASE PROVIDE THE FIRST DATE THE PATIENT WAS UNABLE TO WORK BEFORE THE SURGERY OR PROCEDURE

B28. ICD PROCEDURE CODE(S) ☐ ICD-9 ☐ ICD-10

CPT CODE(S) (DO NOT INCLUDE MODIFIERS)

B29. WAS THIS DISABLING CONDITION CAUSED AND/OR AGGRAVATED BY THE PATIENT'S REGULAR OR CUSTOMARY WORK? ☐ YES ☐ NO

B30. ARE YOU COMPLETING THIS FORM FOR THE SOLE PURPOSE OF REFERRAL/RECOMMENDATION TO AN ALCOHOLIC RECOVERY HOME OR DRUG-FREE RESIDENTIAL FACILITY AS INDICATED BY THE PATIENT IN QUESTION A30? ☐ YES ☐ NO

B31. DATE YOUR PATIENT BECAME A RESIDENT OF A DRUG OR ALCOHOL FACILITY (IF KNOWN) M M D D Y Y Y Y

B32. WOULD DISCLOSURE OF THE INFORMATION ON THIS FORM BE MEDICALLY OR PSYCHOLOGICALLY DETRIMENTAL TO YOUR PATIENT? ☐ YES ☐ NO

B33. **ALL PERSONS AUTHORIZED TO CERTIFY (REQUIRED) (CHECK ONE)**

☐ **ALL PHYSICIANS** (MEDICAL OR OSTEOPATHIC PHYSICIAN, SURGEON, CHIROPRACTOR, DENTIST, PODIATRIST, OPTOMETRIST OR PSYCHOLOGIST)

I CERTIFY UNDER PENALTY OF PERJURY THAT THE PATIENT IS UNABLE TO PERFORM HIS/HER REGULAR OR CUSTOMARY WORK BECAUSE OF THE DISABLING CONDITION(S) LISTED ABOVE AND I HAVE TREATED THE PATIENT WITHIN MY SCOPE OF PRACTICE.

☐ **NURSE PRACTITIONER**

I CERTIFY UNDER PENALTY OF PERJURY THAT THE PATIENT IS UNABLE TO PERFORM HIS/HER REGULAR OR CUSTOMARY WORK BECAUSE OF THE DISABLING CONDITION(S) LISTED ABOVE AND I HAVE TREATED THE PATIENT WITHIN MY SCOPE OF PRACTICE. IF FOR A CONDITION OTHER THAN A NORMAL PREGNANCY OR DELIVERY, I CERTIFY THAT I HAVE PERFORMED A PHYSICAL EXAMINATION AND HAVE COLLABORATED WITH A PHYSICIAN OR SURGEON.

☐ **REGISTRAR OF A COUNTY HOSPITAL IN CALIFORNIA OR MEDICAL OFFICER OF A US GOVERNMENT MEDICAL FACILITY**

I CERTIFY UNDER PENALTY OF PERJURY THAT THE PATIENT IS UNABLE TO PERFORM HIS/HER REGULAR OR CUSTOMARY WORK BECAUSE OF THE DISABLING CONDITION(S) LISTED ABOVE AND THESE CONDITIONS ARE SHOWN BY THE PATIENT'S HOSPITAL CHART.

☐ **OTHER:** TITLE OF PERSON IF NOT COVERED ABOVE: (MUST BE ABLE TO LEGALLY CERTIFY TO A DISABILITY)

PHYSICIAN/PRACTITIONER'S ORIGINAL SIGNATURE - **RUBBER STAMP IS NOT ACCEPTABLE**	DATE SIGNED	AREA CODE/PHONE NUMBER
	M M D D Y Y Y Y	

UNDER SECTIONS 2116 AND 2122 OF THE CALIFORNIA UNEMPLOYMENT INSURANCE CODE, IT IS A VIOLATION FOR ANY INDIVIDUAL WHO, WITH INTENT TO DEFRAUD, FALSELY CERTIFIES THE MEDICAL CONDITION OF ANY PERSON IN ORDER TO OBTAIN DISABILITY INSURANCE BENEFITS, WHETHER FOR THE MAKER OR FOR ANY OTHER PERSON, AND IS PUNISHABLE BY IMPRISONMENT AND/OR A FINE NOT EXCEEDING $20,000. SECTION 1143 REQUIRES ADDITIONAL ADMINISTRATIVE PENALTIES.

DE 2501 Rev. 78 (4-12)

OSP 12 127141

Figure 16-5, cont'd

2525XX03121

Mailing Date

RETURN TO: →

EDD Employment Development Department State of California

PHYSICIAN/PRACTITIONER'S SUPPLEMENTARY CERTIFICATE

EDD Customer Account Number (EDDCAN)	CLAIM ID	SSN/ECN	CED

Claimant Instructions: If you are still disabled, contact your physician/practitioner immediately for completion of the Physician/Practitioner's Supplementary Certificate which must be submitted within twenty (20) days of the mailing date shown above or you may lose additional benefits.

Instrucciones al Solicitante de Beneficios: Si Ud. aun sigue incapacitado. comuniquese con su Médico/Profesional (Medico) lo más pronto posible para completar el documento titlado en inglés "Physician/Practitioner Supplementary Certificats" el cual debe ser presentado dentro de un plazo de veinte (20) días de la fecha de envio indicada arriba o de lo contrario es posible que pueda perder beneficios adicionales.

Physician/ Practitioner Instructions: For faster processing, the physician/practitioner may complete and submit this form online at www.edd.ca.gov. If this form is submitted online, you do not have to mail this form back to EDD. When completing this form, **PLEASE PRINT WITH BLACK INK.**

1. ARE YOU STILL TREATING THE PATIENT? YES NO DATE OF LAST TREATMENT

2. WHAT CURRENT CONDITION(S) CONTINUES TO MAKE THE PATIENT DISABLED? (DIAGNOSIS REQUIRED, IF MADE)

3. DAT OF NEXT APPOINTMENT

4. ICD DIAGNOSIS CODE(S) FOR DISABLING CONDITION THAT PREVENT THE PATIENT FROM PERFORMING HIS/HER REGULAR OR CUSTOMARY WORK (REQUIRED)

EXAMPLE OF HOW TO COMPLETE ICD CODES

ICD-9 3 2 0 • 1

ICD-10 G 0 0 • 1

(Check only one box)

☐ ICD-9

☐ ICD-10

PRIMARY •

SECONDARY •

SECONDARY •

SECONDARY •

ADDITIONAL QUESTIONS ON FOLLOWING PAGES

DE 2525XX Rev. 3 (3-12) Page 1 of 3 CU

Figure 16-6

Continued

2525XX03121

5. DESCRIBE HOW THE PATIENT'S PRESENT CONDITION/IMPAIRMENT PREVENTS HIM/HER FROM RETURNING TO HIS/HER REGULAR OR CUSTOMARY WORK.

6. WHAT FACTORS OR COMPLICATIONS ARE DISABLING THE PATIENT LONGER THAN PREVIOUSLY ESTIMATED?

7. IF PATIENT WAS HOSPITALIZED, PROVIDE DATES OF ENTRY AND DISCHARGE M M D D Y Y Y Y TO M M D D Y Y Y Y

☐ CHECK HERE TO INDICATE THE PATIENT IS STILL HOSPITALIZED

8. DATE AND TYPE OF SURGERY/PROCEDURE PERFORMED OR TO BE PERFORMED

M M D D Y Y Y Y

9A. ICD PROCEDURE CODE(S) ☐ ICD-9 ☐ ICD-10

9B. CPT CODE(S) (DO NOT INCLUDE MODIFIERS)

10. CURRENT ESTIMATED DATE PATIENT (EVEN IF STILL UNDER TREATMENT) WILL BE ABLE TO PERFORM HIS/HER REGULAR OR CUSTOMARY WORK ("UNKNOWN," "INDEFINITE," ETC., NOT ACCEPTABLE)

M M D D Y Y Y Y

☐ CHECK HERE TO INDICATE PATIENT'S DISABILITY IS PERMANENT AND YOU NEVER ANTICIPATE RELEASING PATIENT TO RETURN TO HIS/HER REGULAR OR CUSTOMARY WORK

11. WOULD DISCLOSURE OF THE INFORMATION ON THIS FORM BE MEDICALLY OR PSYCHOLOGICALLY DETRIMENTAL TO YOUR PATIENT? YES NO

ADDITIONAL QUESTIONS ON FOLLOWING PAGES

DE 2525XX Rev. 3 (3-12) Page 2 of 3 OSP 12 127858

Figure 16-6, cont'd

2525XX03121

12. PHYSICIAN/PRACTITIONER'S LICENSE NUMBER

13. STATE OR COUNTRY (IF NOT U.S.A.) THAT ISSUED THE LICENSE NUMBER ENTERED IN QUESTION 12

STATE COUNTRY

14. PHYSICIAN/PRACTITIONER'S NAME

(FIRST) (MI) (LAST) (SUFFIX)

15. PHYSICIAN/PRACTITIONER LICENSE TYPE

16. SPECIALTY, IF ANY

17. PHYSICIAN/PRACTITIONER'S ADDRESS

MAILING ADDRESS, PO BOX, OR NUMBER/STREET/SUITE#

CITY STATE ZIP OR POSTAL CODE COUNTRY (IF NOT U.S.A.)

18. COUNTY HOSPITAL/GOVERNMENT FACILITY ADDRESS

FACILITY NAME (IF APPLICABLE)

FACILITY ADDRESS, NUMBER/STREET/SUITE#

CITY STATE ZIP OR POSTAL CODE COUNTRY (IF NOT U.S.A.)

ALL PERSONS AUTHORIZED TO CERTIFY (REQUIRED)

☐ **All Physicians** (Medical or Osteopathic Physician, Surgeon, Chiropractor, Dentist, Podiatrist, Optometrist or Psychologist)
I certify under penalty of perjury that the patient is unable to perform his/her regular or customary work because of the disabling condition(s) listed above and I have treated the patient within my scope of practice.

☐ **Nurse Practitioner**
I certify under penalty of perjury that the patient is unable to perform his/her regular or customary work because of the disabling condition(s) listed above and I have treated the patient within my scope of practice. If for a condition other than a normal pregnancy or delivery, I certify that I have performed a physical examination and have collaborated with a physician or surgeon.

☐ **Registrar of a County Hospital in California or Medical Officer of a U.S. Government Medical Facility**
I certify under penalty of perjury that the patient is unable to perform his/her regular or customary work because of the disabling condition(s) listed above and these conditions are shown by the patient's hospital chart.

☐ **Other**: Title of person if not covered above: (must be able to legally certify to a disability)

19. PHYSICIAN/PRACTITIONER'S ORIGINAL SIGNATURE – RUBBER STAMP IS NOT ACCEPTABLE

SIGNATURE

DATE SIGNED
M M D D Y Y Y Y

AREA CODE/PHONE NUMBER

Under sections 2116 and 2122 of the California Unemployment Insurance Code, it is a violation for any individual who, with intent to defraud, falsely certifies the medical condition of any person in order to obtain Disability Insurance benefits, whether for the maker or for any other person, and is punishable by imprisonment and/or a fine not exceeding $20,000. Section 1143 requires additional administrative penalties.

DE 2525XX Rev. 3 (3-12) Page 3 of 3

Figure 16-6, cont'd

ASSIGNMENT 16-4 COMPLETE A STATE DISABILITY INSURANCE FORM

Performance Objective

Task: Complete a state disability insurance form and define patient record abbreviations.

Conditions: Use the patient's record (Figure 16-7), a Doctor's Certificate form (Figure 16-8), and a computer.

Standards: Time: ______________ minutes

Accuracy: ______________

(Note: The time element and accuracy criteria may be given by your instructor.)

Directions:

1. Assume that the Claim Statement of Employee has been completed satisfactorily by Mr. James T. Fujita (see Figure 16-7). Complete the Doctor's Certificate form (see Figure 16-8) and date it December 15. Remember that this is not a claim for payment to the physician, and so no ledger card has been furnished for this patient.

2. Refer to Chapter 16 and Figure 16-4 of the *Handbook* to assist you in completing this form.

After the instructor has returned your work to you, either make the necessary corrections and place your work in a three-ring notebook for future reference or, if you received a high score, place it in your portfolio for reference when applying for a job.

Abbreviations pertinent to this record:

pt	______________	exam	______________
hx	______________	neg	______________
WBC	______________	imp	______________
wk	______________	SDI	______________

PATIENT RECORD NO. 16-4

Fujita	James	T	03-27-54	M	555-677-2881
LAST NAME	FIRST NAME	MIDDLE NAME	BIRTH DATE	SEX	HOME PHONE

3538 South A Street	Woodland Hills	XY	12345
ADDRESS	CITY	STATE	ZIP CODE

555-499-6556	555-988-4100	555-677-2881	fujita@wb.net
CELL PHONE	PAGER NO.	FAX NO.	E-MAIL ADDRESS

567-XX-8898	M4387931
PATIENT'S SOC. SEC. NO.	DRIVER'S LICENSE

electrician Payoll No. 8834	Macy Electric Company
PATIENT'S OCCUPATION	NAME OF COMPANY

2671 North C Street, Woodland Hills, XY 12345	555-677-2346
ADDRESS OF EMPLOYER	PHONE

Mary J. Fujita	homemaker
SPOUSE OR PARENT	OCCUPATION

EMPLOYER	ADDRESS	PHONE

Atlantic Mutual Insurance Company, 111 South Main Street, Woodland Hills, XY 12345
NAME OF INSURANCE

F20015		James T. Fujita
POLICY/CERTIFICATE NO.	GROUP NO.	INSURED OR SUBSCRIBER

REFERRED BY: Cherry Hotta (aunt)

DATE	PROGRESS NOTES
12-07-XX	Today pt could not go to work and came for exam complaining of pain in abdomen, nausea, and no vomiting. Pt has hx of mesentery adenopathy. Exam neg except abdomen showed tenderness all over with voluntary guarding. WBC 10,000. Imp: Mesenteric adenitis. Advised strict bed rest at home and bland diet. To return in 1 wk. Will file for SDI benefits. Pt states illness is not work connected and he receives sick leave pay of $150/wk.
	GI/mtf Gaston Input, MD
12-15-xx	Exam showed normal nontender abdomen. No nausea. Pt tolerating food well. WBC 7,500. Pt will be capable of returning to work 12-22-xx.
	GI/mtf Gaston Input, MD

Figure 16-7

Claim for Disability Insurance (DI) Benefits - Physician/Practitioner's Certificate
PLEASE PRINT WITH BLACK INK.

250104125

PART B - PHYSICIAN/PRACTITIONER'S CERTIFICATE

B1. PATIENT'S SOCIAL SECURITY NUMBER

B2. PATIENT'S FILE NUMBER

B3. IF YOU KNOW THE PATIENT'S ELECTRONIC RECEIPT NUMBER, ENTER IT HERE:
R

B4. PATIENT'S DATE OF BIRTH
M M D D Y Y Y Y

B5. PATIENT'S NAME (FIRST) (MI) (LAST)

B6. PHYSICIAN/PRACTITIONER'S LICENSE NUMBER

B7. STATE **OR** COUNTRY (IF NOT U.S.A.) THAT ISSUED LICENSE NUMBER ENTERED IN B6
STATE COUNTRY

B8. PHYSICIAN/PRACTITIONER LICENSE TYPE

B9. SPECIALTY (IF ANY)

B10. PHYSICIAN/PRACTITIONER'S NAME AS SHOWN ON LICENSE
(FIRST) (MI) (LAST) SUFFIX

B11. PHYSICIAN/PRACTITIONER'S ADDRESS
MAILING ADDRESS, PO BOX OR NUMBER/STREET/SUITE#
CITY STATE ZIP OR POSTAL CODE COUNTRY (IF NOT U.S.A.)

COUNTY HOSPITAL/GOVERNMENT FACILITY ADDRESS
FACILITY NAME (IF APPLICABLE)
FACILITY ADDRESS, NUMBER/STREET/SUITE#
CITY STATE ZIP OR POSTAL CODE COUNTRY (IF NOT U.S.A.)

B12. THIS PATIENT HAS BEEN UNDER MY CARE AND TREATMENT FOR THIS MEDICAL PROBLEM
FROM M M D D Y Y Y Y TO M M D D Y Y Y Y ☐ CHECK HERE TO INDICATE YOU ARE STILL TREATING THE PATIENT

AT INTERVALS OF: ☐ DAILY ☐ WEEKLY ☐ MONTHLY ☐ AS NEEDED ☐ OTHER

B13. AT ANY TIME DURING YOUR ATTENDANCE FOR THIS MEDICAL PROBLEM, HAS THE PATIENT BEEN INCAPABLE OF PERFORMING HIS/HER REGULAR OR CUSTOMARY WORK?
☐ YES - ENTER DATE DISABILITY BEGAN M M D D Y Y Y Y ☐ NO - SKIP TO B33

WAS THE DISABILITY CAUSED BY AN ACCIDENT OR TRAUMA? ☐ YES ☐ NO

M M D D Y Y Y Y IF YES, INDICATE THE DATE THE ACCIDENT OR TRAUMA OCCURRED.

B14. DATE YOU RELEASED OR ANTICIPATE RELEASING PATIENT TO RETURN TO HIS/HER REGULAR OR CUSTOMARY WORK
("UNKNOWN", "INDEFINITE", ETC., NOT ACCEPTABLE.) M M D D Y Y Y Y

☐ CHECK HERE TO INDICATE PATIENT'S DISABILITY IS PERMANENT AND YOU NEVER ANTICIPATE RELEASING PATIENT TO RETURN TO HIS/HER REGULAR OR CUSTOMARY WORK

B15. IF PATIENT IS NOW PREGNANT OR HAS BEEN PREGNANT, PLEASE CHECK THE APPROPRIATE BOX AND ENTER THE FOLLOWING:
☐ ESTIMATED DELIVERY DATE: M M D D Y Y Y Y ☐ DATE PREGNANCY ENDED: M M D D Y Y Y Y

TYPE OF DELIVERY, IF PATIENT HAS DELIVERED: ☐ VAGINAL ☐ CESAREAN

DE 2501 Rev. 78 (4-12)

Figure 16-8

Continued

250104126

PART B - PHYSICIAN/PRACTITIONER'S CERTIFICATE - CONTINUED

B16. PLEASE RE-ENTER PATIENT'S SOCIAL SECURITY NUMBER

B17. IF THE PATIENT HAS NOT DELIVERED AND YOU DO NOT ANTICIPATE RELEASING THE PATIENT TO RETURN TO REGULAR OR CUSTOMARY WORK PRIOR TO THE ESTIMATED DELIVERY DATE, ENTER THE **NUMBER OF DAYS** THAT THE PATIENT WILL BE DISABLED POSTPARTUM, FOR EACH DELIVERY TYPE:

VAGINAL DELIVERY ☐☐ CESAREAN DELIVERY ☐☐

B18. IN CASE OF AN ABNORMAL PREGNANCY AND/OR DELIVERY, STATE THE COMPLICATION(S) CAUSING MATERNAL DISABILITY

B19. ICD DIAGNOSIS CODE(S) FOR DISABLING CONDITION THAT PREVENT THE PATIENT FROM PERFORMING HIS/HER REGULAR OR CUSTOMARY WORK (REQUIRED)

PRIMARY ☐☐☐.☐☐☐☐

(Check only one box)

☐ ICD-9

☐ ICD-10

SECONDARY ☐☐☐.☐☐☐☐

SECONDARY ☐☐☐.☐☐☐☐

SECONDARY ☐☐☐.☐☐☐☐

EXAMPLE OF HOW TO COMPLETE ICD CODES

ICD-9	3 2 0 . 1
ICD-10	G 0 0 . 1

B20. DIAGNOSIS (REQUIRED) - IF NO DIAGNOSIS HAS BEEN DETERMINED, ENTER A DETAILED STATEMENT OF SYMPTOMS

B21. FINDINGS - STATE NATURE, SEVERITY, AND EXTENT OF THE INCAPACITATING DISEASE OR INJURY, INCLUDE ANY OTHER DISABLING CONDITIONS

B22. TYPE OF TREATMENT/MEDICATION RENDERED TO PATIENT

B23. IF PATIENT WAS HOSPITALIZED, PROVIDE DATES OF ENTRY AND DISCHARGE M M D D Y Y Y Y TO M M D D Y Y Y Y

☐ CHECK HERE TO INDICATE THE PATIENT IS STILL HOSPITALIZED

B24. ☐ CHECK HERE IF PATIENT IS DECEASED, PLEASE PROVIDE DATE OF DEATH M M D D Y Y Y Y

CITY COUNTY STATE

DE 2501 Rev. 78 (4-12)

Figure 16-8, cont'd

250104127

PART B - PHYSICIAN/PRACTITIONER'S CERTIFICATE - CONTINUED

B25. PLEASE RE-ENTER PATIENT'S SOCIAL SECURITY NUMBER

B26. WAS THE PATIENT SEEN PREVIOUSLY BY ANOTHER PHYSICIAN/PRACTITIONER OR MEDICAL FACILITY FOR THE CURRENT DISABILITY/ILLNESS/INJURY?

☐ YES ☐ NO ☐ UNKNOWN — IF YES, WHAT WAS THE DATE OF FIRST TREATMENT? M M D D Y Y Y Y

B27. DATE AND TYPE OF SURGERY/PROCEDURE MOST RECENTLY PERFORMED OR TO BE PERFORMED

M M D D Y Y Y Y

WAS THE PATIENT UNABLE TO WORK IMMEDIATELY PRIOR TO THE SURGERY OR PROCEDURE? ☐ YES ☐ NO

M M D D Y Y Y Y — IF YES, PLEASE PROVIDE THE FIRST DATE THE PATIENT WAS UNABLE TO WORK BEFORE THE SURGERY OR PROCEDURE

B28. ICD PROCEDURE CODE(S) ☐ ICD-9 ☐ ICD-10

CPT CODE(S) (DO NOT INCLUDE MODIFIERS)

B29. WAS THIS DISABLING CONDITION CAUSED AND/OR AGGRAVATED BY THE PATIENT'S REGULAR OR CUSTOMARY WORK? ☐ YES ☐ NO

B30. ARE YOU COMPLETING THIS FORM FOR THE SOLE PURPOSE OF REFERRAL/RECOMMENDATION TO AN ALCOHOLIC RECOVERY HOME OR DRUG-FREE RESIDENTIAL FACILITY AS INDICATED BY THE PATIENT IN QUESTION A30? ☐ YES ☐ NO

B31. DATE YOUR PATIENT BECAME A RESIDENT OF A DRUG OR ALCOHOL FACILITY (IF KNOWN) M M D D Y Y Y Y

B32. WOULD DISCLOSURE OF THE INFORMATION ON THIS FORM BE MEDICALLY OR PSYCHOLOGICALLY DETRIMENTAL TO YOUR PATIENT? ☐ YES ☐ NO

B33. **ALL PERSONS AUTHORIZED TO CERTIFY (REQUIRED) (CHECK ONE)**

☐ **ALL PHYSICIANS** (MEDICAL OR OSTEOPATHIC PHYSICIAN, SURGEON, CHIROPRACTOR, DENTIST, PODIATRIST, OPTOMETRIST OR PSYCHOLOGIST)

I CERTIFY UNDER PENALTY OF PERJURY THAT THE PATIENT IS UNABLE TO PERFORM HIS/HER REGULAR OR CUSTOMARY WORK BECAUSE OF THE DISABLING CONDITION(S) LISTED ABOVE AND I HAVE TREATED THE PATIENT WITHIN MY SCOPE OF PRACTICE.

☐ **NURSE PRACTITIONER**

I CERTIFY UNDER PENALTY OF PERJURY THAT THE PATIENT IS UNABLE TO PERFORM HIS/HER REGULAR OR CUSTOMARY WORK BECAUSE OF THE DISABLING CONDITION(S) LISTED ABOVE AND I HAVE TREATED THE PATIENT WITHIN MY SCOPE OF PRACTICE. IF FOR A CONDITION OTHER THAN A NORMAL PREGNANCY OR DELIVERY, I CERTIFY THAT I HAVE PERFORMED A PHYSICAL EXAMINATION AND HAVE COLLABORATED WITH A PHYSICIAN OR SURGEON.

☐ **REGISTRAR OF A COUNTY HOSPITAL IN CALIFORNIA OR MEDICAL OFFICER OF A US GOVERNMENT MEDICAL FACILITY**

I CERTIFY UNDER PENALTY OF PERJURY THAT THE PATIENT IS UNABLE TO PERFORM HIS/HER REGULAR OR CUSTOMARY WORK BECAUSE OF THE DISABLING CONDITION(S) LISTED ABOVE AND THESE CONDITIONS ARE SHOWN BY THE PATIENT'S HOSPITAL CHART.

☐ **OTHER:** TITLE OF PERSON IF NOT COVERED ABOVE: (MUST BE ABLE TO LEGALLY CERTIFY TO A DISABILITY)

PHYSICIAN/PRACTITIONER'S ORIGINAL SIGNATURE - **RUBBER STAMP IS NOT ACCEPTABLE**	DATE SIGNED	AREA CODE/PHONE NUMBER
	M M D D Y Y Y Y	

UNDER SECTIONS 2116 AND 2122 OF THE CALIFORNIA UNEMPLOYMENT INSURANCE CODE, IT IS A VIOLATION FOR ANY INDIVIDUAL WHO, WITH INTENT TO DEFRAUD, FALSELY CERTIFIES THE MEDICAL CONDITION OF ANY PERSON IN ORDER TO OBTAIN DISABILITY INSURANCE BENEFITS, WHETHER FOR THE MAKER OR FOR ANY OTHER PERSON, AND IS PUNISHABLE BY IMPRISONMENT AND/OR A FINE NOT EXCEEDING $20,000. SECTION 1143 REQUIRES ADDITIONAL ADMINISTRATIVE PENALTIES.

DE 2501 Rev. 78 (4-12)

OSP 12 127141

Figure 16-8, cont'd

ASSIGNMENT 16-5 COMPLETE A STATE DISABILITY INSURANCE FORM

Performance Objective

Task: Complete a state disability insurance form and define patient record abbreviations.

Conditions: Use the patient's record (Figure 16-9), a Doctor's Certificate form (Figure 16-10), and a computer.

Standards: Time: ______________ minutes

Accuracy: ______________

(Note: The time element and accuracy criteria may be given by your instructor.)

Directions:

1. Mr. Vincent P. Michael (see Figure 16-9) is applying for state disability benefits. Complete the Doctor's Certificate form (see Figure 16-10) and date it September 22. Assume that the Claim Statement of Employee has been completed satisfactorily by Mr. Michael. Remember that this is not a claim for payment to the physician, and so no ledger card has been furnished for this patient.

2. Refer to Chapter 16 and Figure 16-4 of the *Handbook* to assist you in completing this form.

After the instructor has returned your work to you, either make the necessary corrections and place your work in a three-ring notebook for future reference or, if you received a high score, place it in your portfolio for reference when applying for a job.

Abbreviations pertinent to this record:

Pt	______________________	exam	______________________
ESR	______________________	mm	______________________
hr	______________________	imp	______________________
CVA	______________________	adv	______________________
retn	______________________	wk	______________________
approx	______________________	L	______________________

PATIENT RECORD NO. 16-5

LAST NAME	FIRST NAME	MIDDLE NAME	BIRTH DATE	SEX	HOME PHONE
Michael	Vincent	P	05-17-55	M	555-567-9001

ADDRESS	CITY	STATE	ZIP CODE
1529 1/2 Thompson Boulevard	Woodland Hills	XY	12345

CELL PHONE	PAGER NO.	FAX NO.	E-MAIL ADDRESS
555-398-5677	555-311-0098	555-567-9001	michael@wb.net

PATIENT'S SOC. SEC. NO.	DRIVER'S LICENSE
562-XX-8888	E0034578

PATIENT'S OCCUPATION	NAME OF COMPANY
assembler "A"	Burroughs Corporation

ADDRESS OF EMPLOYER	PHONE
5411 North Lindero Canyon Road, Woodland Hills, XY 12345	555-560-9008

SPOUSE OR PARENT	OCCUPATION
Helen J. Michael	homemaker

EMPLOYER	ADDRESS	PHONE

NAME OF INSURANCE	INSURED OR SUBSCRIBER
Blue Shield	Vincent P. Michael

POLICY/CERTIFICATE NO.	GROUP NO.
T8411981A	677899AT

REFERRED BY: Robert T. Smith (friend)

DATE	PROGRESS NOTES
9-20-xx	Patient calls the office complaining of having had the flu, headache, dizziness, and of being tired. Pt unable to go to work today. Exam shows weakness of L hand. Pt exhibits light dysphasia and confusion. Pt is referred to XYZ Radiology for chest x-ray, frontal and lateral, and to the lab at College Hospital for ESR. Pt to return tomorrow at 11 AM for results.
	BC/mtf Brady Coccidioides, MD
9-21-xx	Chest x-rays show cardiomegaly and slight pulmonary congestion. ESR 46 mm/hr. Imp. Post flu syndrome, transient ischemic attack, possible CVA. Prescribed medication for the congestion and adv. pt. to take aspirin 1/day. Pt to stay off work and retn in 1 week. Approx. date of retn to work 10-16-xx.
	BC/mtf Brady Coccidioides, MD

Figure 16-9

Claim for Disability Insurance (DI) Benefits - Physician/Practitioner's Certificate
PLEASE PRINT WITH BLACK INK.

250104125

PART B - PHYSICIAN/PRACTITIONER'S CERTIFICATE

B1. PATIENT'S SOCIAL SECURITY NUMBER

B2. PATIENT'S FILE NUMBER

B3. IF YOU KNOW THE PATIENT'S ELECTRONIC RECEIPT NUMBER, ENTER IT HERE:
R

B4. PATIENT'S DATE OF BIRTH
M M D D Y Y Y Y

B5. PATIENT'S NAME (FIRST) (MI) (LAST)

B6. PHYSICIAN/PRACTITIONER'S LICENSE NUMBER

B7. STATE **OR** COUNTRY (IF NOT U.S.A.) THAT ISSUED LICENSE NUMBER ENTERED IN B6
STATE COUNTRY

B8. PHYSICIAN/PRACTITIONER LICENSE TYPE

B9. SPECIALTY (IF ANY)

B10. PHYSICIAN/PRACTITIONER'S NAME AS SHOWN ON LICENSE
(FIRST) (MI) (LAST) SUFFIX

B11. PHYSICIAN/PRACTITIONER'S ADDRESS
MAILING ADDRESS, PO BOX OR NUMBER/STREET/SUITE#
CITY STATE ZIP OR POSTAL CODE COUNTRY (IF NOT U.S.A.)

COUNTY HOSPITAL/GOVERNMENT FACILITY ADDRESS
FACILITY NAME (IF APPLICABLE)
FACILITY ADDRESS, NUMBER/STREET/SUITE#
CITY STATE ZIP OR POSTAL CODE COUNTRY (IF NOT U.S.A.)

B12. THIS PATIENT HAS BEEN UNDER MY CARE AND TREATMENT FOR THIS MEDICAL PROBLEM
FROM M M D D Y Y Y Y TO M M D D Y Y Y Y ☐ CHECK HERE TO INDICATE YOU ARE STILL TREATING THE PATIENT
AT INTERVALS OF: ☐ DAILY ☐ WEEKLY ☐ MONTHLY ☐ AS NEEDED ☐ OTHER

B13. AT ANY TIME DURING YOUR ATTENDANCE FOR THIS MEDICAL PROBLEM, HAS THE PATIENT BEEN INCAPABLE OF PERFORMING HIS/HER REGULAR OR CUSTOMARY WORK?
☐ YES - ENTER DATE DISABILITY BEGAN M M D D Y Y Y Y ☐ NO - SKIP TO B33
WAS THE DISABILITY CAUSED BY AN ACCIDENT OR TRAUMA? ☐ YES ☐ NO
M M D D Y Y Y Y IF YES, INDICATE THE DATE THE ACCIDENT OR TRAUMA OCCURRED.

B14. DATE YOU RELEASED OR ANTICIPATE RELEASING PATIENT TO RETURN TO HIS/HER REGULAR OR CUSTOMARY WORK
("UNKNOWN", "INDEFINITE", ETC., NOT ACCEPTABLE.) M M D D Y Y Y Y
☐ CHECK HERE TO INDICATE PATIENT'S DISABILITY IS PERMANENT AND YOU NEVER ANTICIPATE RELEASING PATIENT TO RETURN TO HIS/HER REGULAR OR CUSTOMARY WORK

B15. IF PATIENT IS NOW PREGNANT OR HAS BEEN PREGNANT, PLEASE CHECK THE APPROPRIATE BOX AND ENTER THE FOLLOWING:
☐ ESTIMATED DELIVERY DATE: M M D D Y Y Y Y ☐ DATE PREGNANCY ENDED: M M D D Y Y Y Y
TYPE OF DELIVERY, IF PATIENT HAS DELIVERED: ☐ VAGINAL ☐ CESAREAN

DE 2501 Rev. 78 (4-12)

Figure 16-10

Continued

250104126

PART B - PHYSICIAN/PRACTITIONER'S CERTIFICATE - CONTINUED

B16. PLEASE RE-ENTER PATIENT'S SOCIAL SECURITY NUMBER

B17. IF THE PATIENT HAS NOT DELIVERED AND YOU DO NOT ANTICIPATE RELEASING THE PATIENT TO RETURN TO REGULAR OR CUSTOMARY WORK PRIOR TO THE ESTIMATED DELIVERY DATE, ENTER THE **NUMBER OF DAYS** THAT THE PATIENT WILL BE DISABLED POSTPARTUM, FOR EACH DELIVERY TYPE:

VAGINAL DELIVERY ☐☐ CESAREAN DELIVERY ☐☐

B18. IN CASE OF AN ABNORMAL PREGNANCY AND/OR DELIVERY, STATE THE COMPLICATION(S) CAUSING MATERNAL DISABILITY

B19. ICD DIAGNOSIS CODE(S) FOR DISABLING CONDITION THAT PREVENT THE PATIENT FROM PERFORMING HIS/HER REGULAR OR CUSTOMARY WORK (REQUIRED)

PRIMARY ☐☐☐.☐☐☐☐

(Check only one box)

SECONDARY ☐☐☐.☐☐☐☐

EXAMPLE OF HOW TO COMPLETE ICD CODES

ICD-9	3 2 0 . 1
ICD-10	G 0 0 . 1

☐ ICD-9

☐ ICD-10

SECONDARY ☐☐☐.☐☐☐☐

SECONDARY ☐☐☐.☐☐☐☐

B20. DIAGNOSIS (REQUIRED) - IF NO DIAGNOSIS HAS BEEN DETERMINED, ENTER A DETAILED STATEMENT OF SYMPTOMS

B21. FINDINGS - STATE NATURE, SEVERITY, AND EXTENT OF THE INCAPACITATING DISEASE OR INJURY, INCLUDE ANY OTHER DISABLING CONDITIONS

B22. TYPE OF TREATMENT/MEDICATION RENDERED TO PATIENT

B23. IF PATIENT WAS HOSPITALIZED, PROVIDE DATES OF ENTRY AND DISCHARGE M M D D Y Y Y Y TO M M D D Y Y Y Y

☐ CHECK HERE TO INDICATE THE PATIENT IS STILL HOSPITALIZED

B24. ☐ CHECK HERE IF PATIENT IS DECEASED, PLEASE PROVIDE DATE OF DEATH M M D D Y Y Y Y

CITY COUNTY STATE

DE 2501 Rev. 78 (4-12)

Figure 16-10, cont'd

250104127

PART B - PHYSICIAN/PRACTITIONER'S CERTIFICATE - CONTINUED

B25. PLEASE RE-ENTER PATIENT'S SOCIAL SECURITY NUMBER

B26. WAS THE PATIENT SEEN PREVIOUSLY BY ANOTHER PHYSICIAN/PRACTITIONER OR MEDICAL FACILITY FOR THE CURRENT DISABILITY/ILLNESS/INJURY?

☐ YES ☐ NO ☐ UNKNOWN IF YES, WHAT WAS THE DATE OF FIRST TREATMENT? M M D D Y Y Y Y

B27. DATE AND TYPE OF SURGERY/PROCEDURE MOST RECENTLY PERFORMED OR TO BE PERFORMED

M M D D Y Y Y Y

WAS THE PATIENT UNABLE TO WORK IMMEDIATELY PRIOR TO THE SURGERY OR PROCEDURE? ☐ YES ☐ NO

M M D D Y Y Y Y IF YES, PLEASE PROVIDE THE FIRST DATE THE PATIENT WAS UNABLE TO WORK BEFORE THE SURGERY OR PROCEDURE

B28. ICD PROCEDURE CODE(S) ☐ ICD-9 ☐ ICD-10

CPT CODE(S) (DO NOT INCLUDE MODIFIERS)

B29. WAS THIS DISABLING CONDITION CAUSED AND/OR AGGRAVATED BY THE PATIENT'S REGULAR OR CUSTOMARY WORK? ☐ YES ☐ NO

B30. ARE YOU COMPLETING THIS FORM FOR THE SOLE PURPOSE OF REFERRAL/RECOMMENDATION TO AN ALCOHOLIC RECOVERY HOME OR DRUG-FREE RESIDENTIAL FACILITY AS INDICATED BY THE PATIENT IN QUESTION A30? ☐ YES ☐ NO

B31. DATE YOUR PATIENT BECAME A RESIDENT OF A DRUG OR ALCOHOL FACILITY (IF KNOWN) M M D D Y Y Y Y

B32. WOULD DISCLOSURE OF THE INFORMATION ON THIS FORM BE MEDICALLY OR PSYCHOLOGICALLY DETRIMENTAL TO YOUR PATIENT? ☐ YES ☐ NO

B33. **ALL PERSONS AUTHORIZED TO CERTIFY (REQUIRED) (CHECK ONE)**

☐ **ALL PHYSICIANS** (MEDICAL OR OSTEOPATHIC PHYSICIAN, SURGEON, CHIROPRACTOR, DENTIST, PODIATRIST, OPTOMETRIST OR PSYCHOLOGIST)

I CERTIFY UNDER PENALTY OF PERJURY THAT THE PATIENT IS UNABLE TO PERFORM HIS/HER REGULAR OR CUSTOMARY WORK BECAUSE OF THE DISABLING CONDITION(S) LISTED ABOVE AND I HAVE TREATED THE PATIENT WITHIN MY SCOPE OF PRACTICE.

☐ **NURSE PRACTITIONER**

I CERTIFY UNDER PENALTY OF PERJURY THAT THE PATIENT IS UNABLE TO PERFORM HIS/HER REGULAR OR CUSTOMARY WORK BECAUSE OF THE DISABLING CONDITION(S) LISTED ABOVE AND I HAVE TREATED THE PATIENT WITHIN MY SCOPE OF PRACTICE. IF FOR A CONDITION OTHER THAN A NORMAL PREGNANCY OR DELIVERY, I CERTIFY THAT I HAVE PERFORMED A PHYSICAL EXAMINATION AND HAVE COLLABORATED WITH A PHYSICIAN OR SURGEON.

☐ **REGISTRAR OF A COUNTY HOSPITAL IN CALIFORNIA OR MEDICAL OFFICER OF A US GOVERNMENT MEDICAL FACILITY**

I CERTIFY UNDER PENALTY OF PERJURY THAT THE PATIENT IS UNABLE TO PERFORM HIS/HER REGULAR OR CUSTOMARY WORK BECAUSE OF THE DISABLING CONDITION(S) LISTED ABOVE AND THESE CONDITIONS ARE SHOWN BY THE PATIENT'S HOSPITAL CHART.

☐ **OTHER:** TITLE OF PERSON IF NOT COVERED ABOVE: (MUST BE ABLE TO LEGALLY CERTIFY TO A DISABILITY)

PHYSICIAN/PRACTITIONER'S ORIGINAL SIGNATURE - **RUBBER STAMP IS NOT ACCEPTABLE**	DATE SIGNED	AREA CODE/PHONE NUMBER
	M M D D Y Y Y Y	

UNDER SECTIONS 2116 AND 2122 OF THE CALIFORNIA UNEMPLOYMENT INSURANCE CODE, IT IS A VIOLATION FOR ANY INDIVIDUAL WHO, WITH INTENT TO DEFRAUD, FALSELY CERTIFIES THE MEDICAL CONDITION OF ANY PERSON IN ORDER TO OBTAIN DISABILITY INSURANCE BENEFITS, WHETHER FOR THE MAKER OR FOR ANY OTHER PERSON, AND IS PUNISHABLE BY IMPRISONMENT AND/OR A FINE NOT EXCEEDING $20,000. SECTION 1143 REQUIRES ADDITIONAL ADMINISTRATIVE PENALTIES.

DE 2501 Rev. 78 (4-12)

OSP 12 127141

Figure 16-10, cont'd

17 Hospital Billing

Payel Madero

KEY TERMS

Your instructor may wish to select some words pertinent to this chapter for a test. For definitions of the terms, further study, and/or reference, the words, phrases, and abbreviations may be found in the glossary at the end of the Handbook. *Key terms for this chapter follow.*

admission review
ambulatory payment classifications
appropriateness evaluation protocols
benefit summary sheets
capitation
case rate
charge description master
charges
clinical outliers
code sequence
comorbidity
cost outlier
cost outlier review
day outlier review
diagnosis-related groups
DRG creep
DRG validation
elective surgery
grouper
inpatient
International Classification of Diseases, Ninth Revision, Clinical Modification
International Classification of Diseases, Tenth Revision, Procedure Classification System
looping
major diagnostic categories
outpatient
percentage of revenue
per diem
preadmission testing
principal diagnosis
procedure review
Quality Improvement Organizations
readmission review
reason for encounter
scrubbing
stop loss
transfer review
Uniform Bill CMS-1450 (UB-04)
utilization review

KEY ABBREVIATIONS

See how many abbreviations and acronyms you can translate and then use this as a handy reference list. Definitions for the key abbreviations are located near the back of the Handbook *in the glossary.*

AEP ______________________
APC ______________________
APG ______________________
ASC ______________________
AVG ______________________
CC ______________________
CDM ______________________
CMHC ______________________
CMS-1450 (UB-04) ______________________
DRG ______________________
FL ______________________
GAO ______________________
HSI ______________________
ICD-9-CM ______________________

ICD-10-PCS ______________________

LOS ______________________

MCC ______________________

MCE ______________________

MDC ______________________

MS-DRG ______________________

OCE ______________________

OPPS ______________________

PAT ______________________

QIO program ______________________

RHIA ______________________

RHIT ______________________

RN ______________________

TJC ______________________

UR ______________________

PERFORMANCE OBJECTIVES

The student will be able to:

- Define and spell the key terms and key abbreviations for this chapter, given the information from the *Handbook* glossary, within a reasonable time period and with enough accuracy to obtain a satisfactory evaluation.
- After reading the chapter, answer the fill-in-the-blank, mix and match, multiple choice, and true/false review questions after reading the chapter, with enough accuracy to obtain a satisfactory evaluation.
- Answer questions about the insurance verification process by reviewing a couple of health insurance cards within a reasonable time period and with enough accuracy to obtain a satisfactory evaluation.
- Use ICD-10-PCS tables to determine appropriate procedure codes and define the various character meanings, within a reasonable time period and with enough accuracy to obtain a satisfactory evaluation.
- Given CMS-1450 (UB-04) claim forms, state the reasons why claims may be rejected or delayed or why incorrect payment is received; state these reasons within a reasonable time period and with enough accuracy to obtain a satisfactory evaluation. Analyze DRG codes to determine if the reimbursement was appropriate for the treatment rendered.
- Answer questions about the CMS-1450 (UB-04) claim form to learn which hospital departments input data for different blocks on this form, within a reasonable time period and with enough accuracy to obtain a satisfactory evaluation.
- Answer questions about the CMS-1450 (UB-04) claim form to become familiar with the data it contains and which data are assigned to which fields, within a reasonable time period and with enough accuracy to obtain a satisfactory evaluation.
- After practicing completing some CMS-1450 (UB-04) forms, troubleshoot and critically analyze potential errors that can occur, within a reasonable time period and with enough accuracy to obtain a satisfactory evaluation.

STUDY OUTLINE

Health Insurance Reimbursement
Patient Account Representative
- Qualifications
- Primary Functions and Competencies
- Principal Responsibilities

Admissions Procedures
- Appropriateness Evaluation Protocols
- Admitting Procedures for Major Insurance Programs
- Preadmission Testing
- Present on Admission

Utilization Review
- Quality Improvement Organization Program

Coding Hospital Diagnoses and Procedures
- Principal Diagnosis

Coding Inpatient Procedures

Procedural Coding Systems
- *International Classification of Diseases,* Tenth Revision, Procedure Coding System

Coding Hospital Outpatient Procedures
- HCPCS Level I CPT Coding System
- Modifiers

Inpatient Medical Billing Process
- Admitting Clerk
- Insurance Verifier
- The Admission Process
- Discharge Process
- Charge Description Master
- Coding Specialist
- Electronic Claims Submission
- Nurse Auditor

ASSIGNMENT 17-1 REVIEW QUESTIONS

Part I Fill in the Blank

Review the objectives, key terms, glossary definitions of key terms, chapter information, and figures before completing the following review questions.

1. You are reviewing a computer-generated insurance claim before it is sent to the insurance carrier and you notice the patient's name as being that of an old friend. You quickly read the code for the diagnosis. Is this a breach of confidentiality?

____

____

____

2. You are coding in a medical records department when an agent from the Federal Bureau of Investigation walks in and asks for a patient's address. You ask, "Why do you need Mrs. Doe's address? Do you have a signed authorization from Mrs. Doe for release of information from our facility?" The FBI agent responds, "I'm trying to locate this person because of counterfeiting charges. No, I don't have a signed authorization form." Would there be any breach of confidentiality if you release the patient's address? Explain.

____

____

3. List three instances of breaching confidentiality in a hospital setting.

   a. ____

   b. ____

   c. ____

   d. ____

   e. ____

4. What is the purpose of appropriateness evaluation protocols (AEPs)?

____

____

____

5. If a patient under a managed care plan goes to a hospital that is under contract with the plan for nonemergency admission, what is necessary for inpatient admission?

____

____

6. When a patient receives diagnostic tests and hospital outpatient services before admission to the hospital and these charges are combined with inpatient services, becoming part of the diagnostic-related group payment, this regulation in hospital billing is known as

____

____.

7. The diagnosis established after study and listed for admission to the hospital for an illness or injury is called a/an ______________ diagnosis.

8. For reviewing an inpatient medical record, terminology and/or phrases to look for that relate to uncertain diagnoses are

____.

9. From the list of International Classification of Diseases, Tenth Revision, Clinical Modification (ICD-10-CM) descriptions shown, place these items in correct sequential order (1, 2, 3) for billing purposes. In this case, the medical procedure is a repair of other hernia of the anterior abdominal wall, incisional hernia repair with prosthesis, ICD-10-PCS code 0WUF4JZ.

	Diagnosis	*ICD-10-CM Code*
____________	Chronic liver disease, liver damage unspecified	K70.0
____________	Alcohol dependence syndrome (other and unspecified)	F10.20
____________	Other hernia of abdominal cavity without mention of obstruction or gangrene (incisional hernia)	K45.8

10. Mrs. Benson, a Medicare patient, is admitted by Dr. Dalton to the hospital on January 4 and is seen in consultation by Dr. Frank on January 5. On January 6, Mrs. Benson is discharged with a diagnosis of coronary atherosclerosis. State some of the problems regarding payment and Medicare policies that would affect this case.

____

____

____

11. Name five payment types under managed care contracts.

a. ____

b. ____

c. ____

d. ____

e. ____

12. Baby Stephens falls from a high chair, cutting his head. His mother rushes him to St. Joseph's Medical Center for emergency care. The physician examines the baby, uses two stitches to close the laceration, sends the child for skull radiographs, and then discharges him to home. Will the emergency care be billed as inpatient or outpatient services?

____

____

13. Name the seven variables that affect Medicare reimbursement under the DRG system.

a. ____

b. ____

c. ____

d. ____

e. ____

f. ____

g. ____

14. You can determine whether a CMS-1450 (UB-04) claim form is for an inpatient or an outpatient by the following observations:

 a. For an inpatient, block number 4 shows three-digit billing code/codes ______________.

 b. For an outpatient, block number 4 shows three-digit billing code/codes ______________.

 c. Revenue codes and block number/numbers ______________ indicate type of service rendered.

15. Describe the significance of Field Locators 42, 43, 44, 46, and 47 of the CMS-1450 (UB-04) claim form.

 a. FL 42 ______________________________

 b. FL 43 ______________________________

 c. FL 44 ______________________________

 d. FL 46 ______________________________

 e. FL 47 ______________________________

Part II Mix and Match

16. Match the words or phrases used for managed care reimbursement methods in the left column with the definitions in the right column. Write the correct letters in the blanks.

_______	Sliding scales for discounts and per diems	a. Reimbursement method that pays more for the first day in the hospital than for subsequent days
_______	Discounts in the form of sliding scale	b. Reimbursement to the hospital on a per member per month basis
_______	Stop loss	c. Plan advances cash to cover expected claims to the hospital
_______	Withhold	d. Fixed percentage paid to the hospital to cover charges
_______	Charges	e. Single charge for a day in the hospital regardless of actual cost
_______	Ambulatory payment classifications	f. Interim per diem paid for each day in the hospital
_______	Case rate	g. Classification system categorizing patients who are medically related with regard to diagnosis and treatment and are statistically similar in lengths of hospital stay
_______	Diagnosis-related groups	h. Hospital receives a flat per admission payment for the particular service to which the patient is admitted
_______	Differential by service type	i. An averaging after a flat rate is given to certain categories of procedures
_______	Periodic interim payments	j. Outpatient classification based on procedures rather than on diagnoses
_______	Bed leasing	k. Hospital buys insurance to protect against lost revenue and receives less of a capitation fee
_______	Differential by day in hospital	l. Method in which part of plan's payment to the hospital may be withheld and paid at the end of the year
_______	Capitation	m. When a managed care plan leases beds from a hospital and pays per bed whether used or not
_______	Per diem	n. A percentage reduction in charges for total bed days per year
_______	Percentage of revenue	o. Dollar amount that a hospital bills a case for services rendered

Part III Multiple Choice

Choose the best answer.

17. Hospital inpatient cases that cannot be assigned to an appropriate DRG because of atypical situations are referred to as
    a. evaluation protocols.
    b. cost outliers.
    c. clinical outliers.
    d. day outliers.

18. An individual who receives medical service in a section or department of the hospital and goes home the same day is called a/an
    a. inpatient.
    b. day patient.
    c. outpatient.
    d. ambulatory patient.

19. A surgical procedure that may be scheduled in advance, is not an emergency, and is discretionary on the part of the physician and patient is called
    a. nonemergency surgery.
    b. inpatient surgery.
    c. outpatient surgery.
    d. elective surgery.

20. A preexisting condition that will, because of its effect on the specific principal diagnosis, require more intensive therapy or cause an increase in length of stay (LOS) by at least 1 day in approximately 75% of cases is called a
    a. chronic condition.
    b. coexisting condition.
    c. comorbid condition.
    d. complicated condition.

Part IV True/False

Write "T" or "F" in the blank to indicate whether you think the statement is true or false.

________ 21. A patient would not have an insurance identification card if he or she was injured while at work.

________ 22. The inpatient and outpatient hospital billing department uses a summary form for submitting an insurance claim to an insurance plan called the Uniform Bill Claim Form (CMS-1450).

________ 23. Medicare implemented the diagnosis-related groups (DRG)–based system of reimbursement to hold down rising health care costs.

Part V ICD-10-PCS Root Operations Review

Review Appendix C in the *Workbook* to match the following root operations to surgical examples.

a. Alteration	________	Face Lift
b. Bypass	________	Coronary Artery Bypass
c. Detachment	________	Below Knee Amputation
d. Excision	________	Partial Nephrectomy
e. Extirpation	________	Thrombectomy
f. Fragmentation	________	Transurethral Lithotripsy
g. Occlusion	________	Fallopian Tube Ligation
h. Release	________	Carpel Tunnel Release
i. Replacement	________	Total Hip Replacement
j. Resection	________	Total Nephrectomy
k. Supplement	________	Herniorraphy Using Mesh
l. Transplantation	________	Kidney Transplant

ASSIGNMENT 17-2 PATIENT ACCOUNT REPRESENTATIVE JOB DESCRIPTIONS

Performance Objective

Task: To review job descriptions and eligibility requirements to become a hospital patient account representative for the local geographic area.

Conditions: Do an Internet search on a major career seeking site such as Careerbuilder.com or Monster.com for positions available near student's home.

Standards: Time: ______________ minutes

Accuracy: ______________

(Note: The time element and accuracy criteria may be given by your instructor.)

Directions: Review Figure 17-1 in Chapter 17 of the *Handbook* for the position description for the patient account representative. Using an Internet search engine (Yahoo, Google, Bing), complete a job search for similar positions in the student's geographic area and answer the following questions.

1. List at least two positions that meet the minimum criteria as outlined in the position description in Figure 17-1.

   a. ____

   b. ____

2. Does this position title have any different names with the same responsibilities as listed? If so, what are some other position names?

   ____

3. Do you feel that you are qualified for any of the positions listed? What are some ways to gain experience needed to qualify for this position?

   ____

   ____

   ____

4. Have you found that there are more job duties that are specific to your geographic area? If so, explain.

   ____

   ____

   ____

ASSIGNMENT 17-3 REVIEW THE INSURANCE VERIFICATION PROCESS

Performance Objective

Task: Answer questions relating to insurance verification in reference to an insurance identification card for Case A.

Conditions: Use an insurance identification card (Figure 17-1 and Figure 17-2), the questions presented, and pen or pencil.

Standards: Time: ______________ minutes

Accuracy: ______________

(Note: The time element and accuracy criteria may be given by your instructor.)

Directions: A health insurance identification card contains information that should be verified by the patient account representative. Both sides of the card should be copied and placed in patient records. To complete the verification process, information such as the subscriber, the subscriber's date of birth, subscriber's employer, the managed care plan type, medical group name, the primary care physician (PCP), copays, and coverages should be identified. Without accurate insurance verification, reimbursements may be reduced or claims may be denied.

CASE A

John Smith made an appointment to see Dr. Richard Weather, a family practitioner, for 11/12/20XX at 3:00 PM. He says that he has Anthem Blue Cross and he proceeded to give the appointment intake clerk at Dr. Richard Weather's office his Member ID number, Date of Birth, his address and phone number. John Smith is in the office on 11/12/20XX for his appointment. Review John Smith's insurance ID card in Figure 17-1 and answer the following questions:

1. What type of insurance does John Smith have? What medical group does John belong to?

____

____

2. Where will the insurance verifier call to confirm benefits and coverage?

____

3. What information is missing from the card that the insurance verifier should confirm?

____

____

4. Based on this type of insurance, will John's office visit be covered? Why or why not?

____

5. Will John Smith be denied at an Emergency Department for care? Explain.

____

____

CASE B

Jessica T. Smith was brought to the Emergency Room at ABC Hospital by her father, John R. Smith for a possible sprained ankle on 11/24/20xx at 4:23 PM. Review Figure 17-2 for the insurance card and answer the following questions.

1. What is the name and type of insurance Jessica has?

____

____

2. Who is the subscriber? What subscriber information is needed to correctly submit the insurance claim?

____

____

3. Is preauthorization needed? Where would admissions call to verify benefits?

____

____

4. Since Jessica T. Smith was admitted through the emergency room, what must John R. Smith do to ensure benefits?

____

____

5. Is the PCP listed on the card? Why would it be important for the hospital to have information about the PCP?

____

____

Anthem

John Smith
Member ID: **FGA784A46927**

Group: **275020H001**
Plan: **040**
BIN: **610053**
PCN: **7700630**
PCP: **DAVIS, RICK (SAN DIEGO MEDICAL GROUP)**
MED Office: **(909) 920-5555**
BLUE CROSS HMO
77 E 7TH ST STE B
SAN DIEGO, CA 75682
Member is enrolled in: **BLUE CROSS HMO**

This temporary ID Card is good through
11/06/2012

℞

Fold line

Anthem

This is your temporary health plan Identification Card. Present it to the provider of healthcare when you or your eligible dependents receive services. See your certificate(s) or booklet(s) for a description of the benefits, terms, conditions, limitations and exclusions of coverage. When submitting inquiries always include your member number from the face of this card. Possession or use of this card does not guarantee payment.

Providers inside California: Please call the Customer Service phone number on the face of this card for eligibility and benefit information.
Providers outside California: Please submit claims to your local Blue Cross and/or Blue Shield Plan. To ensure prompt claims processing, please include the 3-digit alpha prefix that precedes the patient's identification number listed on the front of this card.

anthem.com/ca

Customer Service: (800) 227-5555
Claims & Inquiries:
P.O. BOX 60007
SAN DIEGO, CA 90060-0007

Anthem Blue Cross is the trade name of Blue Cross of California. Anthem Blue Cross and Anthem Blue Cross Life and Health Insurance Company are independent licensees or the Blue Cross Association.

Figure 17-1

Aetna® NAP   Beech Street. A VIANT NETWORK   STERLING JEWELERS

CHOICE POS II
REFERRALS NOT REQUIRED

ID W1665 270 25 GRP: 478599-010-00001
01 JOHN R SMITH
02 JESSICA T SMITH

MEMBER SERVICES	1 - 800 - 331 - 6910	PCP $ 25.00
PROVIDERS CALL	1 - 888 - 632 - 3862	

PAYOR NUMBER 60054 0048

Fold line

www.aetna.com

Benefits are administered by Aetna Life Insurance Company or affiliates. This card does not guarantee coverage. For questions on mental health/substance abuse coverage, or to precertify, call 1 - 800 - 424 - 4047. You do not have to choose a primary care physician (PCP) or obtain referrals. The plan describes what you need to precertify. If you do not precertify, your benefits will be reduced.
EMERGENCY: Call 911 or go to nearest emergency facility. Notify Member Services as soon as possible after treatment.

We recommend you use a Primary Doctor to coordinate your care.

AETNA
P.O. BOX 981106
EL PASO TX 79998 - 1106

AT0152

Figure 17-2

ASSIGNMENT 17-4 UNDERSTANDING HIPAA SECURITY AND CONFIDENTIALITY ISSUES

Performance Objectives

Conditions: Reference Figure 17-3 in the *Handbook* to discuss and analyze the following HIPAA breach cases.

Standards: Time: ______________ minutes

Accuracy: ______________

(Note: The time element and accuracy criteria may be given by your instructor.)

Directions: Review the following examples of HIPAA breaches. Refer to HIPAA Compliance Alert: Legal Confidentiality Issues in the *Handbook* and explain how these cases violate confidentiality standards and what can be done, if anything, to prevent these types of breaches.

Scenario 1: Medical Record

An insurance billing specialist working at home has a sister who was hospitalized to undergo major surgery and wants to help his or her parents better understand the medical condition. The specialist calls a friend in the hospital billing department and asks that person to make photocopies of a document in the medical record.

Analysis

____

____

____

Scenario 2: Financial Record

An experienced insurance billing specialist applies for a job. At an interview, he or she presents some samples of typed insurance claims that include hospital and patient names.

Analysis

____

____

____

Scenario 3: Verbal Breach of Confidentiality

A coding clerk overhears two hospital employees discussing a patient by name. Because the clerk had been working on the medical record of that patient and is now familiar with the patient's history, he or she realizes that the information being discussed is not accurate. The coding clerk then interrupts, making a comment about the patient's diagnosis.

Analysis

____

____

____

Scenario 4: Verbal Breach of Confidentiality

A Marilyn Monroe impersonator is discharged from the hospital after receiving plastic surgery. Over dinner at home, an insurance billing specialist relates the diagnosis and name of the surgery to his or her spouse.

Analysis

___

___

___

Scenario 5: Verbal Breach of Confidentiality

In reviewing an insurance claim before it is mailed, the insurance billing specialist realizes that he or she knows the individual who has a diagnosis that indicates a mental condition. The specialist discusses this with a co-worker.

Analysis

___

___

___

Scenario 6: Verbal Breach of Confidentiality

A physician in private practice calls via cellular telephone to the billing clerk to answer a question about the diagnosis to be listed on a patient's insurance claim.

Analysis

___

___

___

1

2

3a PAT. CNTL #
b. MED. REC. #

4 TYPE OF BILL

5 FED. TAX NO.
6 STATEMENT COVERS PERIOD FROM THROUGH
7

8 PATIENT NAME a
b
9 PATIENT ADDRESS a
b c d e

10 BIRTHDATE | 11 SEX | ADMISSION 12 DATE 13 HR 14 TYPE 15 SRC | 16 DHR | 17 STAT | CONDITION CODES 18 19 20 21 22 23 24 25 26 27 28 | 29 ACDT STATE | 30

31 OCCURRENCE CODE DATE | 32 OCCURRENCE CODE DATE | 33 OCCURRENCE CODE DATE | 34 OCCURRENCE CODE DATE | 35 OCCURRENCE SPAN CODE FROM THROUGH | 36 OCCURRENCE SPAN CODE FROM THROUGH | 37
a
b

38

39 VALUE CODES CODE AMOUNT | 40 VALUE CODES CODE AMOUNT | 41 VALUE CODES CODE AMOUNT
a
b
c
d

42 REV. CD.	43 DESCRIPTION	44 HCPCS / RATE / HIPPS CODE	45 SERV. DATE	46 SERV. UNITS	47 TOTAL CHARGES	48 NON-COVERED CHARGES	49
1							
2							
3							
4							
5							
6							
7							
8							
9							
10							
11							
12							
13							
14							
15							
16							
17							
18							
19							
20							
21							
22							
23	**PAGE ____ OF ____**	**CREATION DATE**		**TOTALS**			

50 PAYER NAME | 51 HEALTH PLAN ID | 52 REL. INFO | 53 ASG. BEN. | 54 PRIOR PAYMENTS | 55 EST. AMOUNT DUE | 56 NPI
A B C
57 OTHER PRV ID

58 INSURED'S NAME | 59 P. REL | 60 INSURED'S UNIQUE ID | 61 GROUP NAME | 62 INSURANCE GROUP NO.
A B C

63 TREATMENT AUTHORIZATION CODES | 64 DOCUMENT CONTROL NUMBER | 65 EMPLOYER NAME
A B C

66 DX | 67 A B C D E F G H | 68
I J K L M N O P Q

69 ADMIT DX | 70 PATIENT REASON DX a b c | 71 PPS CODE | 72 ECI a b c | 73

74 PRINCIPAL PROCEDURE CODE DATE | a. OTHER PROCEDURE CODE DATE | b. OTHER PROCEDURE CODE DATE | 75
c. OTHER PROCEDURE CODE DATE | d. OTHER PROCEDURE CODE DATE | e. OTHER PROCEDURE CODE DATE

76 ATTENDING NPI QUAL
LAST FIRST
77 OPERATING NPI QUAL
LAST FIRST

80 REMARKS | 81CC a b c d

78 OTHER NPI QUAL
LAST FIRST
79 OTHER NPI QUAL
LAST FIRST

UB-04 CMS-1450 APPROVED OMB NO. 0938-0997 NUBC National Uniform Billing Committee

THE CERTIFICATIONS ON THE REVERSE APPLY TO THIS BILL AND ARE MADE A PART HEREOF.

Figure 17-3

ASSIGNMENT 17-5 REVIEWING THE INSURANCE CLAIM LIFE CYCLE

Performance Objective

Conditions: Use a pen or pencil to fill in the blanks to the life cycle of an insurance claim and answer the following questions.

Standards: Time: ____________ minutes

Accuracy: ____________

(Note: The time element and accuracy criteria may be given by your instructor.)

Directions: Match the numbers from the boxes in the illustration to the numbered lines below. Provide two activities that are important in each stage of the life cycle of an insurance claim.

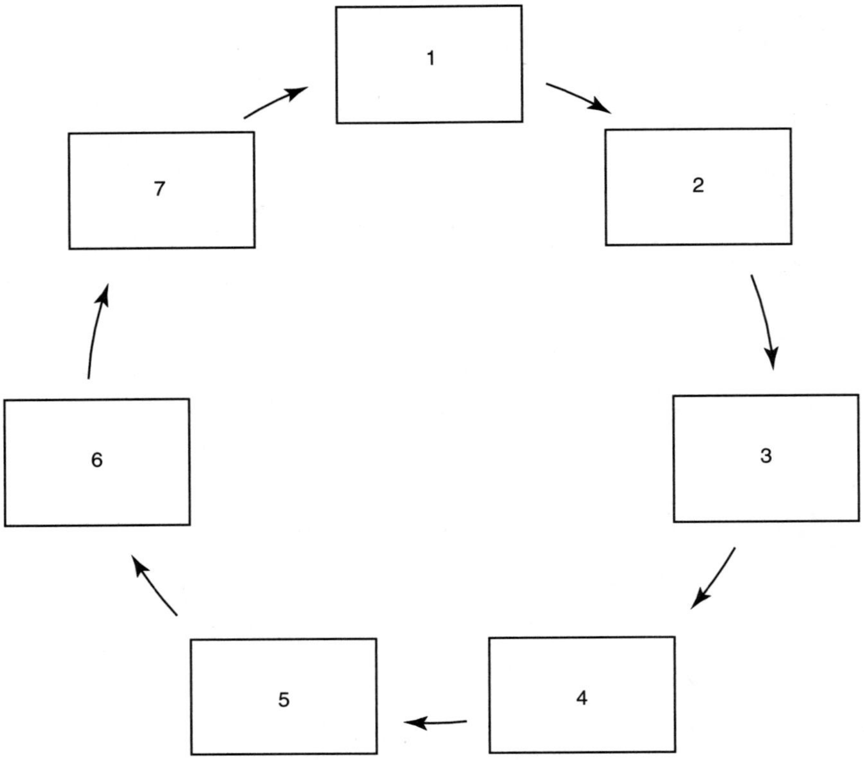

1	2	3	4
________	________	________	________
________	________	________	________
________	________	________	________

5	6	7	8
________	________	________	________
________	________	________	________
________	________	________	________

ASSIGNMENT 17-6 ASSIGN THE ICD-10-PCS CODE USING TABLES

Performance Objective

Task: Determine the correct ICD-10-PCS procedure code for each diagnosis listed for five cases.

Conditions: Use a pen or pencil and the assigned Tables 1 through 5 below.

Standards: Time: ______________

Accuracy: ______________

(Note: The time element and accuracy criteria may be given by your instructor.)

Directions: Review appendices C and D in the *Workbook* which provide the definitions for root operations and various approaches in ICD-10-PCS. Code the following procedures using the included PCS tables. The first three characters are provided for you.

1. **Procedure:** Sciatic Nerve Release

Section **0** Medical and surgical Body system **1** Peripheral nervous system Operation **N** Release: Freeing a body part from an abnormal physical constraint by cutting or by the use of force			
Body part	Approach	Device	Qualifier
0 Cervical plexus **1** Cervical nerve **2** Phrenic nerve **3** Brachial plexus **4** Ulnar nerve **5** Median nerve **6** Radial nerve **8** Thoracic nerve **9** Lumbar plexus **A** Lumbosacral plexus **B** Lumbar nerve **C** Pudendal nerve **D** Femoral nerve **F** Sciatic nerve **G** Tibial nerve **H** Peroneal nerve **K** Head and neck sympathetic nerve **L** Thoracic sympathetic nerve **M** Abdominal sympathetic nerve **N** Lumbar sympathetic nerve **P** Sacral sympathetic nerve **Q** Sacral plexus **R** Sacral nerve	**0** Open **3** Percutaneous **4** Percutaneous endoscopic	**Z** No device	**Z** No qualifier

0 1 N _ _ _ _ _ _ _

2. **Procedure:** Coronary Artery Bypass Graft for five sites, an intraluminal drug-eluting device was sent percutaneous with an endoscopy to the coronary vein

Section **0** Medical and surgical Body system **2** Heart and great vessels Operation **1** Bypass: Altering the route of passage of the contents of a tubular body part			
Body part	Approach	Device	Qualifier
0 Coronary artery, one site **1** Coronary artery, two sites **2** Coronary artery, three sites **3** Coronary artery, four or more sites	**0** Open	**9** Autologous venous tissue **A** Autologous arterial tissue **J** Synthetic substitute **K** Nonautologous tissue substitute	**3** Coronary artery **8** Internal mammary, right **9** Internal mammary, left **C** Thoracic artery **F** Abdominal artery **W** Aorta
0 Coronary artery, one site **1** Coronary artery, two sites **2** Coronary artery, three sites **3** Coronary artery, four or more sites	**0** Open	**Z** No device	**3** Coronary artery **8** Internal mammary, right **9** Internal mammary, left **C** Thoracic artery **F** Abdominal artery
0 Coronary artery, one site **1** Coronary artery, two sites **2** Coronary artery, three sites **3** Coronary artery, four or more sites	**3** Percutaneous	**4** Intraluminal device, drug-eluting **D** Intraluminal device	**4** Coronary vein
0 Coronary artery, one site **1** Coronary artery, two sites **2** Coronary artery, three sites **3** Coronary artery, four or more sites	**4** Percutaneous endoscopic	**4** Intraluminal device, drug-eluting **D** Intraluminal device	**4** Coronary vein
0 Coronary artery, one site **1** Coronary artery, two sites **2** Coronary artery, three sites **3** Coronary artery, four or more sites	**4** Percutaneous endoscopic	**9** Autologous venous tissue **A** Autologous arterial tissue **J** Synthetic substitute **K** Nonautologous tissue substitute	**3** Coronary artery **8** Internal mammary, right **9** Internal mammary, left **C** Thoracic artery **F** Abdominal artery **W** Aorta
0 Coronary artery, one site **1** Coronary artery, two sites **2** Coronary artery, three sites **3** Coronary artery, four or more sites	**4** Percutaneous endoscopic	**Z** No device	**3** Coronary artery **8** Internal mammary, right **9** Internal mammary, left **C** Thoracic artery **F** Abdominal artery
6 Atrium, right	**0** Open **4** Percutaneous endoscopic	**9** Autologous venous tissue **A** Autologous arterial tissue **J** Synthetic substitute **K** Nonautologous tissue substitute	**P** Pulmonary trunk **Q** Pulmonary artery, right **R** Pulmonary artery, left

0 2 1 _ _ _ _ _ _ _

3. **Procedure:** Lymph node removal from right axillary with an endoscope

Section **0** Medical and surgical Body system **7** Lymphatic and hemic systems Operation **T** Resection: Cutting out or off, without replacement, all of a body part			
Body part	Approach	Device	Qualifier
0 Lymphatic, head **1** Lymphatic, right neck **2** Lymphatic, left neck **3** Lymphatic, right upper extremity **4** Lymphatic, left upper extremity **5** Lymphatic, right axillary **6** Lymphatic, left axillary **7** Lymphatic, thorax **8** Lymphatic, internal mammarym right **9** Lymphatic, internal mammarym left **B** Lymphatic, mesenteric **C** Lymphatic, pelvis **D** Lymphatic, aortic **F** Lymphatic, right lower extremity **G** Lymphatic, left lower extremity **H** Lymphatic, right inguinal **J** Lymphatic, left inguinal **K** Thoracic duct **L** Cisterna chyli **M** Thymus **P** Spleen	**0** Open **4** Percutaneous endoscopic	**Z** No device	**Z** No qualifier

0 7 T _ _ _ _ _ _ _

4. **Procedure:** Lens replacement in left eye using a cadaver lens

Section **0** Medical and surgical Body system **8** Eye Operation **R** Replacement: Putting in or on biological or synthetic material that physically takes the place and/or function of all or a portion of a body part			
Body part	Approach	Device	Qualifier
0 Eye, right **1** Eye, left **A** Choroid, right **B** Choroid, left	**0** Open **3** Percutaneous	**7** Autologous tissue substitute **J** Synthetic substitute **K** Nonautologous tissue substitute	**Z** No qualifier
4 Vitreous, right **5** Vitreous, left **C** Iris, right **D** Iris, left **G** Retinal vessel, right **H** Retinal vessel, left	**3** Percutaneous	**7** Autologous tissue substitute **J** Synthetic substitute **K** Nonautologous tissue substitute	**Z** No qualifier
6 Sclera, right **7** Sclera, left **S** Conjunctiva, right **T** Conjunctiva, left	**X** External	**7** Autologous tissue substitute **J** Synthetic substitute **K** Nonautologous tissue substitute	**Z** No qualifier
8 Cornea, right **9** Cornea, left	**3** Percutaneous **X** External	**7** Autologous tissue substitute **J** Synthetic substitute **K** Nonautologous tissue substitute	**Z** No qualifier
J Lens, right **K** Lens, left	**3** Percutaneous	**0** Synthetic substitute, intraocular telescope **7** Autologous tissue substitute **J** Synthetic substitute **K** Nonautologous tissue substitute	**Z** No qualifier
N Upper eyelid, right **P** Upper eyelid, left **Q** Lower eyelid, right **R** Lower eyelid, left	**0** Open **3** Percutaneous **X** External	**7** Autologous tissue substitute **J** Synthetic substitute **K** Nonautologous tissue substitute	**Z** No qualifier
X Lacrimal duct, right **Y** Lacrimal duct, left	**0** Open **3** Percutaneous **7** Via natural or artificial opening **8** Via natural or artificial opening endoscopic	**7** Autologous tissue substitute **J** Synthetic substitute **K** Nonautologous tissue substitute	**Z** No qualifier

0 8 R _ _ _ _ _ _ _

5. **Procedure:** Foreign Body Removal from nasal turbinate via natural opening

Section **0** Medical and surgical Body system **9** Ear, nose, sinus Operation **B** Excision: Cutting out or off, without replacement, a portion of a body part			
Body part	Approach	Device	Qualifier
0 External ear, right **1** External ear, left **K** Nose	**0** Open **3** Percutaneous **4** Percutaneous endoscopic **X** External	**7** No device	**X** Diagnostic **Z** No qualifier
3 External auditory canal, right **4** External auditory canal, left	**0** Open **3** Percutaneous **4** Percutaneous endoscopic **7** Via natural or artificial opening **8** Via natural or artificial opening endoscopic **X** External	**7** No device	**X** Diagnostic **Z** No qualifier
5 Middle ear, right **6** Middle ear, left **9** Auditory ossicle, right **A** Auditory ossicle, left **D** Inner ear, right **E** Inner ear, left	**0** Open	**7** No device	**X** Diagnostic **Z** No qualifier
7 Tympanic membrane, right **8** Tympanic membrane, left **F** Eustachian tube, right **G** Eustachian tube, left **L** Nasal turbinate **N** Nasopharynx	**0** Open **3** Percutaneous **4** Percutaneous endoscopic **7** Via natural or artificial opening **8** Via natural or artificial opening endoscopic	**7** No device	**X** Diagnostic **Z** No qualifier
B Mastoid sinus, right **C** Mastoid sinus, left **M** Nasal septum **P** Accessory sinus **Q** Maxillary sinus, right **R** Maxillary sinus, left **S** Frontal sinus, right **T** Frontal sinus, left **U** Ethmoid, right **V** Ethmoid, left **W** Sphenoid sinus, right **X** Sphenoid sinus, left	**0** Open **3** Percutaneous **4** Percutaneous endoscopic	**7** No device	**X** Diagnostic **Z** No qualifier

0 9 B _ _ _ _ _ _ _

ASSIGNMENT 17-7 STUDY CMS-1450 (UB-04) CLAIM FORM BLOCK OR FIELD FORM LOCATOR (FL) DATA

Performance Objective

Task: Answer questions about the CMS-1450 (UB-04) claim form blocks.

Conditions: Use an ink pen.

Standards: Time: ____________ minutes

Accuracy: ____________

(Note: The time element and accuracy criteria may be given by your instructor.)

Directions: Depending on your instructor's preference, you may complete this exercise with or without notes or other material.

You have learned about a number of reimbursement methods, confidentiality issues, evaluation protocols, and the utilization review process. This information is necessary for processing an insurance claim to obtain maximum reimbursement. To complete the CMS-1450 (UB-04) claim form in Figure 17-3, you must become familiar with the data it contains, including codes and the location of various types of information. Answer the following questions.

1. In FL 4, state the correct billing codes for
   a. Inpatient services ____________
   b. Outpatient services ____________
2. What is listed in FL 7?

   ____
3. What insurance carriers or programs require FL 9 to be completed?

   ____

   ____
4. What format is required in FL 10 for the patient's date of birth? ____________
5. If a patient was in the hospital for the delivery of a premature infant, what code would be used in FL 15? ______
6. If a patient was discharged from inpatient care at 2:15 PM, how would this be noted in FL 16? ____________
7. What is the correct code to use in FL 17 if a patient was discharged to a home hospice situation? ____________
8. If neither the patient nor spouse was employed, what code would be used to indicate this in FL 18 through 28? ____
9. State the reason for the codes used in FL 31 through 34.

   ____

   ____
10. What revenue code must be shown on all bills as a final entry, and in what block or field form locator (FL) does it occur? ____________

ASSIGNMENT 17-8 LOCATE ERRORS ON A CMS-1450 (UB-04) CLAIM FORM

Performance Objective

Task: Locate the blocks on the computer-generated insurance claim form that need completion of missing information or have data that need to be corrected before submission to the insurance company.

Conditions: Use Mary J. Torre's completed insurance claim (Figure 17-4), the checklist for editing a CMS-1450 (UB-04) claim form, and a red ink pen.

Standards: Time: ____________ minutes

Accuracy: ____________

(Note: The time element and accuracy criteria may be given by your instructor.)

Directions: Refer to Figure 17-5 in the *Handbook* to use the step-by-step approach while editing the computer-generated CMS-1450 (UB-04) claim form (see Figure 17-4). Use the checklist to help you when reviewing the claim form. Locate the blocks on the claim form that need completion of missing information or that have data to be corrected before submission to the insurance company. Highlight all errors you discover. Insert all corrections and missing information in red. If you cannot locate the necessary information but know it is mandatory, write "NEED" in the corresponding form locator block/field.

In addition, you notice that the second line entry for pharmacy shows a total of $6806. However, you know from reviewing the case that one injection of a drug known as TPA (revenue code 259 and fee $5775), which dissolves clots and opens vessels when a patient has a myocardial infarction, was not broken out of the fee. Handwrite this final entry. On line 2, cross out the total charge $6806 and insert the correct pharmacy-reduced amount.

Checklist for Editing a Uniform Bill (CMS-1450)

Claim Form: Mary J. Torre

Steps	*Form Locator Blocks/Fields*
1	FL 1 ____________ and 5 ____________
2	FL 4: Inpatient ____________ Outpatient ____________
3	FL 8b ____________, 38 ____________, 58 ____________, and 59 ____________
4	FL 10 ____________
5	FL 8b ____________ and 11 ____________
6	FL 50 ____________, 60 ____________, 61 ____________, 62 ____________, and 65 ____________
7	FL 66-67 A-Q ____________ and 69 ____________
8	FL 74 ____________ and 74 a-e ____________
9	FL 76 ____________
10	FL 6 ____________, 12 ____________, and 31 ____________
11	Inpatient: FL 42-47: 13 ____________, 16 ____________, and 46 ____________
12	FL 47 ____________
13	FL 42 ____________ and 46 ____________
14	Outpatient: FL 43 ____________, 44 ____________, and 45 ____________
15	Detailed record to be checked
16	FL 42 ____________, 43 ____________, and 47 ____________
17	FL 55 ____________

1 COLLEGE HOSPITAL
4500 BROAD AVENUE
WOODLAND HILLS XY 12345-0001
555-487-6789

2

3a PAT. CNTL # 10687127
b. MED. REC. # 2018856

4 TYPE OF BILL 0111

5 FED. TAX NO. 95-0731067

6 STATEMENT COVERS PERIOD FROM 071120XX THROUGH 071420XX

7

8 PATIENT NAME a
b TORRE, MARY J.

9 PATIENT ADDRESS a 452 JEME STREET
b WOODLAND HILLS c XY d 12345-0001 e

10 BIRTHDATE	11 SEX	ADMISSION 12 DATE	13 HR	14 TYPE	15 SRC	16 DHR	17 STAT	CONDITION CODES 18	19	20	21	22	23	24	25	26	27	28	29 ACDT STATE	30
12031918	F	071120XX	21	2	7	17	01	C5	04											

31 OCCURRENCE CODE	DATE	32 OCCURRENCE CODE	DATE	33 OCCURRENCE CODE	DATE	34 OCCURRENCE CODE	DATE	35 OCCURRENCE SPAN CODE	FROM	THROUGH	36 OCCURRENCE SPAN CODE	FROM	THROUGH	37
11	071120XX													

38
TORRE, MARY J.
452 JEME STREET
WOODLAND HILLS, XY 12345-0001

	39 VALUE CODES CODE	AMOUNT	40 VALUE CODES CODE	AMOUNT	41 VALUE CODES CODE	AMOUNT
a	01	650 00				
b						
c						
d						

	42 REV. CD.	43 DESCRIPTION	44 HCPCS / RATE / HIPPS CODE	45 SERV. DATE	46 SERV. UNITS	47 TOTAL CHARGES	48 NON-COVERED CHARGES	49	
1	210	ROOM AND CARE CCU	1600.00		3	4800 00			1
2	250	PHARMACY			121	6806 00			2
3	270	MED-SUR SUPPLIES			31	700 50			3
4	300	LABORATORY			45	1710 50			4
5	310	PATHOLOGY LABORATORY			1	99 50			5
6	320	RADIOLOGY			3	159 00			6
7	450	EMERGENCY ROOM SERVICE			5	196 00			7
8	730	ELECTROCARDIOLOGY			7	700 00			8
9	001	TOTAL				15171 50			9
10									10
11									11
12									12
13									13
14									14
15									15
16									16
17									17
18									18
19									19
20									20
21									21
22									22
23		PAGE ____ OF ____	CREATION DATE		TOTALS				23

	50 PAYER NAME	51 HEALTH PLAN ID	52 REL. INFO	53 ASG. BEN.	54 PRIOR PAYMENTS	55 EST. AMOUNT DUE	56 NPI 950731067	
A	MEDPRIME - HPR		Y	Y			57	A
B							OTHER	B
C							PRV ID	C

	58 INSURED'S NAME	59 P. REL	60 INSURED'S UNIQUE ID	61 GROUP NAME	62 INSURANCE GROUP NO.	
A	TORRE, MARY J	01	54626897101		6500-0000	A
B						B
C						C

	63 TREATMENT AUTHORIZATION CODES	64 DOCUMENT CONTROL NUMBER	65 EMPLOYER NAME	
A			RETIRED 080184	A
B				B
C				C

66 DX 9: 41011 | 4589 | 5780 | | | | E9344 | E8497 | | 68

69 ADMIT DX 41011 | 70 PATIENT REASON DX | 71 PPS CODE | 72 ECI E9444 | E9424 | E8490 | 73

74 PRINCIPAL PROCEDURE CODE DATE | a. OTHER PROCEDURE CODE DATE | b. OTHER PROCEDURE CODE DATE | 75
c. OTHER PROCEDURE CODE DATE | d. OTHER PROCEDURE CODE DATE | e. OTHER PROCEDURE CODE DATE

76 ATTENDING NPI 642110670 QUAL
LAST CARDI FIRST PERRY
77 OPERATING NPI QUAL
LAST FIRST
78 OTHER NPI QUAL
LAST FIRST
79 OTHER NPI QUAL
LAST FIRST

80 REMARKS
81CC a
b
c
d

UB-04 CMS-1450 APPROVED OMB NO.
THE CERTIFICATIONS ON THE REVERSE APPLY TO THIS BILL AND ARE MADE A PART HEREOF.
NUBC National Uniform Billing Committee
LIC9213257

Figure 17-4

ASSIGNMENT 17-9 LOCATE ERRORS ON A CMS-1450 (UB-04) CLAIM FORM

Performance Objective

Task: Locate the Form Locator blocks/fields on the computer-generated insurance claim form that need completion of missing information or have data that need to be corrected before submission to the insurance company.

Conditions: Use Henry M. Cosby's completed insurance claim (Figure 17-5), the checklist for editing a CMS-1450 (UB-04) claim form, and a red ink pen.

Standards: Time: ________ minutes

Accuracy: ________

(Note: The time element and accuracy criteria may be given by your instructor.)

Directions: Refer to Figure 17-5 in the *Handbook* to employ the step-by-step approach while editing the computer-generated CMS-1450 (UB-04) claim form (see Figure 17-5). Use the checklist to help you when reviewing the claim form. Locate the Form Locator blocks/fields on the claim form that need completion of missing information or that have data to be corrected before submission to the insurance company. Highlight all errors you discover. Insert all corrections and missing information in red. If you cannot locate the necessary information but know it is mandatory, write "NEED" in the corresponding Form Locator block/field. State the reason or reasons why the claim may be rejected or delayed or why incorrect payment may be generated because of one or more errors discovered.

Checklist for Editing a Uniform Bill (CMS-1450)
Claim Form: Henry M. Cosby

Steps	*Form Locator Blocks/Fields*
1	FL 1 ________ and 5 ________
2	FL 4: Inpatient ________ Outpatient ________
3	FL 8b ________, 38 ________, 58 ________, and 59 ________
4	FL 10 ________
5	FL 8b ________ and 11 ________
6	FL 50 ________, 60 ________, 61 ________, 62 ________, and 65 ________
7	FL 66 ________ and 69 ________
8	FL 74 ________ and 74 a-e ________
9	FL 76 ________
10	FL 6 ________, 12 ________, and 31 ________
11	Inpatient: FL 42-47: 13 ________, 16 ________, and 46 ________
12	FL 47 ________
13	FL 42 ________ and 46 ________
14	Outpatient: FL 43 ________, 44 ________, and 45 ________
15	Detailed record to be checked
16	FL 42 ________, 43 ________, and 47 ________
17	FL 55 ________

1	COLLEGE HOSPITAL 4500 BROAD AVENUE WOODLAND HILLS XY 12345-0001 555-487-6789
2	
3a PAT. CNTL #	10687127
b. MED. REC. #	2084100
4 TYPE OF BILL	0131
5 FED. TAX NO.	95-0731067
6 STATEMENT COVERS PERIOD FROM / THROUGH	031520XX / 031520XX
7	
8 PATIENT NAME a / b	COSBY, HENRY M
9 PATIENT ADDRESS a	1501 PACIFIC WAY
b	WOODLAND HILLS
c / d / e	XY / 12345-0001
10 BIRTHDATE	03101956
11 SEX	M
ADMISSION 12 DATE	031520XX
13 HR	13
14 TYPE	3
15 SRC	2
16 DHR	99
17 STAT	01
CONDITION CODES 18	C5
19–28	
29 ACDT STATE	
30	
31 OCCURRENCE CODE / DATE	05 / 072120XX
32, 33, 34 OCCURRENCE CODE / DATE	
35, 36 OCCURRENCE SPAN CODE / FROM / THROUGH	
37	
38	COSBY, HENRY M 1501 PACIFIC WAY WOODLAND HILLS XY 12345
39, 40, 41 VALUE CODES CODE / AMOUNT (a–d)	

	42 REV. CD.	43 DESCRIPTION	44 HCPCS / RATE / HIPPS CODE	45 SERV. DATE	46 SERV. UNITS	47 TOTAL CHARGES	48 NON-COVERED CHARGES	49	
1	110	ROOM-BOARD/SEMI/PVT	650.00		1	650 00			1
2	250	PHARMACY			11	207 20			2
3	270	MED-SUR SUPPLIES			4	1041 28			3
4	360	OPERATING ROOM				865 00			4
5	370	ANESTHESIA				64 50			5
6	730	ELECTROCARDIOGRAM	93000	031320XX	031320XX	100 00			6
7	001	Total				2927 98			7
8									8
9									9
10									10
11									11
12									12
13									13
14									14
15									15
16									16
17									17
18									18
19									19
20									20
21									21
22									22
23		**PAGE ____ OF ____**	**CREATION DATE**		**TOTALS**				23

	50 PAYER NAME	51 HEALTH PLAN ID	52 REL. INFO	53 ASG. BEN.	54 PRIOR PAYMENTS	55 EST. AMOUNT DUE
A	BLUE SHIELD OF CA	Z22C49122	Y	Y		
B						
C						

56 NPI: 950731067

57 OTHER PRV ID:

	58 INSURED'S NAME	59 P. REL	60 INSURED'S UNIQUE ID	61 GROUP NAME	62 INSURANCE GROUP NO.
A	COSBY, HENRY M	01	564729922		PA 0132
B					
C					

	63 TREATMENT AUTHORIZATION CODES	64 DOCUMENT CONTROL NUMBER	65 EMPLOYER NAME
A			DBA: COSBY AUTO BODY
B			
C			

66 DX: 9

67: 8408

68:

69 ADMIT DX:

70 PATIENT REASON DX:

71 PPS CODE:

72 ECI:

73:

74 PRINCIPAL PROCEDURE CODE / DATE: 8301 / 031520XX

a. OTHER PROCEDURE CODE / DATE:

b. OTHER PROCEDURE CODE / DATE:

c. OTHER PROCEDURE CODE / DATE:

d. OTHER PROCEDURE CODE / DATE:

e. OTHER PROCEDURE CODE / DATE:

75:

76 ATTENDING NPI 126785470 QUAL

LAST SKELETON FIRST RAYMOND

77 OPERATING NPI QUAL

LAST FIRST

78 OTHER NPI QUAL

LAST FIRST

79 OTHER NPI QUAL

LAST FIRST

80 REMARKS: FELL WATERSKIING 7/21/20XX

81CC a / b / c / d:

UB-04 CMS-1450 APPROVED OMB NO.

THE CERTIFICATIONS ON THE REVERSE APPLY TO THIS BILL AND ARE MADE A PART HEREOF.

NUBC National Uniform Billing Committee LIC9213257

Figure 17-5

ASSIGNMENT 17-10 LOCATE ERRORS ON A CMS-1450 (UB-04) CLAIM FORM

Performance Objective

Task: Locate the blocks on the computer-generated insurance claim form that need completion of missing information or have data that need to be corrected before submission to the insurance company.

Conditions: Use Harold M. McDonald's completed insurance claim (Figure 17-6), the checklist for editing a CMS-1450 (UB-04) claim form, and a red ink pen.

Standards: Time: ________________ minutes

Accuracy: ________________

(Note: The time element and accuracy criteria may be given by your instructor.)

Directions: Refer to Figure 17-5 in the *Handbook* to use the step-by-step approach while editing the computer-generated CMS-1450 (UB-04) claim form (see Figure 17-6). Use the checklist to help you when reviewing the claim form. Locate the blocks on the claim form that need completion of missing information or that have data to be corrected before submission to the insurance company. Highlight all errors you discover. Insert all corrections and missing information in red. If you cannot locate the necessary information but know it is mandatory, write "NEED" in the corresponding block.

You notice that the seventh CPT/Healthcare Common Procedure Coding System (HCPCS) code 43450 for operating room is missing. On hospital claims, the entry for operating room is usually blank and must be handwritten in, because this is the code for the surgical procedure.

Checklist for Editing a Uniform Bill (CMS-1450) Claim Form: Harold M. McDonald

Steps	*Form Locator Blocks/Fields*
1	FL 1 ________________ and 5 ________________
2	FL 4: Inpatient ________________ Outpatient ________________
3	FL 8b ________________, 38 ________________, 58 ________________, and 59 ________________
4	FL 10 ________________
5	FL 8b ________________ and 11 ________________
6	FL 50 ________________, 60 ________________, 61 ________________, 62 ________________, and 65 ________________
7	FL 66-67 A-Q ________________ and 69 ________________
8	FL 74 ________________ and 74 a-e ________________
9	FL 76 ________________
10	FL 6 ________________, 12 ________________, and 31 ________________
11	Inpatient: FL 42-47: 13 ________________, 16 ________________, and 46 ________________
12	FL 47 ________________
13	FL 42 ________________ and 46 ________________
14	Outpatient: FL 43 ________________, 44 ________________, and 45 ________________
15	Detailed record to be checked
16	FL 42 ________________, 43 ________________, and 47 ________________
17	FL 55 ________________

1 COLLEGE HOSPITAL
4500 BROAD AVENUE
WOODLAND HILLS XY 12345-0001
555-487-6789

2

3a PAT. CNTL # 10670685
b. MED. REC. # 2071307
4 TYPE OF BILL 0131
5 FED. TAX NO. 95-0731067
6 STATEMENT COVERS PERIOD FROM 070520XX THROUGH 070520XX
7

8 PATIENT NAME a
b MCDONALD HAROLD M

9 PATIENT ADDRESS a 22 BEACON ROAD
b WOODLAND HILLS c XY d 12345-0001 e

10 BIRTHDATE	11 SEX	12 ADMISSION DATE	13 HR	14 TYPE	15 SRC	16 DHR	17 STAT	18 CONDITION CODES	19	20	21	22	23	24	25	26	27	28	29 ACDT STATE	30
04261929	M	070520XX	12	3	1	99	01	C5												

31 OCCURRENCE CODE DATE | 32 OCCURRENCE CODE DATE | 33 OCCURRENCE CODE DATE | 34 OCCURRENCE CODE DATE | 35 OCCURRENCE SPAN CODE FROM THROUGH | 36 OCCURRENCE SPAN CODE FROM THROUGH | 37

38
MCDONALD HAROLD M
22 BEACON ROAD
WOODLAND HILLS XY 12345-0001

39 VALUE CODES CODE AMOUNT | 40 VALUE CODES CODE AMOUNT | 41 VALUE CODES CODE AMOUNT
a
b
c
d

	42 REV. CD.	43 DESCRIPTION	44 HCPCS / RATE / HIPPS CODE	45 SERV. DATE	46 SERV. UNITS	47 TOTAL CHARGES	48 NON-COVERED CHARGES	49	
1	250	PHARMACY			5	90 90			1
2	270	MED - SUR SUPPLIES			16	2519 50			2
3	300	DRAWING BLOOD	36415	070520XX	1	8 50			3
4	300	13-16 BLOOD/URINE TESTS	80016	070520XX	1	28 00			4
5	300	CREATININE CLEARANCE TEST	82575	070520XX	1	20 00			5
6	300	CBC	85025 24	070520XX	1	16 50			6
7	320	CONTRAST XRAY EXAM, ESOPH	74220	070520XX	1	114 00			7
8	320	X-RAY GUIDE, GI DILATION	74360	070520XX	1	750 00			8
9	360	OPERATING ROOM				500 00			9
10	410	CONT OXIMETER HOURS	82805 22	070520XX	1	8 00			10
11	001	Total				4055 40			11
12									12
13									13
14									14
15									15
16									16
17									17
18									18
19									19
20									20
21									21
22									22
23		PAGE ____ OF ____	CREATION DATE		TOTALS				23

	50 PAYER NAME	51 HEALTH PLAN ID	52 REL. INFO	53 ASG. BEN.	54 PRIOR PAYMENTS	55 EST. AMOUNT DUE	56 NPI 950731067	
A	HEALTH PLAN REDWOOD	278654901	Y	Y			57	A
B							OTHER	B
C							PRV ID	C

	58 INSURED'S NAME	59 P. REL	60 INSURED'S UNIQUE ID	61 GROUP NAME	62 INSURANCE GROUP NO.	
A	MCDONALD HAROLD M	01	31424435401		1320-0000 PLAN GO	A
B						B
C						C

	63 TREATMENT AUTHORIZATION CODES	64 DOCUMENT CONTROL NUMBER	65 EMPLOYER NAME	
A			WC PEDERSON FORD	A
B				B
C				C

66 DX 9 | 1509 | V725 | 68

69 ADMIT DX | 70 PATIENT REASON DX | 71 PPS CODE | 72 ECI | 73

74 PRINCIPAL PROCEDURE CODE DATE | a. OTHER PROCEDURE CODE DATE | b. OTHER PROCEDURE CODE DATE | 75
c. OTHER PROCEDURE CODE DATE | d. OTHER PROCEDURE CODE DATE | e. OTHER PROCEDURE CODE DATE

76 ATTENDING NPI 124589770 QUAL
LAST ANTRUM FIRST CONCHA
77 OPERATING NPI QUAL
LAST FIRST
78 OTHER NPI QUAL
LAST FIRST
79 OTHER NPI QUAL
LAST FIRST

80 REMARKS
HPR

81CC a b c d

UB-04 CMS-1450 APPROVED OMB NO.

THE CERTIFICATIONS ON THE REVERSE APPLY TO THIS BILL AND ARE MADE A PART HEREOF.

NUBC National Uniform Billing Committee LIC9213257

Figure 17-6

ASSIGNMENT 17-11 LOCATE ERRORS ON A CMS-1450 (UB-04) CLAIM FORM

Performance Objective

Task: Locate the blocks on the computer-generated insurance claim form that need completion of missing information or have data that need to be corrected before submission to the insurance company.

Conditions: Use Pedro Martinez's completed insurance claim (Figure 17-7), the checklist for editing a CMS-1450 (UB-04) claim form, and a red ink pen.

Standards: Time: ____________ minutes

Accuracy: ____________

(Note: The time element and accuracy criteria may be given by your instructor.)

Directions: Refer to Figure 17-5 in the *Handbook* to use the step-by-step approach while editing the computer-generated CMS-1450 (UB-04) claim form (see Figure 17-7). Use the checklist to help you when reviewing the claim form. Locate the blocks on the claim form that need completion of missing information or that have data to be corrected before submission to the insurance company. Highlight all errors you discover. Insert all corrections and missing information in red. If you cannot locate the necessary information but know it is mandatory, write "NEED" in the corresponding block. Then write a list of reasons why the claim may be rejected or delayed or why incorrect payment may be generated because of errors discovered.

Checklist for Editing a Uniform Bill (CMS-1450)
Claim Form: Pedro Martinez

Steps	*Form Locator Blocks/Fields*
1	FL 1 ____________ and 5 ____________
2	FL 4: Inpatient ____________ Outpatient ____________
3	FL 8b ____________, 38 ____________, 58 ____________, and 59 ____________
4	FL 10 ____________
5	FL 8b ____________ and 11 ____________
6	FL 50 ____________, 60 ____________, 61 ____________, 62 ____________, and 65 ____________
7	FL 66-67 A-Q ____________ and 69 ____________
8	FL 74 ____________ and 74 a-e ____________
9	FL 76 ____________
10	FL 6 ____________, 12 ____________, and 32 ____________
11	Inpatient: FL 42-47: 13 ____________, 16 ____________, and 46 ____________
12	FL 47 ____________,
13	FL 42 ____________, and 46 ____________,
14	Outpatient: FL 43 ____________, 44 ____________, and 45 ____________
15	Detailed record to be checked
16	FL 42 ____________, 43 ____________, and 47 ____________
17	FL 55 ____________

1 COLLEGE HOSPITAL	2	3a PAT. CNTL # 10630911	4 TYPE OF BILL
4500 BROAD AVENUE		b. MED. REC. # 3567811	0111
WOODLAND HILLS XY 12345-0001		5 FED. TAX NO. 95-0731067	6 STATEMENT COVERS PERIOD FROM 06120XX THROUGH 06120XX
555-487-6789			7

8 PATIENT NAME a	9 PATIENT ADDRESS a 7821 SENSOR AVE
b MARTINEZ PEDRO	b WOODLAND HILLS c XY d 12345-0001 e

10 BIRTHDATE	11 SEX	12 ADMISSION DATE	13 HR	14 TYPE	15 SRC	16 DHR	17 STAT	18 CONDITION CODES	19	20	21	22	23	24	25	26	27	28	29 ACDT STATE	30
092218	M	061120XX	20	1	7	19	03	C5	04											

31 OCCURRENCE CODE DATE | 32 OCCURRENCE CODE DATE | 33 OCCURRENCE CODE DATE | 34 OCCURRENCE CODE DATE | 35 OCCURRENCE SPAN CODE FROM THROUGH | 36 OCCURRENCE SPAN CODE FROM THROUGH | 37

38
MARTINEZ PEDRO
7821 SENSOR AVENUE
WOODLAND HILLS XY 12345-0001

	39 VALUE CODES CODE	AMOUNT	40 VALUE CODES CODE	AMOUNT	41 VALUE CODES CODE	AMOUNT
a	01	650 00				
b						
c						
d						

	42 REV. CD.	43 DESCRIPTION	44 HCPCS / RATE / HIPPS CODE	45 SERV. DATE	46 SERV. UNITS	47 TOTAL CHARGES	48 NON-COVERED CHARGES	49	
1	110	ROOM - BOARD/SEMI/PVT	650.00		1	650 00			1
2	120	ROOM AND CARE SEMI	650.00		1	650 00			2
3	210	ROOM AND CARE CCU	1600.00		8	12800 00			3
4	250	PHARMACY			500	7133 90			4
5	270	MED - SUR SUPPLIES			149	3689 50			5
6	300	LABORATORY			97	5399 33			6
7	320	RADIOLOGY			27	1544 00			7
8	350	CT SCAN			1	622 00			8
9	410	RESPIRATORY THERAPY			240	6698 50			9
10	420	PHYSICAL THERAPY			9	470 00			10
11	450	EMERGENCY ROOM SERV			6	197 00			11
12	460	PULMONARY FUNCTION				29 00			12
13	730	ELECTROCARDIOLOGY			1	100 00			13
14	942	EDUCATION			6	82 50			14
15	001	Total				40065 73			15
16									16
17									17
18									18
19									19
20									20
21									21
22									22
23		PAGE ____ OF ____	CREATION DATE		TOTALS				23

	50 PAYER NAME	51 HEALTH PLAN ID	52 REL. INFO	53 ASG. BEN.	54 PRIOR PAYMENTS	55 EST. AMOUNT DUE	56 NPI 950731067	
A	MEDIPRIME-HPR		Y	Y			57	A
B							OTHER	B
C							PRV ID	C

	58 INSURED'S NAME	59 P. REL	60 INSURED'S UNIQUE ID	61 GROUP NAME	62 INSURANCE GROUP NO.	
A	MARTINEZ PEDRO	01	55025897001		6500-0000	A
B						B
C						C

	63 TREATMENT AUTHORIZATION CODES	64 DOCUMENT CONTROL NUMBER	65 EMPLOYER NAME	
A			RETIRED 1975	A
B				B
C				C

66 DX 9 | 4169 | 51881 | 49121 | 68

69 ADMIT DX | 70 PATIENT REASON DX | 71 PPS CODE | 72 ECI | 73

74 PRINCIPAL PROCEDURE CODE DATE | a. OTHER PROCEDURE CODE DATE | b. OTHER PROCEDURE CODE DATE | 75

c. OTHER PROCEDURE CODE DATE | d. OTHER PROCEDURE CODE DATE | e. OTHER PROCEDURE CODE DATE

76 ATTENDING NPI 642110670 QUAL
LAST COCCIDIOIDES FIRST BRADY

77 OPERATING NPI QUAL
LAST FIRST

78 OTHER NPI QUAL
LAST FIRST

79 OTHER NPI QUAL
LAST FIRST

80 REMARKS | 81CC a b c d

UB-04 CMS-1450 APPROVED OMB NO.

THE CERTIFICATIONS ON THE REVERSE APPLY TO THIS BILL AND ARE MADE A PART HEREOF.

NUBC National Uniform Billing Committee LIC9213257

Figure 17-7

18 Seeking a Job and Attaining Professional Advancement

Marilyn T. Fordney

KEY TERMS

Your instructor may wish to select some words pertinent to this chapter for a test. For definitions of the terms, further study, and/or reference, the words, phrases, and abbreviations may be found in the glossary at the end of the Handbook. *Key terms for this chapter follow.*

alien
application form
blind mailing
business associate agreement
certification
Certified Coding Specialist
Certified Coding Specialist-Physician
Certified Medical Assistant
Certified Medical Billing Specialist
Certified Professional Coder
chronologic résumé
claims assistance professional
combination résumé
continuing education
cover letter
employment agencies
functional résumé
interview
mentor
National Certified Insurance and Coding Specialist
networking
portfolio
Professional Association of Health Care Office Management
Registered Medical Assistant
Registered Medical Coder
registration
résumé
self-employment
service contract

KEY ABBREVIATIONS

See how many abbreviations and acronyms you can translate and then use this as a handy reference list. Definitions for the key abbreviations are located near the back of the Handbook *in the glossary.*

AAPC ______________________

AHIMA ______________________

CAP ______________________

CCAP ______________________

CCS ______________________

CCS-P ______________________

CECP ______________________

CMA ______________________

CMBS ______________________

CMRS ______________________

CPC ______________________

CPC-A ______________________

CPC-H ______________________

ECP ______________________

EEOC ______________________

HRS ______________________

NCICS ______________________

PAHCOM ______________________

RMA ______________________

RMC ______________________

USCIS ______________________

PERFORMANCE OBJECTIVES

The student will be able to:

- Define and spell the key terms and key abbreviations for this chapter, given the information from the *Handbook* glossary, within a reasonable time period and with enough accuracy to obtain a satisfactory evaluation.
- After reading the chapter, answer the fill-in-the-blank, multiple choice, and true/false review questions with enough accuracy to obtain a satisfactory evaluation.
- Research information in preparation for typing a résumé, given a worksheet to complete, within a reasonable time period and with enough accuracy to obtain a satisfactory evaluation.
- Type an accurate résumé in attractive format, using plain typing paper, within a reasonable time period, to obtain a satisfactory evaluation.
- Compose and type a letter of introduction to go with the résumé and place it in a typed envelope, using one sheet of plain typing paper and a number 10 envelope, within a reasonable time period, to obtain a satisfactory evaluation.
- Complete an application form for a job, given an application for position form, within a reasonable time period and with enough accuracy to obtain a satisfactory evaluation.
- Compose and type a follow-up thank-you letter and place it in a typed envelope, using one sheet of plain typing paper and a number 10 envelope, within a reasonable time period, to obtain a satisfactory evaluation.
- Access the Internet and visit websites to research and/or obtain data, within a reasonable time period and with enough accuracy to obtain a satisfactory evaluation.

STUDY OUTLINE

Employment Opportunities
- Insurance Billing Specialist
- Claims Assistance Professional

Job Search
- Online Job Search
- Job Fairs
- Application
- Letter of Introduction
- Résumé
- Interview
- Follow-up Letter

Self-Employment
- Setting Up an Office
- Finances to Consider
- Marketing, Advertising, Promotion, and Public Relations
- Documentation
- Mentor and Business Incubator Services
- Networking

Procedure 18-1: Creating an Electronic Résumé

ASSIGNMENT 18-1 REVIEW QUESTIONS

Part I Fill in the Blank

Review the objectives, key terms, glossary definitions of key terms, chapter information, and figures before completing the following review questions.

1. You have just completed a 1-year medical insurance billing course at a college. Name some preliminary job search contacts to make on campus.

   a. ____________________

   b. ____________________

   c. ____________________

   d. ____________________

2. Name skills that may be listed on an application form or in a résumé when a person is seeking a position as an insurance billing specialist.

   a. ____________________

   b. ____________________

   c. ____________________

   d. ____________________

   e. ____________________

   f. ____________________

3. A question appears on a job application form about salary. Two ways in which to handle this question are

   a. ____________________

   b. ____________________

4. State the chief purpose of a cover letter when a résumé is sent to a prospective employer.

   ____

5. List the items to be compiled in a portfolio.

   a. ____________________

   b. ____________________

   c. ____________________

   d. ____________________

   e. ____________________

   f. ____________________

   g. ____________________

   h. ____________________

   i. ____________________

6. You are being interviewed for a job and the interviewer asks this question: "What is your religious preference?" How would you respond?

____

____

7. If a short period of time elapses after an interview and the applicant has received no word from the prospective employer, what follow-up steps may be taken?

   a. ____

   b. ____

8. If an individual creates a billing company and coding services are to be part of the offerings, the coding professional should have what type of professional status?

____

9. Hugh Beason was the owner of XYZ Medical Reimbursement Service. A fire occurred, damaging some of the equipment and part of the office premises and requiring him to stop his work for a month so that repairs could be made. What type/types of insurance would be helpful for this kind of problem?

____

10. Gwendolyn Stevens has an insurance billing company and is attending a professional meeting where she has given business cards to a few attendees. Give two reasons for using this business marketing strategy.

    a. ____

    b. ____

11. State the difference between *certification* and *registration*.

    a. Certification: ____

    ____

    b. Registration: ____

    ____

12. Name some ways an insurance billing specialist may seek to keep knowledge current.

    a. ____

    b. ____

    c. ____

    d. ____

13. Jerry Hahn is pursuing a career as a claims assistance professional. When he markets his business, the target audience should be ________________________________.

14. Jennifer Inouye has been hired as a coding specialist by a hospital and needs to keep documentation when working. This may consist of

a. ______________________________.

b. ______________________________.

c. ______________________________.

15. Give the names of at least two national organizations that certify billers and coders.

a. ______________________________

b. ______________________________

Part II Multiple Choice

Choose the best answer.

16. A résumé format that emphasizes work experience dates is known as
    a. functional.
    b. combination.
    c. business.
    d. chronologic.

17. When an individual plans to start an insurance billing company, he or she should have enough funds to operate the business for a period of
    a. 6 months or more.
    b. 18 months or more.
    c. 1 year or more.
    d. 2 years.

18. Under HIPAA regulations, if a physician's insurance billing is outsourced to a person, this individual is known as a/an ______________ because he or she uses and discloses individuals' identifiable health information.
    a. billing specialist
    b. business associate
    c. outside contractor
    d. outside vendor

19. When insurance billing is outsourced to a company, a document should be created, signed, and notarized by both parties known as a
    a. contract agreement.
    b. business agreement.
    c. service contract.
    d. legal contract.

20. A guide who offers advice, criticism, and guidance to an inexperienced person to help him or her reach a goal is known as a/an
    a. mentor.
    b. counselor.
    c. associate.
    d. instructor.

Part III True/False

Write "T" or "F" in the blank to indicate whether you think the statement is true or false.

________ 21. A résumé format that stresses job skills is known as functional.

________ 22. When job applicants have similar skills and education, surveys have shown that hiring by employers has been based on bilingual skills.

________ 23. Enhancing knowledge and keeping up to date are responsibilities of an insurance billing specialist.

________ 24. Professional status of an insurance billing specialist may be obtained by passing a national examination for a CMRS.

________ 25. Professional status of a claims assistance professional may be obtained by passing a national examination as a CCS.

ASSIGNMENT 18-2 JOB SEARCHING AND JOB SKILLS

Performance Objective

Task: Read these job advertisements. Then read the interests and abilities of the applicants to decide which job title belongs to each job hunter.

Conditions: Use the job advertisements and pen or pencil.

Standards: Time ______________ minutes

Accuracy ______________

(Note: The time element and accuracy criteria may be given by your instructor.)

Directions: These advertisements appeared in your local newspaper. Read the ads and then read the interests and abilities of each job applicant. Insert the job title for each applicant.

Job Titles

Insurance Biller	**Insurance Coder**	**Bilingual Collections Manager**
HS grad, computer exp. typing 40 wpm. Needed for busy outpt clinic, insurance claims knowledge	Detailed oriented individual, Dx and proc coder. 2 yr exp preferred	Self-motivated individual with good communications skills. Bilingual. Enjoys working in health care.

Trudy

Trudy is bilingual in English and Spanish and enjoys working with people. She is especially good with the telephone and likes communications.

Job Title: ____

Walter

Walter wants to work in the health care field. He has taken diagnostic and procedure coding classes, and enjoys problem solving.

Job Title: ____

Ilona

Ilona has experience with inputting patient data and transmitting insurance claims. She says she is honest and dependable.

Job Title: ____

ASSIGNMENT 18-3 COMPLETE A WORKSHEET AND TYPE A RÉSUMÉ

Performance Objective

Task: Respond to a job advertisement by completing a worksheet and typing a résumé by abstracting data from your worksheet.

Conditions: Use two sheets of plain typing paper, a newspaper advertisement (Figure 18-1), and a computer.

Standards: Time: ______________ minutes

Accuracy: ______________

(Note: The time element and accuracy criteria may be given by your instructor.)

Directions: An advertisement appeared in your local newspaper (see Figure 18-1). You decide to apply for the position. Complete a worksheet in preparation for typing your résumé. Some of the information requested on the worksheet should not appear on the résumé but should be available if you are asked to provide it. Ask a classmate to review and comment about the information in your worksheet. Abstract data that you think are relevant from the worksheet, and type a résumé in rough draft. Ask the instructor for suggestions to improve the rough draft. Refer to Chapter 18 and Figure 18-6 in the *Handbook* to help organize your résumé into an attractive format before you type the final copy.

1. Insert title of personal data sheet from worksheet.

2. Insert heading: name, address, telephone number, and so on.

3. Select one of three formats for data.

4. Insert heading and data for education information.

5. Insert heading and data for skill information.

6. Insert heading and data for employment information.

7. Insert reference information.

8. Proofread résumé.

9. Print résumé.

MEDICAL INSURANCE CODING/REIMBURSEMENT SPECIALIST

Mid-Atlantic Clinic, a 20-physician, multi-specialty group practice in Chicago, Illinois, has a need for a coding and reimbursement specialist. Knowledge of medical terminology, CPT and ICD-9-CM coding systems, Medicare regulations, third-party insurance reimbursement and physician billing procedures required. Proficiency in the interpretation and coding of procedural and diagnostic codes is strongly preferred. Successful candidates must have excellent communication and problem-solving skills. This position offers a competitive salary and superior benefits. Please send resume to:

George B. Pason, Personnel Director
Mid-Atlantic Clinic
1230 South Main Street
Chicago, IL 60611

Figure 18-1

ASSIGNMENT 18-4 COMPLETE A COVER LETTER

Performance Objective

Task: Compose a cover letter to accompany your résumé.

Conditions: Use one sheet of plain typing paper, a number 10 envelope, and a computer, printer, thesaurus, and English dictionary.

Standards: Time: ______________ minutes

Accuracy: ______________

(Note: The time element and accuracy criteria may be given by your instructor.)

Directions: Compose a cover letter introducing yourself, and type a rough draft. Consult the instructor for suggestions. Type the cover letter on plain bond paper in a form that can be mailed. Refer to the sample letter in Chapter 18 and Figure 18-5 in the *Handbook* as a guide to help organize your thoughts. Type the name and address of the employer on a number 10 envelope, and insert the letter with the résumé from Assignment 18-3.

ASSIGNMENT 18-5 COMPLETE A JOB APPLICATION FORM

Performance Objective

Task: Complete a job application form by using data from your résumé.

Conditions: Use application form (Figure 18-2), your résumé, and a computer.

Standards: Time: ____________ minutes

Accuracy: ____________

(Note: The time element and accuracy criteria may be given by your instructor.)

Directions: Assume that the employer asked you to come to his or her place of business to complete an application form and make an appointment for an interview. Using your data and résumé, complete an application form (see Figure 18-2).

APPLICATION FOR POSITION/ Medical or Dental Office
AN EQUAL OPPORTUNITY EMPLOYER

(In answering questions, use extra blank sheet if necessary)

No employee, applicant, or candidate for promotion training or other advantage shall be discriminated against (or given preference) because of race, color, religion, sex, age, physical handicap, veteran status, or national origin.
PLEASE READ CAREFULLY AND WRITE OR PRINT ANSWERS TO ALL QUESTIONS. DO NOT TYPE.

Date of application

A. PERSONAL INFORMATION

Name- Last First Middle		Social Security No.	Area Code/Phone No. ( )	
Present Address: -Street (Apt. #) City		State Zip		How long at this address?
Previous Address: -Street Clty State Zip From: To:		Person to notify in case of Emergency or Accident - Name: Address: Telephone:		

B. EMPLOYMENT INFORMATION

For what position are you applying?	☐ Full-time ☐ Part-time ☐ Either	Date available for employment?:	Wage/Salary Expectations:
List hrs./days you prefer to work:	List any hrs./days you are not available: (Except for times required for religious practices or observances)		Can you work overtime, if necessary? ☐ Yes ☐ No
Are you employed now?: ☐ Yes ☐ No	If so, may we inquire of your present employer?: ☐ No ☐ Yes, If yes: Name of employer: Phone number: ( )		
Have you ever been bonded?: ☐ Yes ☐ No	If required for position, are you bondable? ☐ Yes ☐ No ☐ Uncertain	Have you applied for a position with this office before? ☐ No ☐ Yes, If yes, when?:	
Referred by/ or where did you hear of this job?:			
Can you, upon employment, submit verification of your legal right to work in the United States? ☐ Yes ☐ No Submit proof that you meet legal age requirement for employment? ☐ Yes ☐ No		Language(s) applicant speaks or writes (if use of a language other than English is relevant to the job for which applicant is applying):	

C. EDUCATIONAL HISTORY

Name and address of schools attended (Include current)	Dates From	Thru	Highest grade/level completed	Diploma/degree(s) obtained/areas of study:
High school				
College				Degree/Major
Post graduate				Degree/Major
Other				Course/Diploma/License Certificate

Specific training, education, or experiences which will assist you in the job for which you have applied:

Future educational plans:

D. SPECIAL SKILLS

CHECK BELOW THE KINDS OF WORK YOU HAVE DONE:			
		☐ MEDICAL INSURANCE FORMS	☐ RECEPTIONIST
☐ BLOOD COUNTS	☐ DENTAL ASSISTANT	☐ MEDICAL TERMINOLOGY	☐ TELEPHONES
☐ BOOKKEEPING	☐ DENTAL HYGIENIST	☐ MEDICAL TRANSCRIPTION	☐ TYPING
☐ COLLECTIONS	☐ FILING	☐ NURSING	☐ STENOGRAPHY
☐ COMPOSING LETTERS	☐ INJECTIONS	☐ PHLEBOTOMY (Draw Blood)	☐ URINALYSIS
☐ COMPUTER INPUT	☐ INSTRUMENT STERILIZATION	☐ POSTING	☐ X-RAY
OFFICE EQUIPMENT USED: ☐ COMPUTER	☐ DICTATING EQUIPMENT	☐ WORD PROCESSOR	☐ OTHER:
Other kinds of tasks performed or skills that may be applicable to position:		Typing speed:	Shorthand speed:

(PLEASE COMPLETE OTHER SIDE)

Figure 18-2

Continued

E. EMPLOYMENT RECORD

LIST MOST RECENT EMPLOYMENT FIRST — May we contact your previous Employer(s) for a reference? ☐ yes ☐ no

1) Employer	Work performed. Be specific.
Address Street City State Zip code	
Phone number ( )	
Type of business — Dates From Mo. Yr. To Mo. Yr.	
Your position — Hourly rate/Salary Starting Final	
Supervisor's name	
Reason for leaving	
2) Employer	Work performed. Be specific.
Address Street City State Zip code	
Phone number ( )	
Type of business — Dates From Mo. Yr. To Mo. Yr.	
Your position — Hourly rate/Salary Starting Final	
Supervisor's name	
Reason for leaving	
3) Employer	Work performed. Be specific.
Address Street City State Zip code	
Phone number ( )	
Type of business — Dates From Mo. Yr. To Mo. Yr.	
Your position — Hourly rate/Salary Starting Final	
Supervisor's name	
Reason for leaving	

F. REFERENCES: FRIENDS/ACQUAINTANCES NON-RELATED

	Name	Address	Telephone Number (☐ Work ☐ Home)	Occupation	Years acquainted
1)					
2)					

Please feel free to add any information which you feel will help us consider you for employment.

READ THE FOLLOWING CAREFULLY, THEN SIGN AND DATE THE APPLICATION

I certify that all answers given by me on this application are true, correct and complete to the best of my knowledge. I acknowledge notice that the information contained in this application is subject to check. I agree that, if hired, my continued employment may be contingent upon the accuracy of that information. If employed, I further agree to comply with company/office rules and regulations.

Signature ______________________ Date: ______________

RM NO. 72-110 ©1976 BIBBERO SYSTEMS INC. PETALUMA, CA (MB-CO) # 6-7 (REV. 4/92) TO REORDER CALL 800-BIBBERO (800) 242-2376

Figure 18-2, cont'd

ASSIGNMENT 18-6 PREPARE A FOLLOW-UP THANK-YOU LETTER

Performance Objective

Task: Prepare a follow-up thank-you letter after the interview, sending it to the interviewer.

Conditions: Use one sheet of plain typing paper, a number 10 envelope, and a computer, printer, thesaurus, and English dictionary.

Standards: Time: ______________ minutes

Accuracy: ______________

(Note: The time element and accuracy criteria may be given by your instructor.)

Directions: After the interview, you decide to send a follow-up thank-you letter to the person who interviewed you. Type a letter and address a number 10 envelope. Refer to Chapter 18 and Figure 18-11 in the *Handbook* to help organize your thoughts.

ASSIGNMENT 18-7 VISIT WEBSITES FOR JOB OPPORTUNITIES

Performance Objective

Task: Access the Internet and visit several websites of the World Wide Web.

Conditions: Use a computer with printer and/or a pen or pencil to make notes.

Standards: Time: ______________ minutes

Accuracy: ______________

(Note: The time element and accuracy criteria may be given by your instructor.)

Directions: Visit at least five websites by using either a search engine (Yahoo, Google, Bing) or a job search website. Some suggestions are:

www.healthcarejobs.org
www.indeed.com
www.job-search-engine.com
www.flipdog.com
www.topusajobs.com
www.monster.com

Enter a keyword or job title, such as "medical billing specialist" or "medical coder." Enter your city and state to locate listings near you. Click on the search button. If you get some results, print the listings that appeal to you for sharing and discussing in class.

ASSIGNMENT 18-8 CRITICAL THINKING

Performance Objective

Task: Write a paragraph describing the benefits of becoming certified in this field.

Conditions: Use a computer with printer and/or a pen or pencil.

Standards: Time: ______________ minutes

Accuracy: ______________

(Note: The time element and accuracy criteria may be given by your instructor.)

Directions: Write a paragraph or two describing why you would like to become certified in this field, and incorporate a numbered list of benefits. Make sure grammar, punctuation, and spelling are correct.

Tests

TEST 1: PROCEDURE (E/M AND MEDICINE SECTIONS) AND DIAGNOSTIC PROCEDURE CODE TEST

Directions: Using a *Current Procedural Terminology* (CPT) code book or Appendix A in this *Workbook*, insert the correct code numbers and modifiers for each service rendered. Give a brief description for each professional service rendered, although this is not needed for completing the CMS-1500 (02-12) claim form. An optional exercise is to abstract the pertinent data from each case, then use the *International Classification of Diseases, Ninth Revision, Clinical Modification* (ICD-9-CM) or ICD-10-CM draft code book to insert the diagnosis code.

Insert year of the CPT code book used:

____

Insert year of the ICD-9-CM and/or ICD-10-CM code book used:

____

1. Dr. Input sees a new patient, Mrs. Post, in the office for acute abdominal distress. The physician spends approximately 1 hour obtaining a comprehensive history and physical examination with high-complexity decision making. Several diagnostic studies are ordered, and Mrs. Post is given an appointment to return in 1 week.

Description

______________________________ CPT # ________

______________________________ ICD-9-CM # ________

______________________________ ICD-10-CM # ________

2. Mr. Nakahara, an established patient, sees Dr. Practon in the office on January 11 for a reevaluation of his type 2 diabetic condition. Dr. Practon takes a detailed history and performs a detailed examination. Decision making is moderately complex.

Description

______________________________ CPT # ________

______________________________ ICD-9-CM # ________

______________________________ ICD-10-CM # ________

3. Dr. Cardi sees Mrs. Franklin for a follow-up office visit for her hypertension. A problem-focused history and examination of her cardiovascular system are obtained and reveal a blood pressure of 140/100. Decision making is straightforward, with medication being prescribed. The patient is advised to return in 2 weeks to have her blood pressure checked by the nurse. Mrs. Franklin returns 2 weeks later, and the nurse checks her blood pressure.

Description

______________________________ CPT # ________

______________________________ ICD-9-CM # ________

______________________________ ICD-10-CM # ________

______________________________ CPT # ________

______________________________ ICD-9-CM # ________

______________________________ ICD-10-CM # ________

4. Dr. Skeleton receives a call at 7 PM from Mrs. Snyder. Her husband, a patient of Dr. Skeleton's, has been very ill for 2 hours with profuse vomiting. Dr. Skeleton goes to their home to see Mr. Snyder and spends considerable time obtaining a detailed history and examination. The medical decision making is of a highly complex nature. The physician administers an injection of prochlorperazine (Compazine).

Description

______________________________ CPT # ________

______________________________ CPT # ________

______________________________ ICD-9-CM # ________

______________________________ ICD-10-CM # ________

5. Dr. Cutis sees an established patient, a registered nurse, for determination of pregnancy. A detailed history and examination are obtained, with moderate-complexity medical decision making. A Papanicolaou smear is taken, a blood sample is drawn, and the specimens are sent to an independent laboratory for a qualitative human chorionic gonadotropin (hCG) test. The patient also complains of something she has discovered under her armpit. On examination, there is a furuncle of the left axilla, which is incised and drained during this visit. The laboratory requires CPT coding on the laboratory requisition. List how these laboratory procedures would appear on the requisition sheet. The Papanicolaou smear is processed according to the Bethesda System and under physician supervision.

Professional Service Rendered by Dr. Cutis

______________________________ CPT # ________

______________________________ CPT # ________

______________________________ CPT # ________

______________________________ CPT # ________

____ ICD-9-CM # ________

____ ICD-10-CM # ________

____ ICD-9-CM # ________

____ ICD-10-CM # ________

Laboratory Service on Requisition Sheet

____ CPT # ________

____ CPT # ________

6. Dr. Antrum makes a house call on Betty Mason, an established patient, for a problem-focused history of acute otitis media. A problem-focused examination is performed, with straightforward medical decision making. While there, Dr. Antrum also sees Betty's younger sister, Sandra, whom she has seen previously in the office, for acute tonsillitis. A problem-focused history and examination are performed with low-complexity decision making. In addition to the examinations, Dr. Antrum gives both children injections of penicillin.

Professional Service Rendered to Betty

____ CPT # ________

____ CPT # ________

____ ICD-9-CM # ________

____ ICD-10-CM # ________

Professional Service Rendered to Sandra

____ CPT # ________

____ CPT # ________

____ ICD-9-CM # ________

____ ICD-10-CM # ________

7. Two weeks later, Dr. Antrum is called to the emergency department at College Hospital at 2 AM on Sunday to see Betty Mason for recurrent chronic otitis media with suppuration. A problem-focused history and examination are performed with straightforward decision making. Dr. Antrum administers a second injection of penicillin.

Description

____ CPT # ________

____ CPT # ________

____ ICD-9-CM # ________

____ ICD-10-CM # ________

8. While at the hospital, Dr. Antrum is asked to see another patient in the emergency department, who is new to her. A problem-focused history is taken. She performs a problem-focused examination and straightforward decision making for an intermediate 3.5-cm laceration of the scalp. The laceration is sutured, and the patient is advised to come to the office in 4 days for a dressing change. Four days later, the patient comes into the office for a dressing change by the nurse.

Description

____ CPT # ______

____ CPT # ______

____ ICD-9-CM # ______

____ ICD-10-CM # ______

9. Dr. Menter, a psychiatrist, sees the following patients in the hospital. Code each procedure.

   Ms. Blake: Consultation, expanded problem-focused history and examination and straightforward decision making; referred by Dr. Practon CPT # ______

   Mrs. Clark: Group psychotherapy (50 min) CPT # ______

   Mrs. Samson: Group psychotherapy (50 min) CPT # ______

   Mr. Shoemaker: Group psychotherapy (50 min) CPT # ______

   Miss James: Individual psychotherapy (25 min) CPT # ______

10. Dr. Input, a gastroenterologist, sees Mrs. Chan in the hospital at the request of Dr. Practon for an esophageal ulcer. In addition to the detailed history and examination and the low-complexity decision making, Dr. Input performs an esophageal intubation and washings, and prepares slides for cytology. Two days later, he sees Mrs. Chan in a follow-up hospital visit and obtains a problem-focused interval history and examination with low-complexity decision making. He performs a gastric intubation and collects washings for cytologic evaluation for a gastric ulcer.

Description

____ CPT # ______

____ CPT # ______

____ ICD-9-CM # ______

____ ICD-10-CM # ______

____ CPT # ______

____ CPT # ______

____ ICD-9-CM # ______

____ ICD-10-CM # ______

11. Mrs. Galati, a new patient, goes to Dr. Cardi because of chest pain (moderate to severe), weakness, fatigue, and dizziness. Dr. Cardi takes a comprehensive history and performs a comprehensive examination, followed by a treadmill ECG with interpretation and report. He also performs a vital capacity test and dipstick urinalysis, and draws blood for triiodothyronine (T_3) testing and for analysis by sequential multiple analyzer computer (SMAC) (16 panel tests, including complete blood cell count [CBC]), which are sent to and billed by a laboratory. Medical decision making is of high complexity.

Description

______________________________ CPT # ________

______________________________ CPT # ________

______________________________ CPT # ________

______________________________ CPT # ________

______________________________ CPT # ________

______________________________ CPT # ________

______________________________ ICD-9-CM # ________

______________________________ ICD-10-CM # ________

______________________________ ICD-9-CM # ________

______________________________ ICD-10-CM # ________

______________________________ ICD-9-CM # ________

______________________________ ICD-10-CM # ________

12. Jake Wonderhill has not had his eyes examined by Dr. Lenser for about 5 years. He is seen by Dr. Lenser, who performs the following ophthalmologic procedures in addition to a comprehensive eye examination: fluorescein angioscopy and electroretinography. Mr. Wonderhill receives a diagnosis of retinitis pigmentosa.

Description

______________________________ CPT # ________

______________________________ CPT # ________

______________________________ CPT # ________

______________________________ ICD-9-CM # ________

______________________________ ICD-10-CM # ________

13. Dr. Practon is making rounds at the College Hospital and answers an urgent call on 3rd Floor East. He performs cardiopulmonary resuscitation on Mr. Sanchez for cardiac arrest and orders the patient taken to the critical care unit. Chest radiographs, laboratory work, blood gas measurements, and ECG are performed. The physician is detained 2 hours in constant attendance on the patient.

Description

____ CPT # _______

____ CPT # _______

____ CPT # _______

____ ICD-9-CM # _______

____ ICD-10-CM # _______

14. Mrs. Powers, a new patient, sees Dr. Skeleton for low sciatica. Dr. Skeleton takes a detailed history and performs a detailed examination of the patient's lower back and extremities. Medical decision making is of low complexity. Diathermy (30 minutes) is given. The next day the patient comes in for therapeutic exercises in the Hubbard tank (30 minutes).

Description

____ CPT # _______

____ CPT # _______

____ ICD-9-CM # _______

____ ICD-10-CM # _______

____ CPT # _______

____ ICD-9-CM # _______

____ ICD-10-CM # _______

15. a. Mrs. Garcia, a new patient, is seen by Dr. Caesar for occasional vaginal spotting (detailed history/examination and low-complexity decision making). The doctor determines that the bleeding is coming from the cervix and asks her to return in 3 days for cryocauterization of the cervix. During the initial examination, Mrs. Garcia asks for an evaluation for possible infertility. Dr. Caesar advises her to wait 2 to 3 weeks and make an appointment for two infertility tests.
    b. When the patient returns in 3 days for cryocauterization, the doctor also takes a wet mount for bacteria/fungi, which is sent to and billed by a laboratory.
    c. Three weeks later, an injection procedure for hysterosalpingography and endometrial biopsy are performed.

Description

a. ______________________________ CPT # ______

______________________________ ICD-9-CM # ______

______________________________ ICD-10-CM # ______

b. ______________________________ CPT # ______

______________________________ CPT # ______

______________________________ ICD-9-CM # ______

______________________________ ICD-10-CM # ______

c. ______________________________ CPT # ______

______________________________ CPT # ______

______________________________ ICD-9-CM # ______

______________________________ ICD-10-CM # ______

Multiple Choice

After reading the boxed codes with descriptions, select the answer/answers that is/are best in each case.

59120	surgical treatment of ectopic pregnancy; tubal or ovarian, requiring salpingectomy and/or oophorectomy, abdominal or vaginal approach
59121	tubal or ovarian, without salpingectomy and/or oophorectomy
59130	abdominal pregnancy
59135	interstitial, uterine pregnancy requiring total hysterectomy
59136	interstitial, uterine pregnancy with partial resection of uterus
59140	cervical, with evacuation

16. In regard to this section of CPT codes, which of the following statements is true about codes 59120 through 59140? Mark all that apply.
    a. They refer to abdominal hysterotomy.
    b. They involve laparoscopic treatment of ectopic pregnancy.
    c. They refer to treatment of ectopic pregnancy by surgery.
    d. They involve tubal ligation.

17. In regard to this section of CPT codes, for treatment of a tubal ectopic pregnancy, necessitating oophorectomy, the code to select is
    a. 59121.
    b. 59120.
    c. 59135.
    d. 59136.
    e. 59130.

18. In regard to this section of CPT codes, for treatment of an ectopic pregnancy (interstitial, uterine) requiring a total hysterectomy, the code/codes to select is/are
    a. 59135.
    b. 59135 and 59120.
    c. 59120.
    d. 59130 and 59120.
    e. 59121.

TEST 2: PROCEDURE CODE WITH MODIFIERS AND DIAGNOSTIC CODE TEST

Directions: Match the description given in the right column with the procedure code/modifier combination in the left column. Write the letter in the blank.

Procedure With Modifier		*Description*
1. 99214-25	____________	a. Dr. Practon assisted Dr. Caesar with a total abdominal hysterectomy and bilateral salpingo-oophorectomy.
2. 99204-57	____________	b. Dr. Skeleton interprets a thoracolumbar x-ray film that was taken at College Hospital.
3. 58150-80	____________	c. Mrs. Ulwelling saw Dr. Antrum for an office visit as a new patient, and she recommended that the patient undergo a laryngoscopy, with stripping of vocal cords to be done the following day.
4. 32440-55	____________	d. Mrs. Gillenbach walked through a plate glass window and underwent a rhinoplasty, performed by Dr. Graff on February 16, 20xx. On February 26, 20xx, she came to see Dr. Graff for a consultation regarding reconstructive surgery on her right leg.
5. 72080-26	____________	e. An established patient, Mrs. Mercado, is seen in a follow-up exam for type 2 diabetes. The patient asks Dr. Langerhans to look at some skin tags. The doctor examines them and says they need to be removed (11200). The evaluation and management service was detailed and of a moderate complexity.
6. 29425-58	____________	f. Dr. Cutler performed a bilateral orchiopexy (inguinal approach) on baby Kozak.
7. 54640-50	____________	g. Dr. Skeleton applied a short leg walking cast to Mrs. Belchere's right leg 4 weeks after his initial treatment of her fractured tibia.
8. 99253-24	____________	h. Dr. Cutler went on vacation, and Dr. Coccidioides took care of Mrs. Ash during the postoperative period after her total pneumonectomy.

Directions: Using a *Current Procedural Terminology* (CPT) code book or Appendix A in this Workbook, insert the correct code numbers and modifiers for each service rendered. Give a brief description for each professional service rendered, although this is not needed for completing the CMS-1500 (02-12) claim form.

9. Dr. Input performs a gastrojejunostomy for carcinoma in situ of the duodenum and calls in Dr. Scott to administer the anesthesia and Dr. Cutler to assist. This intraperitoneal surgery takes 2 hours, 30 minutes. The patient is otherwise normal and healthy. List the procedure and diagnostic code numbers with appropriate modifiers for each physician.

Professional Service Rendered by Dr. Input

____ CPT # ________

____ ICD-9-CM # ________

____ ICD-10-CM # ________

Professional Service Rendered by Dr. Scott

____ CPT # ______

____ ICD-9-CM # ______

____ ICD-10-CM # ______

Professional Service Rendered by Dr. Cutler

____ CPT # ______

____ ICD-9-CM # ______

____ ICD-10-CM # ______

10. Dr. Rumsey assists Dr. Cutler with a total colectomy (intraperitoneal procedure) with ileostomy. Dr. Scott is the anesthesiologist. Surgery takes 2 hours, 55 minutes. The patient has a secondary malignant neoplasm of the colon (severe systemic disease). List the procedure code numbers with appropriate modifiers and diagnostic code numbers for each physician.

Professional Service Rendered by Dr. Rumsey

____ CPT # ______

____ ICD-9-CM # ______

____ ICD-10-CM # ______

Professional Service Rendered by Dr. Scott

____ CPT # ______

____ ICD-9-CM # ______

____ ICD-10-CM # ______

Professional Service Rendered by Dr. Cutler

____ CPT # ______

____ ICD-9-CM # ______

____ ICD-10-CM # ______

11. Dr. Cutis removes a malignant tumor from a patient's back (1.5 cm) and does the local anesthesia herself.

Description

____ CPT # ______

____ ICD-9-CM # ______

____ ICD-10-CM # ______

12. Dr. Skeleton sees Mr. Richmond, a new patient worked into the office schedule on an emergency basis after a motor vehicle traffic accident with another car. Mr. Richmond has multiple lacerations of the face, arm, and chest and a fracture of the left tibia. The physician takes a comprehensive history and performs a comprehensive examination. Decision making is moderately complex. Dr. Skeleton orders bilateral radiographs of the tibia and fibula and two views of the chest and left wrist to be taken in his office. Then he closes the following lacerations: 2.6 cm, simple, face; 2.0 cm, intermediate, face; 7.5 cm, intermediate, right arm; 4.5 cm, intermediate, chest. All radiographs are negative except that of the left tibia. Dr. Skeleton performs a manipulative reduction of the left tibial shaft and applies a cast. Code this case as if you were actually listing the codes on the CMS-1500 (02-12) claim form.

Description

Description	Code
______________________________	CPT # ______ and ______
______________________________	CPT # ______
______________________________	CPT # ______
______________________________	CPT # ______
______________________________	CPT # ______
______________________________	CPT # ______
______________________________	CPT # ______
______________________________	CPT # ______
______________________________	CPT # ______
______________________________	CPT # ______
______________________________	ICD-9-CM # ______
______________________________	ICD-10-CM # ______
______________________________	ICD-9-CM # ______
______________________________	ICD-10-CM # ______
______________________________	ICD-9-CM # ______
______________________________	ICD-10-CM # ______
______________________________	ICD-9-CM # ______
______________________________	ICD-10-CM # ______
______________________________	ICD-9-CM # ______
______________________________	ICD-10-CM # ______

Six weeks later, Dr. Skeleton sees the same patient for an office visit and obtains radiographs (two views) of the left tibia and fibula. Treatment involves application of a cast below the patient's left knee to the toes, including a walking heel.

Description

_______________ CPT # _______

_______________ CPT # _______

_______________ CPT # _______

_______________ ICD-9-CM # _______

_______________ ICD-10-CM # _______

13. Dr. Cutler performs an incisional biopsy of a patient's breast for a breast lump, which requires 40 minutes of anesthesia. Dr. Scott is the anesthesiologist. The patient is otherwise normal and healthy. List the procedure and diagnostic code numbers for each physician.

Professional Service Rendered by Dr. Cutler

_______________ CPT # _______

_______________ ICD-9-CM # _______

_______________ ICD-10-CM # _______

Professional Service Rendered by Dr. Scott

_______________ CPT # _______

_______________ ICD-9-CM # _______

_______________ ICD-10-CM # _______

14. Mrs. DeBeau is aware that Dr. Input will be out of town for 6 weeks; however, she decides to have him perform the recommended combined anterior-posterior colporrhaphy with enterocele repair for vaginal enterocele. Dr. Practon agrees to perform the follow-up care and assist. Dr. Scott is the anesthesiologist. The anesthesia time is 2 hours, 15 minutes. The patient is normal and healthy. List the procedure and diagnostic code numbers for each physician. Note: Emphasis for this problem should be placed on the choice of CPT modifiers.

Professional Service Rendered by Dr. Input

_______________ CPT # _______

_______________ ICD-9-CM # _______

_______________ ICD-10-CM # _______

Professional Service Rendered by Dr. Practon

_______________ CPT # _______

_______________ CPT modifier _______

_______________ CPT modifier _______

_______________ ICD-9-CM # _______

_______________ ICD-10-CM # _______

Professional Service Rendered by Dr. Scott

____ CPT # _______

____ ICD-9-CM # _______

____ ICD-10-CM # _______

15. Mr. Wong, a new patient, is seen in the College Hospital and undergoes a comprehensive history and physical examination (H & P) with moderately complex decision making. Dr. Coccidioides performs a bronchoscopy with biopsy. Results of the biopsy confirm the diagnosis: malignant neoplasm of upper left lobe of lung. The following day the physician performs a total pneumonectomy. Dr. Cutler assists on the total pneumonectomy (pulmonary resection), and Dr. Scott is the anesthesiologist. Surgery takes 3 hours, 45 minutes. The patient has mild systemic disease. List the procedure and diagnostic code numbers for each physician.

Professional Service Rendered by Dr. Coccidioides

____ CPT # _______

____ CPT # _______

____ CPT # _______

____ ICD-9-CM # _______

____ ICD-10-CM # _______

Professional Service Rendered by Dr. Cutler

____ CPT # _______

____ ICD-9-CM # _______

____ ICD-10-CM # _______

Professional Service Rendered by Dr. Scott

____ CPT # _______

____ ICD-9-CM # _______

____ ICD-10-CM # _______

When completing the CMS-1500 (02-12) claim form for Dr. Scott, in which block would you list anesthesia minutes? ____________________________

TEST 3: PROCEDURE (RADIOLOGY AND PATHOLOGY SECTIONS) AND DIAGNOSTIC CODE TEST

Directions: Using a CPT code book or Appendix A in this *Workbook*, insert the correct procedure code numbers and modifiers and diagnostic codes for each service rendered. Give a brief description for each professional service rendered, although this is not needed for completing the CMS-1500 (02-12) claim form.

1. Mrs. Cahn sees Dr. Skeleton because of severe pain in her right shoulder. She is a new patient. Dr. Skeleton takes a detailed history and performs a detailed examination. A complete x-ray study of the right shoulder is done. Decision making is of low complexity. A diagnosis of bursitis is made, and an injection into the bursa is administered.

Description

____ CPT # ________

____ CPT # ________

____ CPT # ________

____ ICD-9-CM # ________

____ ICD-10-CM # ________

2. John Murphy comes into the Broxton Radiologic Group, Inc., for an extended radiation therapy consultation for prostatic cancer. The radiologist takes a detailed history and does a detailed examination. Decision making is of low complexity. The physician determines a simple treatment plan involving simple simulation-aided field settings. Basic dosimetry calculations are done, and the patient returns the following day and receives radiation therapy to a single treatment area (6 to 10 MeV).

Description

____ CPT # ________

____ CPT # ________

____ CPT # ________

____ CPT # ________

____ CPT # ________

Diagnosis:

____ ICD-9-CM # ________

____ ICD-10-CM # ________

3. Dr. Input refers Mrs. Horner to the Nuclear Medicine department of the Broxton Radiologic Group, Inc., for a bone marrow imaging of the whole body and imaging of the liver and spleen. List the procedure code numbers after each radiologic procedure to show how the radiology group would bill. Also, list the diagnosis of malignant neoplasm of the bone marrow.

Description

Total body bone marrow, imaging CPT # ________

Radiopharmaceuticals, diagnostic (Iodine I-123) HCPCS # ________

Liver and spleen imaging CPT # ________

Radiopharmaceuticals, diagnostic (Iodine I-123) HCPCS # ________

Diagnosis:

____ ICD-9-CM # ________

____ ICD-10-CM # ________

4. Dr. Input also refers Mrs. Horner to XYZ Laboratory for the following tests. List the procedure code numbers to indicate how the laboratory would bill.

Description

CBC, automated and automated differential CPT # ________

Urinalysis, automated with microscopy CPT # ________

Urine culture (quantitative, colony count) CPT # ________

Urine antibiotic sensitivity (microtiter) CPT # ________

5. The general laboratory at College Hospital receives a surgical tissue specimen (ovarian biopsy) for gross and microscopic examination from a patient with Stein-Leventhal syndrome. List the procedure and diagnostic code numbers to indicate what the hospital pathology department would bill.

Description

____ CPT # ________

Diagnosis:

____ ICD-9-CM # ________

____ ICD-10-CM # ________

6. Dr. Langerhans refers Jerry Cramer to XYZ Laboratory for a lipid panel. He has a family history of cardiovascular disease. List the procedure and diagnostic code number or numbers to indicate how the laboratory would bill.

Description

____ CPT # ________

Diagnosis:

____ ICD-9-CM # ________

____ ICD-10-CM # ________

7. Dr. Caesar is an OB/GYN specialist who has her own ultrasound machine. Carmen Cardoza, age 45, is referred to Dr. Caesar for an obstetric consultation and an amniocentesis with ultrasonic guidance. The diagnosis is Rh incompatibility. The doctor performs a detailed history and physical examination, and decision making is of low complexity.

Description

____ CPT # _______

____ CPT # _______

Diagnosis:

____ ICD-9-CM # _______

____ ICD-10-CM # _______

8. Mr. Marcos's medical record indicates that a retrograde pyelogram followed by a percutaneous nephrostolithotomy, with basket extraction of a 1-cm stone, was performed by Dr. Ulibarri for nephrolithiasis.

Description

____ CPT # _______

____ CPT # _______

Diagnosis:

____ ICD-9-CM # _______

____ ICD-10-CM # _______

9. Broxton Radiologic Group, Inc., performs the following procedures on Mrs. Stephens at the request of Dr. Input. List the procedure code numbers after each radiologic procedure. On the laboratory slip, the following congenital diagnoses are listed: Diverticulum of the stomach and colon; cystic lung. Locate the corresponding diagnostic codes.

Barium enema CPT # _______

Evaluation of upper gastrointestinal tract with small bowel CPT # _______

Complete chest x-ray CPT # _______

Diagnosis:

____ ICD # _______

Diagnosis:

____ ICD # _______

Diagnosis:

____ ICD # _______

10. Two weeks later, Mrs. Stephens is referred again for further radiologic studies for flank pain. List the procedure and diagnostic code numbers after each radiologic procedure.

Intravenous pyelogram (IVP) with drip infusion CPT # _______

Oral cholecystography CPT # _______

Diagnosis:

____ ICD # _______

TEST 4: COMPLETE A CMS-1500 (02-12) CLAIM FORM

Performance Objective

Task: Complete a CMS-1500 (02-12) claim form for a private case and post transactions to the patient's financial accounting record.

Conditions: Use the patient's record (Figure 1) and financial statement (Figure 2); one health insurance claim form; a computer or pen; procedural and diagnostic code books; and Appendixes A and B in this *Workbook.*

Standards: Claim Productivity Management

Time: ______________ minutes

Accuracy: ______________

(Note: The time element and accuracy criteria may be given by your instructor.)

Directions

1. Using NUCC guidelines, complete a CMS-1500 (02-12) claim form and direct it to the private carrier. Refer to Jennifer T. Lacey's patient record for information and Appendix A in this *Workbook* to locate the fees to record on the claim, and post them to the financial statement. Date the claim August 15. Dr. Caesar is accepting assignment, and the patient's signatures to release information to the insurance company and to have the payment forwarded directly to the physician are on file.
2. Use your CPT code book or Appendix A in this *Workbook* to determine the correct five-digit code numbers and modifiers for each professional service rendered. Use your HCPCS Level II code book or refer to Appendix B in this *Workbook* for HCPCS procedure codes and modifiers. Use your diagnostic code book to code each active diagnosis. If your instructor tells you to also find the ICD-10-CM codes, a draft version may be downloaded from the following website: http://www.cdc.gov/nchs/icd/icd10cm.htm.
3. Record the proper information on the financial record and claim form, and note the date when you have billed the insurance company.
4. American Commercial Insurance Company sent a check (voucher number 5586) on November 17 in the amount of $880. The patient's responsibility is $220. Post the payment, write off (adjust) the remaining balance, and circle the amount billed to the patient.

PATIENT RECORD NO. T-4

Lacey	Jennifer	T	11-12-55	F	555-549-0098
LAST NAME	FIRST NAME	MIDDLE NAME	BIRTH DATE	SEX	HOME PHONE

451 Roberts Street	Woodland Hills	XY	12345
ADDRESS	CITY	STATE	ZIP CODE

555-443-9899	555-549-0098		lacey@wb.net
CELL PHONE	PAGER NO.	FAX NO.	E-MAIL ADDRESS

430-XX-7709	Y0053498
PATIENT'S SOC. SEC. NO.	DRIVER'S LICENSE

legal secretary	Higgins and Higgins Attorneys at Law
PATIENT'S OCCUPATION	NAME OF COMPANY

430 Second Avenue, Woodland Hills, XY 12345	555-540-6675
ADDRESS OF EMPLOYER	PHONE

SPOUSE OR PARENT	OCCUPATION

EMPLOYER	ADDRESS	PHONE

American Commercial Insurance Company, 5682 Bendix Blvd., Woodland Hills, XY 12345	
NAME OF INSURANCE	INSURED OR SUBSCRIBER

5789022	444
POLICY/CERTIFICATE NO.	GROUP NO.

REFERRED BY: Clarence Cutler, MD

Figure 1

DATE	PROGRESS NOTES No. T-4
8-1-xx	New pt referred by Dr. Cutler, came into office for consultation and additional opinion.
	CC: Full feeling in stomach and low abdominal region.
	Irregular menstruation. Ultrasonic report showed
	leiomyomata uteri and rt ovarian mass; however, visualization of mass poor and type
	cannot be identified. Pap smear Class I. No personal or family hx of CA.
	Comprehensive hx and physical examination performed on healthy appearing white female.
	Wt: 136 lbs. BP 128/60. T 98.6 F. Palpated rt adnexal mass and
	enlarged uterus; vulva and cervix appear normal; LMP 7/16/XX.
	Medical decision making: mod complex
	Tx plan: Adv hospital admit and additional tests to R/O carcinoma.
	Tentatively scheduled abdominal hysterectomy with bilateral salpingo-oophorectomy.
	(M/MDM).
	BC/llf Bertha Caesar, MD
8-2-xx	Adm to College Hosp (C HX/PX M/MDM). Scheduled
	surgery at 7:00 A.M. tomorrow.
	BC/llf Bertha Caesar, MD
8-3-xx	Perf abdominal
	hysterectomy with bilateral salpingo-oophorectomy.
	BC/llf Bertha Caesar, MD
8-4-xx	HV (EPF HX/PX M/MDM) Path report revealed interstitial leiomyomata uteri and corpus
	luteum cyst of rt ovary. Pt C/O PO pain, otherwise doing well.
	BC/llf Bertha Caesar, MD
8-5-xx	HV (EPF HX/PX M/MDM). Pt ambulating well, pain decreased. Dressing changed, wound
	healing well.
	BC/llf Bertha Caesar, MD
8-6-xx	HV (PF HX/PX SF/MDM). Pain minimal. Pt ambulating without assistance.
	Removed staples, no redness or swelling. Pln DC tomorrow.
	BC/llf Bertha Caesar, MD
8-7-xx	Discharge to home; pt doing well. RTO next wk. Disability from 8-1 to 8-23-xx.
	BC/llf Bertha Caesar, MD

Figure 1, cont'd

Acct. No. T-4

STATEMENT

COLLEGE CLINIC
4567 Broad Avenue
Woodland Hills, XY 12345-0001
Tel. 555-486-9002
Fax No. 555-487-8976

Jennifer T. Lacey
451 Roberts Street
Woodland Hills, XY 12345

Phone No. (H) (555) 549-0098 (W) (555) 540-6675 Birthdate 11-12-55

Insurance Co. American Commercial Insurance Company Policy/Group No. 5789022 / 444

DATE	REFERENCE	DESCRIPTION	CHARGES	CREDITS PYMNTS.	CREDITS ADJ.	BALANCE
20XX		BALANCE FORWARD →				
8-1-xx		Consult				
8-2-xx		Admit				
8-3-xx		TAH BSO				
8-4-xx		HV				
8-5-xx		HV				
8-6-xx		HV				
8-7-xx		Discharge				

PLEASE PAY LAST AMOUNT IN BALANCE COLUMN

THIS IS A COPY OF YOUR FINANCIAL ACCOUNT AS IT APPEARS ON OUR RECORDS

Figure 2

TEST 5: COMPLETE A CMS-1500 (02-12) CLAIM FORM

Performance Objective

Task: Complete a CMS-1500 (02-12) claim form for a private case and post transactions to the patient's financial accounting record.

Conditions: Use the patient's record (Figure 3) and financial statement (Figure 4); one health insurance claim form; a computer or pen; procedural and diagnostic code books; and Appendixes A and B in this *Workbook*.

Standards: Claim Productivity Management

Time: ______________ minutes

Accuracy: ______________

(Note: The time element and accuracy criteria may be given by your instructor.)

Directions

1. Using NUCC guidelines, complete a CMS-1500 (02-12) claim form and direct it to the private carrier. Refer to Hortense N. Hope's patient record for information and Appendix A in this *Workbook* to locate the fees to record on the claim, and post them to the financial statement. Date the claim July 31. Dr. Practon is accepting assignment, and the patient's signatures to release information to the insurance company and to have the payment forwarded directly to the physician are on file.

2. Use your CPT code book or Appendix A in this *Workbook* to determine the correct five-digit code numbers and modifiers for each professional service rendered. Use your HCPCS Level II code book or refer to Appendix B in this *Workbook* for HCPCS procedure codes and modifiers. Use your diagnostic code book to code each active diagnosis. If your instructor tells you to also find the ICD-10-CM codes, a draft version may be downloaded from the following website: http://www.cdc.gov/nchs/icd/icd10cm.htm.

3. Record the proper information on the financial record and claim form, and note the date you have billed the insurance company.

PATIENT RECORD NO. T-5

LAST NAME	FIRST NAME	MIDDLE NAME	BIRTH DATE	SEX	HOME PHONE
Hope	Hortense	N	04-12-56	F	555-666-7821

ADDRESS	CITY	STATE	ZIP CODE
247 Lantern Pike	Woodland Hills	XY	12345

CELL PHONE	PAGER NO.	FAX NO.	E-MAIL ADDRESS
	555-323-1687	555-666-7821	hope@wb.net

PATIENT'S SOC. SEC. NO.	DRIVER'S LICENSE
321-XX-8809	N0058921

PATIENT'S OCCUPATION	NAME OF COMPANY
Clerk typist	R and S Manufacturing Company

ADDRESS OF EMPLOYER	PHONE
2271 West 74 Street, Torres, XY 12349	555-466-5890

SPOUSE OR PARENT	OCCUPATION
Harry J. Hope	carpenter

EMPLOYER	ADDRESS	PHONE
Jesse Construction Company	3861 South Orange Street, Torres, XY 12349	555-765-2318

NAME OF INSURANCE	INSURED OR SUBSCRIBER
Ralston Insurance Company, 2611 Hanley Street, Woodland Hills, XY 12345	Hortense N. Hope

POLICY/CERTIFICATE NO.	GROUP NO.
ATC321458809	T8471811A

REFERRED BY: Harry J. Hope (husband)

DATE	PROGRESS NOTES
7-1-xx	New F pt comes in complaining of lt great toe pain. Incised, drained, and cleaned area
	around nail on lt great toe. Dx: onychia and paronychia. Started on antibiotic and adv to
	retn in 2 days for permanent excision of nail plate (EPF HX/PX SF/MDM).
	GP/llf Gerald Practon, MD
7-3-xx	Pt returns for nail excision. Injected procaine in lt great toe; removed entire toenail.
	Drs applied. PTR in 5 days for PO check.
	GP/llf Gerald Practon, MD
7-7-xx	PO check. Dressing changed, nail bed healing well. Pt to continue on AB until gone.
	Retn PRN (PF HX/PX SF/MDM).
	GP/llf Gerald Practon, MD

Figure 3

Acct No. T-5

STATEMENT
Financial Account

COLLEGE CLINIC
4567 Broad Avenue
Woodland Hills, XY 12345-0001
Tel. 555-486-9002
Fax No. 555-487-8976

Hortense N. Hope
247 Lantern Pike
Woodland Hills, XY 12345

Phone No. (H) 555-666-7821 (W) 555-466-5890 Birthdate 4/12/56

Primary Insurance Co. Ralston Insurance Company Policy/Group No. ATC321458809 / T8471811A

Secondary Insurance Co. None Policy/Group No. ______

DATE	REFERENCE	DESCRIPTION	CHARGES	CREDITS PYMNTS.	CREDITS ADJ.	BALANCE
20xx		BALANCE FORWARD →				
7-1-xx		NP OV				
7-1-xx		I & D lt great toe				
7-3-xx		Excision lt great toenail				
7-7-xx		PO check				

PLEASE PAY LAST AMOUNT IN BALANCE COLUMN

THIS IS A COPY OF YOUR FINANCIAL ACCOUNT AS IT APPEARS ON OUR RECORDS

Figure 4

TEST 6: COMPLETE A CLAIM FORM FOR A MEDICARE CASE

Performance Objective

Task: Complete a CMS-1500 (02-12) claim form and post transactions to the patient's financial accounting record.

Conditions: Use the patient's record (Figure 5) and financial statement (Figure 6); one health insurance claim form; a computer or pen; procedural and diagnostic code books; and Appendixes A and B in this *Workbook*.

Standards: Claim Productivity Management

Time: ______________ minutes

Accuracy: ______________

(Note: The time element and accuracy criteria may be given by your instructor.)

Directions

1. Using NUCC guidelines, complete a CMS-1500 (02-12) claim form and direct it to the Medicare fiscal intermediary. To locate your local fiscal intermediary, go to the website http://www.cms.hhs.gov/contacts/incardir.asp. Refer to Frances F. Foote's patient record for information and Appendix A in this *Workbook* to locate the fees to record on the claim, and post them to the financial statement. Date the claim October 31. Dr. Practon is a participating provider, and the patient's signatures to release information to the insurance company and to have the payment forwarded directly to the physician are on file.

2. Use your CPT code book or Appendix A in this *Workbook* to determine the correct five-digit code numbers and modifiers for each professional service rendered. Use your HCPCS Level II code book or refer to Appendix B in this *Workbook* for HCPCS procedure codes and modifiers. Use your diagnostic code book to code each active diagnosis. If your instructor tells you to also find the ICD-10-CM codes, a draft version may be downloaded from the following website: http://www.cdc.gov/nchs/icd/icd10cm.htm.

3. Record the proper information on the patient's financial accounting record and claim form, and note the date when you have billed the insurance company.

PATIENT RECORD NO. T-6

LAST NAME	FIRST NAME	MIDDLE NAME	BIRTH DATE	SEX	HOME PHONE
Foote	Frances	F	08-10-32	F	555-678-0943

ADDRESS	CITY	STATE	ZIP CODE
984 North A Street	Woodland Hills	XY	12345

CELL PHONE	PAGER NO.	FAX NO.	E-MAIL ADDRESS
555-443-9908	555-320-7789	555-678-0943	foote@wb.net

PATIENT'S SOC. SEC. NO.	DRIVER'S LICENSE
578-XX-8924	B4309811

PATIENT'S OCCUPATION	NAME OF COMPANY
retired legal secretary	

ADDRESS OF EMPLOYER	PHONE

SPOUSE OR PARENT	OCCUPATION
Harry L. Foote	roofer

EMPLOYER	ADDRESS	PHONE
BDO Construction Company,	340 North 6th Street, Woodland Hills, XY 12345	555-478-9083

NAME OF INSURANCE	INSURED OR SUBSCRIBER
Medicare	self

POLICY/CERTIFICATE NO.	GROUP NO.
578-XX-8924A	

REFERRED BY: G. U. Curette, MD, 4780 Main Street, Ehrlich, XY 12350 Tel: 555-430-8788 NPI #34216600XX

DATE	PROGRESS NOTES
10-11-xx	NP pt referred by Dr. Curette with a CC of foot pain centering around rt great toe and
	sometimes shooting up her leg. PF history taken. PF exam revealed severe overgrowth
	of nail into surrounding tissues. AP and lat right foot x-rays taken & interpreted which
	indicate no fractures or arthritis. Pt has had a N workup for gout by Dr. Curette.
	DX: Severe onychocryptosis both margins of rt hallux. Adv to sched. OP surgery at
	College Hospital for wedge resection of skin of nail fold to repair ingrown nail.
	No disability from work (SF/MDM).
	NP/llf Nick Pedro, MD
10-13-xx	Pt admitted for OP surgery at College Hospital. Complete wedge resection performed for
	repair of rt hallux ingrown nail. Pt will stay off foot over the weekend and retn next wk for
	PO re ch.
	NP/llf Nick Pedro, MD
10-20-xx	PO visit (PF HX/PX SF/MDM). Rt hallux healing well. RTC as necessary.
	NP/llf Nick Pedro, MD

Figure 5

Acct No. T-6

STATEMENT
Financial Account
COLLEGE CLINIC
4567 Broad Avenue
Woodland Hills, XY 12345-0001
Tel. 555-486-9002
Fax No. 555-487-8976

Frances F. Foote
984 North A Street
Woodland Hills, XY 12345

Phone No. (H) 555-678-0943 (W) Birthdate 8/10/32

Primary Insurance Co. Medicare Policy/Group No. 578-XX-8924A

DATE	REFERENCE	DESCRIPTION	CHARGES	CREDITS PYMNTS.	CREDITS ADJ.	BALANCE
20xx		BALANCE FORWARD →				
10-11-xx		NP OV				
10-11-xx		X-rays				
10-13-xx		Wedge excision/skin of nail fold				
10-20-xx		PO				

PLEASE PAY LAST AMOUNT IN BALANCE COLUMN

THIS IS A COPY OF YOUR FINANCIAL ACCOUNT AS IT APPEARS ON OUR RECORDS

Figure 6

TEST 7: COMPLETE A CLAIM FORM FOR A MEDICARE/MEDIGAP CASE

Performance Objective

Task: Complete two CMS-1500 (02-12) claim forms for a Medicare/Medigap case and post transactions to the patient's financial accounting record.

Conditions: Use patient's record (Figure 7) and financial statement (Figure 8); two health insurance claim forms; a computer or pen; procedural and diagnostic code books; and Appendixes A and B in this *Workbook*.

Standards: Claim Productivity Management

Time: ______________ minutes

Accuracy: ______________

(Note: The time element and accuracy criteria may be given by your instructor.)

Directions

1. Using NUCC guidelines, complete two CMS-1500 (02-12) claim forms and direct them to the Medicare fiscal intermediary. To locate your local fiscal intermediary, go to the website http://www.cms.gov/About-CMS/Contracting-With-CMS/ContractingGeneralInformation/downloads/ICdirectory.pdf. Refer to Charles B. Kamb's patient record for information and Appendix A to locate the fees to record on the claim, and post them to the financial statement. Be sure to include the Medigap information on the claim form so that it will be crossed over (sent to the Medigap insurance carrier) automatically. Date the claim June 30. Dr. Practon is a participating provider with both Medicare and the Medigap program, and the patient's signatures to release information to the insurance companies and to have the payment forwarded directly to the physician are on file.

2. Use your CPT code book or Appendix A in this *Workbook* to determine the correct five-digit code numbers and modifiers for each professional service rendered. Use your HCPCS Level II code book or refer to Appendix B in this *Workbook* for HCPCS procedure codes and modifiers. Use your diagnostic code book to code each active diagnosis. If your instructor tells you to also find the ICD-10-CM codes, a draft version may be downloaded from the following website: http://www.cdc.gov/nchs/icd/icd10cm.htm.

3. Record the proper information on the patient's financial accounting record and claim form, and note the date when you have billed the insurance company.

PATIENT RECORD NO. T-7

LAST NAME	FIRST NAME	MIDDLE NAME	BIRTH DATE	SEX	HOME PHONE
Kamb	Charles	B	01-26-27	M	555-467-2601

ADDRESS	CITY	STATE	ZIP CODE
2600 West Nautilus Street	Woodland Hills	XY	12345

CELL PHONE	PAGER NO.	FAX NO.	E-MAIL ADDRESS

PATIENT'S SOC. SEC. NO.	DRIVER'S LICENSE
454-XX-9569	M3200563

PATIENT'S OCCUPATION	NAME OF COMPANY
Retired TV actor	Amer. Federation of TV & Radio Artists (AFTRA)

ADDRESS OF EMPLOYER	PHONE
30077 Ventura Boulevard, Woodland Hills, XY 12345	555-466-3331

SPOUSE OR PARENT	OCCUPATION
Jane C. Kamb	homemaker

EMPLOYER	ADDRESS	PHONE

NAME OF INSURANCE	INSURED OR SUBSCRIBER	
Medicare (Primary)	self	National Insurance Company (Medigap)

POLICY/CERTIFICATE NO.	GROUP NO.
454-XX-9569A	Medigap Policy No. 5789002

REFERRED BY: Mrs. O. S. Tomy (friend)

National PAYRID NAT234567

DATE	PROGRESS NOTES
6-1-xx	New pt comes into ofc to est new PCP in area; recently moved from Ohio. W obese M c/o
	nasal bleeding for two and a half months c̄ headaches and nasal congestion. Pt states he
	has had HBP for 1 yr. Taking med: Serpasil prescribed by dr in Ohio; does not know dosage.
	Took a C HX and performed a C PX which revealed post nasal hemorrhage. Coagulation
	time (Lee and White) and microhematocrit (spun) done in ofc are WNL. BP 180/100.
	Used nasal cautery and post nasal packs to control hemorrhage. Rx prophylactic antibiotic
	to guard against sinusitis NKA. Adv retn tomorrow, bring hypertensive medication.
	Pt signed authorization to request med records from dr in Ohio. D: Recurrent epistaxis
	due to nonspecific hypertension. No disability from work.
	GP/llf Gerald Practon, MD
6-2-xx	Pt retns and nasal hemorrhage is reevaluated (PF HX/PX SF/MDM). Postnasal packs
	removed and replaced. BP 182/98. Pt forgot medication for hypertension but states he is
	taking it 2 X d. Adv retn in 1 day, bring medication.
	GP/llf Gerald Practon, MD
6-3-xx	Pt retns and nasal hemorrhage is reevaluated (PF HX/PX SF/MDM). Postnasal packs
	removed. BP 178/100. Verified hypertensive medication. Pt to increase dosage to 4 X d.
	Adv retn in 5 days.
	GP/llf Gerald Practon, MD
6-8-xx	Pt retns and nasal hemorrhage is reevaluated (EPF HX/PX L/MDM). Prev medical records
	arrived and reviewed. BP 190/102. Pt referred to Dr. Perry Cardi (int) for future care of
	hypertension.
	GP/llf Gerald Practon, MD

Figure 7

Acct No. T-7

STATEMENT
Financial Account

COLLEGE CLINIC
4567 Broad Avenue
Woodland Hills, XY 12345-0001
Tel. 555-486-9002
Fax No. 555-487-8976

Charles B. Kamb
2600 West Nautilus Street
Woodland Hills, XY 12345

Phone No. (H) 555-467-2601 (W) None/retired Birthdate 1-26-27

Primary Insurance Co. Medicare Policy/Group No. 454-XX-9569A

Secondary Insurance Co. National Insurance Company (Medigap) Policy/Group No. 5789002

DATE	REFERENCE	DESCRIPTION	CHARGES	CREDITS PYMNTS.	CREDITS ADJ.	BALANCE
20xx		BALANCE FORWARD →				
6-1-xx		NP OV				
6-1-xx		Coagulation time				
6-1-xx		Microhematocrit				
6-1-xx		Post nasal pack/cautery				
6-2-xx		OV				
6-2-xx		Subsequent nasal pack				
6-3-xx		OV				
6-8-xx		OV				

PLEASE PAY LAST AMOUNT IN BALANCE COLUMN

THIS IS A COPY OF YOUR FINANCIAL ACCOUNT AS IT APPEARS ON OUR RECORDS

Figure 8

TEST 8: COMPLETE A CLAIM FORM FOR A MEDICAID CASE

Performance Objective

Task: Complete a CMS-1500 (02-12) claim form for a Medicaid case and post transactions to the patient's financial accounting record.

Conditions: Use the patient's record (Figure 9) and financial statement (Figure 10); one health insurance claim form; a computer or pen; procedural and diagnostic code books; and Appendixes A and B in this *Workbook*.

Standards: Claim Productivity Management

Time: ______________ minutes

Accuracy: ______________

(Note: The time element and accuracy criteria may be given by your instructor.)

Directions

1. Using NUCC guidelines, complete a CMS-1500 (02-12) claim form and direct it to the Medicaid fiscal intermediary. Obtain the address of your Medicaid fiscal agent by first going to the website http://www.cms.hhs.gov/medicaid/geninfo and then either sending an e-mail message to the Medicaid contact or using the toll-free number to obtain the Medicaid carrier name and address. An option might be to contact your local state medical society. Refer to Louise K. Herman's patient record for information and Appendix A to locate the fees to record on the claim, and post them to the financial statement. Date the claim May 31.

2. Use your CPT code book or Appendix A in this *Workbook* to determine the correct five-digit code numbers and modifiers for each professional service rendered. Use your HCPCS Level II code book or refer to Appendix B in this *Workbook* for HCPCS procedure codes and modifiers. Use your diagnostic code book to code each active diagnosis. If your instructor tells you to also find the ICD-10-CM codes, a draft version may be downloaded from the following website: http://www.cdc.gov/nchs/icd/icd10cm.htm.

3. Record the proper information on the patient's financial accounting record and claim form and note the date when you have billed the insurance company.

4. Post the payment of $350 (voucher number 4300), received from the Medicaid fiscal intermediary 40 days after claim submission, and write off (adjust) the balance of the account.

PATIENT RECORD NO. T-8

LAST NAME	FIRST NAME	MIDDLE NAME	BIRTH DATE	SEX	HOME PHONE
Herman	Louise	K	11-04-60	F	555-266-9085

ADDRESS	CITY	STATE	ZIP CODE
13453 Burbank Boulevard	Woodland Hills	XY	12345

CELL PHONE	PAGER NO.	FAX NO.	E-MAIL ADDRESS
555-466-7003		555-266-9085	herman@wb.net

PATIENT'S SOC. SEC. NO.	DRIVER'S LICENSE
519-XX-0018	T0943995

PATIENT'S OCCUPATION	NAME OF COMPANY
unemployed budget analyst	

ADDRESS OF EMPLOYER	PHONE

SPOUSE OR PARENT	OCCUPATION
Harold D. Herman	retired salesman

EMPLOYER	ADDRESS	PHONE

NAME OF INSURANCE	INSURED OR SUBSCRIBER
Medicaid	self

MEDICAID NO.	GROUP NO.
0051936001X	

REFERRED BY: Raymond Skeleton, MD

DATE	PROGRESS NOTES
5-6-xx	NP pt referred by Dr. Skeleton. CC: Rectal bleeding. Took a comprehensive history and
	performed a comprehensive physical examination. Diagnostic anoscopy revealed
	bleeding int and ext hemorrhoids and 2 infected rectal polyps. Rx antibiotics. Retn in
	2 days for removal of hemorrhoids and polyps (M/MDM)
	RR/llf Rex Rumsey, MD
5-8-xx	Pt returned to office for simple internal/external hemorrhoidectomy. Rigid
	proctosigmoidoscopy also perf for removal of polyps using snare technique. Adv. sitz
	baths daily. Continue on AB until gone. Retn in 1 wk.
	RR/llf Rex Rumsey, MD
5-15-xx	DNS Telephoned pt and rescheduled.
	Mary Bright, CMA
5-17-xx	PO OV (EPF HX/PX LC/MDM). Pt progressing well. No pain, discomfort or bleeding.
	Discharged from care, retn PRN.
	RR/llf Rex Rumsey, MD

Figure 9

Acct No. T-8

STATEMENT
Financial Account
COLLEGE CLINIC
4567 Broad Avenue
Woodland Hills, XY 12345-0001
Tel. 555-486-9002
Fax No. 555-487-8976

Louise K. Herman
13453 Burbank Boulevard
Woodland Hills, XY 12345

Phone No. (H) 555-266-9085 (W) ______ Birthdate 11/4/60

Primary Insurance Co. Medicaid Policy/Group No. 0051936001X

Secondary Insurance Co. ______ Policy/Group No. ______

DATE	REFERENCE	DESCRIPTION	CHARGES	CREDITS PYMNTS.	CREDITS ADJ.	BALANCE
20xx		BALANCE FORWARD →				
5-6-xx		NP OV				
5-6-xx		Dx anoscopy				
5-8-xx		Int/Ext Hemorrhoidectomy				
5-8-xx		Proctosigmoidoscopy with removal of polyps				
5-17-xx		PO OV				

PLEASE PAY LAST AMOUNT IN BALANCE COLUMN

THIS IS A COPY OF YOUR FINANCIAL ACCOUNT AS IT APPEARS ON OUR RECORDS

Figure 10

TEST 9: COMPLETE A CLAIM FORM FOR A TRICARE CASE

Performance Objective

Task: Complete a CMS-1500 (02-12) claim form for a TRICARE case and post transactions to the patient's financial accounting record.

Conditions: Use the patient's record (Figure 11) and financial statement (Figure 12); one health insurance claim form; a computer or pen; procedural and diagnostic code books; and Appendixes A and B in this *Workbook*.

Standards: Claim Productivity Management

Time: ______________ minutes

Accuracy: ______________

(Note: The time element and accuracy criteria may be given by your instructor.)

Directions

1. Using NUCC guidelines, complete a CMS-1500 (02-12) claim form and direct it to the TRICARE carrier. To locate your local fiscal intermediary, go to the website http://www.tricare.osd.mil. Click on the area of the map you are residing in and then choose a state to access claims information for that state. Refer to Darlene M. Cash's patient record for information and Appendix A to locate the fees to record on the claim, and post them to the financial statement. Date the claim February 27. Dr. Cutler is accepting assignment, and the patient's signatures to release information to the insurance company and to have the payment forwarded directly to the physician are on file.

2. Use your CPT code book or Appendix A in this *Workbook* to determine the correct five-digit code numbers and fees for each professional service rendered. Use your HCPCS Level II code book or refer to Appendix B in this *Workbook* for HCPCS procedure codes and modifiers. Use your diagnostic code book to code each active diagnosis. If your instructor tells you to also find the ICD-10-CM codes, a draft version may be downloaded from the following website: http://www.cdc.gov/nchs/icd/icd10cm.htm.

3. Record the proper information on the patient's financial accounting record and claim form, and note the date when you have billed the insurance company.

PATIENT RECORD NO. T-9

Cash	Darlene	M	3-15-70	F	555-666-8901
LAST NAME	FIRST NAME	MIDDLE NAME	BIRTH DATE	SEX	HOME PHONE

5729 Redwood Avenue	Woodland Hills	XY	12344
ADDRESS	CITY	STATE	ZIP CODE

555-290-5400		555-666-8901	cash@wb.net
CELL PHONE	PAGER NO.	FAX NO.	E-MAIL ADDRESS

298-XX-6754	J3457789
PATIENT'S SOC. SEC. NO.	DRIVER'S LICENSE

Teacher	City Unified School District
PATIENT'S OCCUPATION	NAME OF COMPANY

Century High School, 2031 West Olympic Boulevard, Dorland, XY 12345	555-678-1076
ADDRESS OF EMPLOYER	PHONE

David F. Cash	Navy Petty Officer—Grade 8 (active status)
SPOUSE OR PARENT	OCCUPATION

United States Navy	HHC, 2nd Batt, 26th Infantry, APO New York, NY, 10030	
EMPLOYER	ADDRESS	PHONE

TRICARE Standard	David Cash (DOB 4-22-70)
NAME OF INSURANCE	INSURED OR SUBSCRIBER

767-XX-9080	
POLICY/CERTIFICATE NO.	GROUP NO.

REFERRED BY: Hugh R. Foot, MD, 2010 Main St., Woodland Hills, XY 12345 NPI #61 25099XX

DATE	PROGRESS NOTES
1-4-xx	New pt, referred by Dr. Foot comes in complaining of head pain which began yesterday.
	Performed an EPF history and physical exam. Lt parietal area of skull slightly tender,
	some redness of scalp. Pain localized and not consistent with HA syndromes. Rest of
	exam N. Imp: head pain, undetermined nature, possible cyst. Apply hot compresses and
	observe. Take Ibuprofen for pain prn (200 mg up to 2 q. 4 h). Retn in 1 wk, no disability
	from work (SF/MDM).
	CC/llf Clarence Cutler, MD
1-11-xx	Pt retns and states that the hot compresses have helped but is concerned with some
	swelling in area. On exam noticed slt elevation of skin in lt parietal area of scalp, no
	warmth over area. Slt pain on palpation. Exam otherwise neg. Imp: Subcutaneous nodule.
	Continue with same tx plan: Hot compresses daily and Ibuprofen prn. Retn in 2 to 3 wks
	if not resolved (PF HX/PX SF/MDM).
	CC/llf Clarence Cutler, MD
2-3-xx	Pt retns for reexamination of parietal skull. Elevation of skin still persisting. It has now
	come to a head, is warm to the touch, and consistent with an inflammatory cystic lesion.
	A decision is made to excise the benign lesion. Scalp cyst, 1.5 cm removed under
	procaine block with knife dissection; closed wound with six #000 black silk sutures.
	Adv to retn 1 wk for removal of sutures (EPF HX/PX LC/MDM).
	CC/llf Clarence Cutler, MD
2-10-xx	Pt presents for suture removal. Sutures removed and slight oozing occurs in midsection
	of wound. Wound dressed and pt advised to apply antibacterial cream daily. Retn in 4 to
	5 days for final check (PF HX/PX SF/MDM).
	CC/llf Clarence Cutler, MD
2-15-xx	Pt presents for PO check of head wound. Parietal area healed well. RTO prn
	(PF HX/PX SF/MDM).
	CC/llf Clarence Cutler, MD

Figure 11

Acct No. T-9

STATEMENT
Financial Account

COLLEGE CLINIC
4567 Broad Avenue
Woodland Hills, XY 12345-0001
Tel. 555-486-9002
Fax No. 555-487-8976

Darlene M. Cash
5729 Redwood Avenue
Woodland Hills, XY 12345

Phone No. (H) 555-666-8901 (W) 555-678-1076 Birthdate 3/15/70

Primary Insurance Co. TRICARE Standard Policy/Group No. 767-XX-9080

Secondary Insurance Co. ______ Policy/Group No. ______

DATE	REFERENCE	DESCRIPTION	CHARGES	CREDITS PYMNTS.	CREDITS ADJ.	BALANCE
20xx		**BALANCE FORWARD** →				
1-4-xx		NP OV				
1-11-xx		OV				
2-3-xx		OV				
2-3-xx		Excision inflammatory cystic scalp lesion				
2-10-xx		OV				
2-15-xx		OV				

PLEASE PAY LAST AMOUNT IN BALANCE COLUMN

THIS IS A COPY OF YOUR FINANCIAL ACCOUNT AS IT APPEARS ON OUR RECORDS

Figure 12

TEST 10: COMPLETE TWO CLAIM FORMS FOR A PRIVATE PLAN

Performance Objective

Task: Complete two CMS-1500 (02-12) claim forms for a private case and post transactions to the patient's financial accounting record.

Conditions: Use the patient's record (Figure 13) and financial statement (Figure 14); two health insurance claim forms; a computer or pen; procedural and diagnostic code books; and Appendixes A and B in this *Workbook*.

Standards: Claim Productivity Management

Time: ______________ minutes

Accuracy: ______________

(Note: The time element and accuracy criteria may be given by your instructor.)

Directions

1. Using NUCC guidelines, complete two CMS-1500 (02-12) claim forms and direct them to the private carrier. Refer to Gertrude C. Hamilton's patient record for information and Appendix A in this *Workbook* to locate the fees to record on the claim, and post them to the financial statement. Date the first claim August 15 and the second one October 15. Dr. Cardi is accepting assignment, and the patient's signatures to release information to the insurance company and to have the payment forwarded directly to the physician are on file.

2. Use your CPT code book or Appendix A in this *Workbook* to determine the correct five-digit code numbers and modifiers for each professional service rendered. Use your HCPCS Level II code book or refer to Appendix B in this *Workbook* for HCPCS procedure codes and modifiers. Use your diagnostic code books to code each active diagnosis. Frequently, surgeons wait to receive the pathology report before entering a final diagnosis on the claim form. In this case, the claim was submitted before the pathology report was received. If your instructor tells you to also find the ICD-10-CM codes, a draft version may be downloaded from the following website: http://www.cdc.gov/nchs/icd/icd10cm.htm.

3. Record the proper information on the financial record and claim form, and note the date when you have billed the insurance company.

4. Mrs. Hamilton makes a payment of $200, check number 5362, on her account on October 26. Post the proper entry for this transaction.

PATIENT RECORD NO. T-10

Hamilton	Gertrude	C	03-06-57	F	555-798-3321
LAST NAME	FIRST NAME	MIDDLE NAME	BIRTH DATE	SEX	HOME PHONE
5320 Phillips Street	Woodland Hills	XY	12345		
ADDRESS	CITY	STATE	ZIP CODE		
555-399-4990	555-312-6677	555-798-3321			hamilton@wb.net
CELL PHONE	PAGER NO.	FAX NO.			E-MAIL ADDRESS
540-XX-7677	D9043557				
PATIENT'S SOC. SEC. NO.	DRIVER'S LICENSE				
retired secretary					
PATIENT'S OCCUPATION	NAME OF COMPANY				
ADDRESS OF EMPLOYER	PHONE				
deceased					
SPOUSE OR PARENT	OCCUPATION				
EMPLOYER	ADDRESS				PHONE
Colonial Health Insurance, 1011 Main Street, Woodland Hills, XY 12345			self		
NAME OF INSURANCE			INSURED OR SUBSCRIBER		
540XX7677	4566 (through previous employment)				
POLICY/CERTIFICATE NO.	GROUP NO.				

REFERRED BY: Gerald Practon, MD, 4567 Broad Avenue, Woodland Hills, XY 12345

Figure 13

DATE	PROGRESS NOTES No. T-10
7-29-xx	Dr. Practon asked me to consult on this 57-year-old pt adm to College Hosp today.
	Duplex carotid ultrasonography indicates bilateral carotid stenosis. C/HX: Suffered CVA lt
	hemisphere 1 yr prior to adm. Marked rt arm & leg weakness c̄ weakness of rt face and
	slurring of speech. C/PE revealed lt carotid bruit, II/IV, & right carotid bruit, II/IV.
	Performed hand-held Doppler vascular study on bilateral carotids which indicated
	decreased blood flow. Adv brain scan and lt carotid thromboendarterectomy; rt carotid
	thromboendarterectomy at a later date H/MDM.
	PC/llf Perry Cardi, MD
7-30-xx	HV (EPF HX/PX MC/MDM). Dr. Practon asked me to take over pt's care. Pt had brain scan
	done today, ECG, and lab work.
	PC/llf Perry Cardi, MD
7-31-xx	HV (EPF HX/PX MC/MDM). Brain scan indicates prior CVA; no new findings. ECG, normal
	sinus rhythm with occasional premature ventricular contractions. Lab work WNL.
	Discussed test results with Mrs. Hamilton.
	PC/llf Perry Cardi, MD
8-1-xx	HV (PF HX/PX LC/MDM). Decision made for surgery, to be scheduled tomorrow.
	PC/llf Perry Cardi, MD
8-2-xx	Pt taken to the operative suite. Performed lt carotid thromboendarterectomy by neck
	incision (see op report). Surgery went as planned, pt in recovery.
	PC/llf Perry Cardi, MD
8-3-xx	HV (PF HX/PX SF/MDM). Operative site appears normal. Pt resting comfortably.
	PC/llf Perry Cardi, MD
8-4-xx	DC from hosp. Pt to be seen in ofc in 1 week.
	PC/llf Perry Cardi, MD
8-12-xx	PO OV (D HX/PX M/MDM). Discussed outcome of surgery. Pt making satisfactory
	progress. Adv rt carotid thromboendarterectomy. Pt would like it done as soon as possible;
	next month if there is an operative time. Scheduled surgery for September 16, 20XX at
	College Hospital.
	PC/llf Perry Cardi, MD
9-16-xx	Adm to College Hospital. Performed a D history, D physical examination, and SF medical
	decision making. Rt. carotid thromboendarterectomy performed by neck incision.
	DX: Rt carotid stenosis.
	PC/llf Perry Cardi, MD
9-17-xx	HV (PF HX/PX SF/MDM). Pt stable and doing well. Operative site looks good. Plan for
	discharge tomorrow.
	PC/llf Perry Cardi, MD
9-18-xx	DC from hosp to home. RTC 1 wk.
	PC/llf Perry Cardi, MD
9-25-xx	PO visit (PF HX/PX SF/MDM). Pt making satisfactory recovery. Her neighbor will monitor
	BP daily. Retn 1 month.
	PC/llf Perry Cardi, MD

Figure 13, cont'd

Acct. No . T-10

STATEMENT

COLLEGE CLINIC
4567 Broad Avenue
Woodland Hills, XY 12345-0001
Tel. 555-486-9002
Fax No. 555-487-8976

Gertrude C. Hamilton
5320 Phillips Street
Woodland Hills, XY 12345

Phone No. (H) (555) 798-3321 (W) ______ Birthdate 03-06-57

Insurance Co Colonial Health Insurance Policy/Group No. 540Xx7677 / 4566

	REFERENCE	DESCRIPTION	CHARGES	CREDITS PYMNTS.	CREDITS ADJ.	BALANCE
20xx				**BALANCE FORWARD** →		
7-29-xx		Inpatient consult				
7-30-xx		HV				
7-31-xx		HV				
8-1-xx		HV				
8-2-xx		L carotid thromboendarterectomy				
8-3-xx		HV				
8-4-xx		Discharge				
8-12-xx		PO OV				
9-16-xx		Admit				
9-16-xx		R carotid thromboendarterectomy				
9-17-xx		HV				
9-18-xx		Discharge				
9-25-xx		PO OV				

PLEASE PAY LAST AMOUNT IN BALANCE COLUMN

THIS IS A COPY OF YOUR FINANCIAL ACCOUNT AS IT APPEARS ON OUR RECORDS

Figure 14

A College Clinic Office Policies and Mock Fee Schedule

College Clinic

In this simulation, you are employed as an insurance billing specialist for a group of medical doctors, other allied health specialists, and podiatrists. Each clinic is configured in its own way. The College Clinic has staff physicians that are employed, receive monthly pay checks, and are given Wage and Tax Statements (Form W-2) at the end of the tax year. These doctors are on the staff of a nearby hospital, College Hospital.

Medical practices can have different configurations. For example, individuals or groups can be incorporated. Physicians can be independent contractors, running their own practices outside of the clinic; receive payment by the job and not a salary; and receive a Form 1099 at the end of the tax year.

Reference information to complete insurance claim forms for each assignment follows. Claim forms are to be submitted for the group unless a case involves a physician working as an independent contractor.

Office address:
College Clinic
4567 Broad Avenue
Woodland Hills, XY 12345-0001
Telephone: 555-486-9002
FAX: 555-487-8976
Clinic e-mail: cclinic@cmail.net
Staff e-mail: insert physician's last name followed by a period (.) then cclinic@cmail.net
(example: Pedro Atrics, MD, would have an e-mail address of atrics.cclinic@cmail.net)

Group practice, national provider identifier (NPI): 3664021CC

Medicare Durable Medical Equipment (DME) supplier number: 3400760001

Group tax ID #: XX12210XX

Hospital address:
College Hospital
4500 Broad Avenue
Woodland Hills, XY 12345-0001
Telephone: 555-487-6789
FAX: 555-486-8900

Hospital (NPI) national provider identifier: X950731067.

College Clinic Staff

Patient records in this *Workbook* include the doctors' names, specialties, subspecialties, and physicians' identification numbers of the College Clinic staff. They are shown in Table 1.

Table 1. College Clinic Staff

Name	Specialty (Abbreviation)	Social Security No.*	State License No.	EIN No. or Federal Tax Identification No.	Medicare CMS-Assigned National Provider Identifier (NPI)†
Concha Antrum, MD	Otolaryngologist (OTO) or Ear, Nose, and Throat Specialist (ENT)	082–XX–1707	C 01602X	74–10640XX	12458977XX
Pedro Atrics, MD	Pediatrician (PD)	134–XX–7600	D 06012X	71–32061XX	37640017XX
Bertha Caesar, MD	Obstetrician and Gynecologist (OBG)	230–XX–6700	A 01817X	72–57130XX	43056757XX
Perry Cardi, MD	Internist (I) Subspecialty: Cardiovascular Disease (CD)	557–XX–9980	C 02140X	70–64217XX	67805027XX
Brady Coccidioides, MD	Internist (I) Subspecialty: Pulmonary Disease (PUD)	670–XX–0874	C 04821X	75–67321XX	64211067XX
Vera Cutis, MD	Dermatologist (D)	409–XX–8620	C 06002X	71–80561XX	70568717XX
Clarence Cutler, MD	General Surgeon (GS)	410–XX–5630	B 07600X	71–57372XX	43050047XX
Max Glutens, RPT	Physical Therapist (PT)	507–XX–4300	87610X	79–36500XX	65132277XX
Cosmo Graff, MD	Plastic Surgeon (PS)	452–XX–9899	C 08104X	74–60789XX	50307117XX
Malvern Grumose, MD	Pathologist (Path)	470–XX–2301	A 01602X	72–73651XX	
Gaston Input, MD	Internist (I) Subspecialty: Gastroenterologist (GE)	211–XX–6734	C 08001X	75–67210XX	32783127XX
Adam Langerhans, MD	Endocrinologist	447–XX–6720	C 06051X	60–57831XX	47680657XX
Cornell Lenser, MD	Ophthalmologist (OPH)	322–XX–8963	C 06046X	61–78941XX	54037217XX
Michael Menter, MD	Psychiatrist (P)	210–XX–5302	C 07140X	73–66577XX	67301237XX
Astro Parkinson, MD	Neurosurgeon (NS)	210–XX–8533	C 02600X	75–44530XX	46789377XX
Nick Pedro, DPM	Podiatrist	233–XX–4300	E 08340X	62–74109XX	54022287XX
Gerald Practon, MD	General Practitioner (GP) or Family Practitioner (FP)	123–XX–6789	C 01402X	70–34597XX	46278897XX
Walter Radon, MD	Radiologist (R)	344–XX–6540	C 05001X	95–46137XX	40037227XX
Rex Rumsey, MD	Proctologist (Proct)	337–XX–9743	C 03042X	95–32601XX	01999047XX
Sensitive E. Scott, MD	Anesthesiologist (Anes)	220–XX–5655	C 02041X	72–54203XX	99999267XX
Raymond Skeleton, MD	Orthopedist (ORS, Orthop)	432–XX–4589	C 04561X	74–65412XX	12678547XX
Gene Ulibarri, MD	Urologist (U)	990–XX–3245	C 06430X	77–86531XX	25678831XX

*Social Security numbers are shown in the table because each individual is issued one and this is a realistic picture since they would be on file.
†Providers began using the NPI on May 23, 2007, except for small health plans, whose compliance date was May 23, 2008.

Abbreviations and Symbols

Abbreviations and symbols may appear on patient records, prescriptions, hospital charts, and patient ledger cards. Abbreviation styles differ, but the current trend is to omit periods in capital letter abbreviations except for doctors' academic degrees. For information on official American Hospital Association policy, refer to p. XX in the *Handbook*. Following is a list of abbreviations and symbols used in this *Workbook* and their meanings.

Abbreviations

A	allergy
AB	antibiotics
Abdom	abdomen
abt	about
a.c.	before meals
Adj*	adjustment
adm	admit; admission; admitted
adv	advise(d)
aet	at the age of
agit	shake or stir
$AgNO_3$	silver nitrate
ALL	allergy
AM, a.m.	ante meridian (time—before noon)
ant	anterior
ante	before
AP	anterior-posterior; anteroposterior
approx	approximate
appt	appointment
apt	apartment
ASA	acetylsalicylic acid (aspirin)
ASAP	as soon as possible
ASCVD	arteriosclerotic cardiovascular disease
ASHD	arteriosclerotic heart disease
asst	assistant
auto	automated, automobile
AV	atrioventricular
Ba	barium (enema)
Bal/fwd*	balance forward
BE	barium enema
B/F*	balance forward; brought forward
b.i.d.	two times daily
BM	bowel movement
BMR	basal metabolic rate
BP	blood pressure
Brev	Brevital sodium
BX, bx	biopsy
C	cervical (vertebrae); comprehensive (history/examination)
Ca, CA	cancer, carcinoma
c/a*	cash on account
CABG	coronary artery bypass graft
CAT	computed axial tomography
cau	Caucasian
CBC	complete blood count
CBS	chronic brain syndrome
cc	cubic centimeter
CC	chief complaint
chr	chronic
ck*	check
cm	centimeter
CO, c/o	complains of; care of
compl, comp	complete; comprehensive
Con, CON, Cons	consultation
Cont	continue
CPX	complete physical examination
C&R	compromise and release
Cr*	credit
C&S	culture and sensitivity
cs, CS*	cash on account
C-section	cesarean section
CT	computed or computerized tomography
CVA	cardiovascular accident; cerebrovascular accident
CXR	chest radiograph
cysto	cystoscopy
D, d	diagnosis; detailed (history/examination); day(s)
D & C	dilatation and curettage
dc	discontinue
DC	discharge
DDS	Doctor of Dental Surgery
def*	charge deferred
Del	delivery; obstetrics and gynecology
Dg	diagnosis
dia	diameter
diag	diagnosis; diagnostic
dil	dilate (stretch, expand)
Disch	discharge
DM	diabetes mellitus
DNA	does not apply
DNS	did not show
DPM	Doctor of Podiatric Medicine
DPT	diphtheria, pertussis, and tetanus
Dr	Doctor
Dr*	debit
DRG	diagnosis-related group
Drs	dressing
DUB	dysfunctional uterine bleeding
Dx	diagnosis
E	emergency
EC*	error corrected
ECG, EKG	electrocardiogram; electrocardiograph
echo	echocardiogram; echocardiography
ED	emergency department
EDC	estimated date of confinement
EEG	electroencephalograph
EENT	eye, ear, nose, and throat
EGD	esophagogastroduodenoscopy
EKG, ECG	electrocardiogram; electrocardiograph
E/M	Evaluation and Management (*Current Procedural Terminology* code)
EMG	electromyogram
EPF	expanded problem-focused (history/examination)
epith	epithelial
ER	emergency room
Er, ER*	error corrected

*Bookkeeping abbreviation.

ESR	erythrocyte sedimentation rate
est	established (patient); estimated
Ex, exam	examination
exc	excision
Ex MO*	express money order
ext	external
24F, 28F	French (size of catheter)
F	female
FBS	fasting blood sugar
FH	family history
ft	foot, feet
FU	follow-up (examination)
fwd*	forward
Fx	fracture
gb, GB	gallbladder
GGE	generalized glandular enlargement
GI	gastrointestinal
Grav, grav	gravida, a pregnant woman; used with Roman numerals (I, II, III) to indicate the number of pregnancies
GU	genitourinary
H	hospital call
HA	headache
HBP	high blood pressure
HC	hospital call or consultation; high-complexity (decision-making)
HCD	house call (day)
HCN	house call (night)
Hct	hematocrit
HCVD	hypertensive cardiovascular disease
Hgb	hemoglobin
hist	history
hosp	hospital
H & P	history and physical (examination)
hr, hrs	hour, hours
h.s.	before bedtime
HS	hospital surgery
Ht	height
HV	hospital visit
HX, hx	history
HX PX	history and physical examination
I	injection
IC	initial consultation
I & D	incision and drainage
I/f*	in full
IM	intramuscular (injection)
imp, imp.	impression (diagnosis)
incl.	include; including
inflam	inflammation
init	initial (office visit)
inj, INJ	injection
ins, INS*	insurance
int	internal
intermed	intermediate (office visit)
interpret	interpretation
IUD	intrauterine device
IV	intravenous (injection)
IVP	intravenous pyelogram
K 35	Kolman (instrument used in urology)
KUB	kidneys, ureters, and bladder
L	left; laboratory
lab, LAB	laboratory
lat	lateral; pertaining to the side
lbs	pounds
LC	low-complexity (decision-making)
LMP	last menstrual period
LS	lumbosacral
lt	left
ltd	limited (office visit)
L & W	living and well
M	medication; married
MC	moderate-complexity (decision-making)
MDM	medical decision making
med	medicine
mg	milligram(s)
mg/dL	milligrams per deciliter
MI	myocardial infarction
micro	microscopy
mL, ml	milliliter
mo	month(s)
MO*	money order
N	negative
NA	not applicable
NAD	no appreciable disease
NC, N/C*	no charge
NEC	not elsewhere classifiable
neg	negative
NKA	no known allergies
NOS	not otherwise specified
NP	new patient
NYD	not yet diagnosed
OB, Ob-Gyn	obstetrics and gynecology
OC	office call
occ	occasional
OD	right eye
ofc	office
OP	outpatient
Op, op	operation
OR	operating room
orig	original
OS	office surgery; left eye
OV	office visit
oz	ounce
PA	posterior-anterior; posteroanterior
Pap	Papanicolaou (smear, stain, test)
Para I	woman having borne one child
PC	present complaint
p.c.	after meals
PCP	primary care physician
PD	permanent disability
Pd, PD*	professional discount
PE	physical examination
perf	performed
PF	problem-focused (history/examination)
PFT	pulmonary function test
PH	past history
Ph ex	physical examination
phys	physical

*Bookkeeping abbreviation.

PID	pelvic inflammatory disease
PM, p.m.	post meridian (time—after noon)
PND	postnasal drip
PO, P Op	postoperative
p.o.	by mouth (per os)
post	posterior
postop	postoperative
PPD	purified protein derivative (such as in tuberculin test)
preop	preoperative
prep	prepared
PRN, p.r.n.	as necessary (pro re nata)
Proc	procedure
Prog	prognosis
P & S	permanent and stationary
PSA	prostate-specific antigen (blood test to determine cancer in prostate gland)
Pt, pt	patient
PT	physical therapy
PTR	patient to return
PVC	premature ventricular contraction
PVT ck*	private check received
PX	physical examination
q	every
qd	one time daily, every day
qh	every hour
q.i.d.	four times daily
QNS	quantity not sufficient
qod	every other day
R	right; residence call; report
RBC, rbc	red blood cell (count)
rec	recommend
rec'd	received
re ch	recheck
re-exam	reexamination
Reg	regular
ret, retn, rtn	return
rev	review
RHD	rheumatic heart disease
RN	registered nurse
R/O	rule out
ROA*	received on account
RPT	registered physical therapist
rt	right
RTC	return to clinic
RTO	return to office
RTW	return to work
RX, Rx, R_x	prescribe; prescription; any medication or treatment ordered
S	surgery
SC	subcutaneous
sched.	scheduled
SD	state disability
SE	special examination
SF	straightforward (decision-making)
Sig	directions on prescription
SLR	straight leg raising
slt	slight
Smr	smear
SOB	shortness of breath
Sp gr	specific gravity
SQ	subcutaneous (injection)
STAT	immediately
strep	*Streptococcus*
surg	surgery
Sx	symptom(s)
T	temperature
T & A	tonsillectomy and adenoidectomy
Tb, tb	tuberculosis
TD	temporary disability
tech	technician
temp	temperature
tet. tox.	tetanus toxoid
t.i.d.	three times daily
TPR	temperature, pulse, and respiration
Tr, trt	treatment
TURB	transurethral resection of bladder
TURP	transurethral resection of prostate
TX	treatment
u	units
UA, ua	urinalysis
UCHD	usual childhood diseases
UCR	usual, customary, and reasonable (fees)
UGI	upper gastrointestinal
UPJ	ureteropelvic junction or joint
UR	urinalysis
URI	upper respiratory infection
Urn	urinalysis
UTI	urinary tract infection
W	work; white
WBC, wbc	white blood cell (count); well baby care
WC	workers' compensation
wk	week; work
wks	weeks
WNL	within normal limits
Wr	Wassermann reaction (test for syphilis)
Wt, wt	weight
X	xray, x-ray(s), times (e.g., 3X means three times)
XR	xray, x-ray(s)
yr(s)	year(s)

Symbols

+	positive
#	pound(s)
c̄, /c	with
s̄, /s	without
c̄c, c̄/c	with correction (eye glasses)
s̄c, s̄/c	without correction (eye glasses)
-	negative
ō	negative
⊕, +	positive
(L)	left
(R)	right
♂	male
♀	female
–*	charge already made
⊖*	no balance due
√*	posted
($0.00)*	credit

*Bookkeeping abbreviation.

Laboratory Abbreviations

ABG	arterial blood gas(es)
AcG	factor V (AcG or proaccelerin); a factor in coagulation that converts prothrombin to thrombin
ACTH	adrenocorticotropic hormone
AFB	acid-fast bacilli
A/C ratio	albumin-coagulin ratio
AHB	alpha-hydroxybutyric (dehydrogenase)
AHG	antihemophilic globulin; antihemolytic globulin (factor)
ALA	aminolevulinic acid
ALT	alanine aminotransferase (*see* SGPT)
AMP	adenosine monophosphate
APT test	aluminum-precipitated toxoid test
AST	aspartate aminotransferase (*see* SGOT)
ATP	adenosine triphosphate
BSP	bromsulfophthalein (Bromsulphalein; sodium sulfobromophthalein) (test)
BUN	blood urea nitrogen
CBC	complete blood count
CNS	central nervous system
CO	carbon monoxide
CPB	competitive protein binding: plasma
CPK	creatine phosphokinase
CSF	cerebrospinal fluid
D hemoglobin	hemoglobin fractionation by electrophoresis for hemoglobin D
DAP	direct agglutination pregnancy (Gravindex and DAP)
DEAE	diethylaminoethanol
DHT	dihydrotestosterone
diff	differential
DNA	deoxyribonucleic acid
DRT	test for syphilis
EACA	epsilon-aminocaproic acid (a fibrinolysin)
EMIT	enzyme-multiplied immunoassay technique (for drugs)
ENA	extractable nuclear antigen
esr, ESR	erythrocyte sedimentation (sed) rate
FDP	fibrin degradation products
FIGLU	formiminoglutamic acid
FRAT	free radical assay technique (for drugs)
FSH	follicle-stimulating hormone
FSP	fibrinogen split products
FTA	fluorescent-absorbed treponema antibodies
Gc, Gm, Inv	immunoglobulin typing
GG, gamma G, A, D, G, M	gamma-globulin (immunoglobulin fractionation by electrophoresis)
GG, gamma G E, RIA	immunization E fractionation by radioimmunoassay
GGT	gamma-glutamyl transpeptidase
GLC	gas liquid chromatography
GMP	guanosine monophosphate
GTT	glucose tolerance test
G6PD	glucose-6-phosphate dehydrogenase
HAA	hepatitis-associated agent (antigen)
HBD, HBDH	hydroxybutyrate dehydrogenase
HCT	hematocrit
hemoglobin, electrophoresis	letters of the alphabet used for different types or factors of hemoglobins (includes A_2, S, C, etc.)
Hgb	hemoglobin, qualitative
HGH	human growth hormone
HI	hemagglutination inhibition
HIA	hemagglutination inhibition antibody
HIAA	hydroxyindoleacetic acid (urine), 24-hour specimen
HIV	human immunodeficiency virus
HLA	human leukocyte antigen (tissue typing)
HPL	human placental lactogen

HTLV-III	antibody detection; confirmatory test
HVA	homovanillic acid
ICSH	interstitial cell–stimulating hormone
IFA	intrinsic factor, antibody (fluorescent screen)
IgA, IgE, IgG, IgM	immunoglobulins: quantitative by gel diffusion
INH	isonicotinic hydrazide, isoniazid
LAP	leucine aminopeptidase
LATS	long-acting thyroid-stimulating (hormone)
LDH	lactic dehydrogenase
LE Prep	lupus erythematosus cell preparation
L.E. factor	antinuclear antibody
LH	luteinizing hormone
LSD	lysergic acid diethylamide
L/S ratio	lecithin-sphingomyelin ratio
MC *(Streptococcus)*	antibody titer
MIC	minimum inhibitory concentration
NBT	nitro-blue tetrazolium (test)
OCT	ornithine carbamyl transferase
PAH	para-aminohippuric acid
PBI	protein-bound iodine
pCO_2	arterial carbon dioxide pressure (or tension)
PCP	phencyclidine piperidine
pcv	packed cell volume
pH	symbol for expression of concentration of hydrogen ions (degree of acidity)
PHA	phenylalanine
PIT	prothrombin inhibition test
PKU	phenylketonuria—a metabolic disease affecting mental development
PO_2	oxygen pressure
P & P	prothrombin-proconvertin
PSP	phenolsulfonphthalein
PT	prothrombin time
PTA	plasma thromboplastin antecedent
PTC	plasma thromboplastin component; phenylthiocarbamide
PTT	prothrombin time; partial thromboplastin time (plasma or whole blood)
RBC, rbc	red blood cells (count)
RIA	radioimmunoassay
RISA	radioiodinated human serum albumin
RIST	radioimmunosorbent test
RPR	rapid plasma reagin (test)
RT_3U	resin triiodothyronine uptake
S-D	strength-duration (curve)
SGOT	serum glutamic oxaloacetic transaminase (*see* AST)
SGPT	serum glutamic pyruvic transaminase (*see* ALT)
STS	serologic test for syphilis
T_3	triiodothyronine (uptake)
TB	tubercle bacillus, tuberculosis
TBG	thyroxine-binding globulin
T & B differentiation, lymphocytes	thymus-dependent lymphs and bursa-dependent lymphs
THC	tetrahydrocannabinol (marijuana)
TIBC	total iron-binding capacity, chemical
TLC screen	thin-layer chromatography screen
TRP	tubular reabsorption of phosphates
UA	urinalysis
VDRL	Venereal Disease Research Laboratory (agglutination test for syphilis)
VMA	vanillylmandelic acid
WBC, wbc	white blood cells (count)

Mock Fee Schedule

Refer to the Mock Fee Schedule (Table 2) to complete the financial accounting statements (ledgers) and claim forms in this *Workbook*. The fees listed are hypothetical and are intended only for use in completing the questions. For the cases that are private, Medicaid, TRICARE, and workers' compensation, use the amounts in the column labeled Mock Fees. For Medicare cases, refer to the three columns pertaining to Medicare and use the amounts in the column labeled Limiting Charge. Follow these instructions unless your instructor wishes you to round out the amounts on the fee schedule to the next dollar.

In a real medical practice, some offices round out the amounts to the next dollar unless the physician is nonparticipating with Medicare and then, according to Medicare regulations, the provider can only bill the exact limiting amount on nonassigned claims. Other offices may have two fee schedules. Schedule B is for Medicare participating physicians, and amounts are listed in dollars and cents. Schedule A is used for other plans, and the amounts are rounded to the next dollar. However, if a fee schedule is sent by the insurance plan, then the medical practice may use the dollars and cents provided.

When completing the insurance claim forms, use the latest edition of *Current Procedural Terminology* (CPT), the professional code book published by the American Medical Association, to find the correct code numbers and modifiers for the services rendered. If you do not have access to the latest edition of CPT, you may use the code numbers provided in the Mock Fee Schedule; however, do so with the understanding that the code numbers and descriptions provided in this schedule are not comprehensive. They are based on the information found in CPT; however, students are cautioned not to use it as a substitute for CPT. Because the code numbers are subject to change, every medical office must have on hand the most recent edition of CPT.

The Mock Fee Schedule (Tables 2 and 3) is arranged in the same sequence as the six CPT code book sections (i.e., Evaluation and Management; Anesthesia; Surgery; Radiology, Nuclear Medicine, and Diagnostic Ultrasound; Pathology and Laboratory; and Medicine), with a comprehensive list of modifiers placed at the beginning. An index at the end of the Mock Fee Schedule can assist you in locating code numbers. Mock fees for the modifiers are not listed, because these can vary from one claim to another, depending on the circumstances.

Remember that fees can vary with the region of the United States (West, Midwest, South, East), the specialty of the practitioner, the type of community (urban, suburban, or rural), the type of practice (incorporated or unincorporated, solo, partners, or shareholders), the overhead, and a number of other factors.

Table 2. College Clinic Mock Fee Schedule

Modifier Code Number	Description	Mock Fee ($)
-22	*Unusual Services:* When the service(s) provided is substantially greater than that usually required for the listed procedure, it may be identified by adding modifier -22 to the usual procedure code number. Documentation must support the substantial work and the reason for the additional work. This modifier cannot be appended to an E/M service.	Increase fee
-23	*Unusual Anesthesia:* Occasionally a procedure that usually requires either no anesthesia or local anesthesia must be done under general anesthesia because of unusual circumstances. These circumstances may be reported by adding the modifier -23 to the procedure code number of the basic service.	Increase fee
-24	*Unrelated Evaluation and Management Service by the Same Physician During a Postoperative Period:* The physician may need to indicate that an evaluation and management service was performed during a postoperative period for a reason(s) unrelated to the original procedure. This circumstance may be reported by adding the modifier -24 to the appropriate level of E/M service.	Variable per E/M fee
-25	*Significant, Separately Identifiable Evaluation and Management Service by the Same Physician on the Same Day of a Procedure or Other Service:* The physician may need to indicate that on the day a procedure or service identified by a CPT code was performed, the patient's condition required a significant, separately identifiable E/M service above and beyond the other service provided or beyond the usual preoperative and postoperative care associated with the procedure that was performed. The E/M service may be prompted by the symptom or condition for which the procedure and/or service was provided. As such, different diagnoses are not required for reporting of the E/M services on the same date. This circumstance may be reported by adding the modifier -25 to the appropriate level of E/M service. NOTE: This modifier is not used to report an E/M service that resulted in a decision to perform surgery. See modifier -57.	Variable per E/M fee

Table 2. College Clinic Mock Fee Schedule—cont'd

Modifier Code Number	Description	Mock Fee ($)
-26	*Professional Component:* Certain procedures are a combination of a physician component and a technical component. When the physician component is reported separately, the service may be identified by adding the modifier -26 to the usual procedure code number.	Decrease fee
-32	*Mandated Services:* Services related to mandated consultation and/or related services (e.g., PRO, third-party payer) may be identified by adding the modifier -32 to the basic procedure.	Use standard fee
-33	*Preventive Services:* When the primary purpose of the service is the delivery of an evidence-based service in accordance with a U.S. Preventive Services Task Force A or B rating in effect and other preventive services identified in preventive services mandates (legislative or regulatory), the service may be identified by adding this modifier to the procedure.	Variable
-47	*Anesthesia by Surgeon:* Regional or general anesthesia provided by the surgeon may be reported by adding the modifier -47 to the basic service (this does not include local anesthesia). **Note:** Modifier -47 would not be used as a modifier for the anesthesia procedures 00100 through 01999.	Increase fee
-50	*Bilateral Procedure:* Unless otherwise identified in the listings, bilateral procedures that are performed at the same operative session should be identified by the appropriate five-digit code number describing the first procedure. The second (bilateral) procedure is identified by adding modifier -50 to the procedure code number.	Paid at 50% of standard fee
-51	*Multiple Procedures:* When multiple procedures other than E/M services are performed at the same session by the same provider, the primary procedure or service may be reported as listed. The additional procedure(s) or service(s) may be identified by adding the modifier -51 to the additional procedure or service code(s). **Note**: This modifier should not be appended to designated "add-on" codes.	Second procedure usually paid at 50% of fee. Third procedure usually paid at 25% of fee. Fourth and subsequent procedures usually paid at 10% of fee.
-52	*Reduced Services:* Under certain circumstances, a service or procedure is partially reduced or eliminated at the physician's discretion. Under these circumstances, the service provided can be identified by its usual procedure number and the addition of the modifier -52, signifying that the service is reduced. This provides a means of reporting reduced services without disturbing the identification of the basic service. **Note:** For hospital outpatient reporting of a previously scheduled procedure/service that is partially reduced or canceled as a result of extenuating circumstances or those that threaten the well-being of the patient before or after administration of anesthesia, see modifiers -73 and -74.	Decrease fee
-53	*Discontinued Procedure:* Under certain circumstances, the physician may elect to terminate a surgical or diagnostic procedure. Due to extenuating circumstances or those that threaten the well-being of the patient, it may be necessary to indicate that a surgical or diagnostic procedure was started but discontinued. This circumstance may be reported by adding modifier -53 to the code reported by the physician for the discontinued procedure. **Note:** This modifier is not used to report the elective cancellation of a procedure before the patient's anesthesia induction and/or surgical preparation in the operating suite. For outpatient hospital/ambulatory surgery center (ASC) reporting of a previously scheduled procedure/service that is partially reduced or canceled as a result of extenuating circumstances or those that threaten the well-being of the patient before or after administration of anesthesia, see modifiers -73 and -74 (see modifiers approved for ASC hospital outpatient use).	Decrease fee
-54	*Surgical Care Only:* When one physician performs a surgical procedure and another provides preoperative and/or postoperative management, surgical services may be identified by adding the modifier -54 to the usual procedure number.	Decrease fee

Continued

Table 2. College Clinic Mock Fee Schedule—cont'd

Modifier Code Number	Description	Mock Fee ($)
-55	*Postoperative Management Only:* When one physician performs the postoperative management and another physician performs the surgical procedure, the postoperative component may be identified by adding modifier -55 to the usual procedure number.	Decrease fee
-56	*Preoperative Management Only:* When one physician performs the preoperative care and evaluation and another physician performs the surgical procedure, the preoperative component may be identified by adding the modifier -56 to the usual procedure number.	Decrease fee
-57	*Decision for Surgery:* An evaluation and management service that resulted in the initial decision to perform the surgery may be identified by adding the modifier -57 to the appropriate level of E/M service.	Use standard fee
-58	*Staged or Related Procedure or Service by the Same Physician During the Postoperative Period:* The physician may need to indicate that the performance of a procedure or service during the postoperative period was (a) planned prospectively at the time of the original procedure (staged); (b) more extensive than the original procedure; or (c) for therapy following a diagnostic surgical procedure. This circumstance may be reported by adding the modifier -58 to the staged or related procedure. **Note:** This modifier is not used to report the treatment of a problem that requires a return to the operating room. See modifier -78.	Variable
-59	*Distinct Procedural Service:* Under certain circumstances, the physician may need to indicate that a procedure or service was distinct or independent from other services performed on the same day. Modifier -59 is used to identify procedures/services that are not normally reported together but are appropriate under the circumstances. This may represent a different session or patient encounter, different procedure or surgery, different site or organ system, separate incision/excision, separate lesion, or separate injury (or area of injury in extensive injuries) not ordinarily encountered or performed on the same day by the same physician. However, when another already established modifier is appropriate, it should be used rather than modifier -59. Only if no more descriptive modifier is available, and the use of modifier -59 best explains the circumstances, should modifier -59 be used.	Variable
-62	*Two Surgeons:* Under certain circumstances, the skills of two surgeons (usually with different skills) may be required in the management of a specific surgical procedure. Under such circumstances, the separate services may be identified by adding the modifier -62 to the procedure number used by each surgeon for reporting his or her services. **Note:** If a co-surgeon acts as an assistant in the performance of additional procedure(s) during the same surgical session, those services may be reported using separate procedure code(s) with the modifier -80 or modifier -81 added, as appropriate.	Use standard fee
-63	*Procedure Performed on Infants Less Than 4 kg:* Procedures performed on neonates and infants up to a present body weight of 4 kg may involve significantly increased complexity and physician work commonly associated with these patients. This circumstance may be reported by adding the modifier -63 to the procedure number (20000 through 69990).	Increase fee
-66	*Surgical Team:* Under some circumstances, highly complex procedures (requiring the concomitant services of several physicians, often of different specialties, plus other highly skilled, specially trained personnel and various types of complex equipment) are carried out under the "surgical team" concept. Such circumstances may be identified by each participating physician with the addition of the modifier -66 to the basic procedure code number used for reporting services.	Variable
-76	*Repeat Procedure by Same Physician:* The physician may need to indicate that a procedure or service was repeated subsequent to the original procedure or service. This circumstance may be reported by adding modifier -76 to the repeated service/procedure.	Decrease fee

Table 2. College Clinic Mock Fee Schedule—cont'd

Modifier Code Number	Description	Mock Fee ($)
-77	*Repeat Procedure by Another Physician:* The physician may need to indicate that a basic procedure or service performed by another physician had to be repeated. This situation may be reported by adding modifier -77 to the repeated procedure/service.	Decrease fee
-78	*Unplanned Return to the Operating Room for a Related Procedure During the Postoperative Period by the Same Physician:* The physician may need to indicate that another procedure was performed during the postoperative period of the initial procedure. When this subsequent procedure is related to the first and requires the use of the operating room, it may be reported by adding the modifier -78 to the related procedure. (For repeat procedures on the same day, see -76.)	Decrease fee
-79	*Unrelated Procedure or Service by the Same Physician During the Postoperative Period:* The physician may need to indicate that the performance of a procedure or service during the postoperative period was unrelated to the original procedure. This circumstance may be reported by using the modifier -79. (For repeat procedures on the same day, see -76.)	Use standard fee
-80	*Assistant Surgeon:* Surgical assistant services may be identified by adding the modifier -80 to the usual procedure number(s).	Billed and/or paid at approximately 20% of surgeon's fee
-81	*Minimum Assistant Surgeon:* Minimum surgical assistant services are identified by adding the modifier -81 to the usual procedure number.	Billed and/or paid at approximately 10% of surgeon's fee
-82	*Assistant Surgeon When Qualified Resident Surgeon Not Available:* The unavailability of a qualified resident surgeon is a prerequisite for use of modifier -82 appended to the usual procedure code number(s).	Decrease fee
-90	*Reference (Outside) Laboratory:* When laboratory procedures are performed by a party other than the treating or reporting physician and billed by the treating physician, the procedure may be identified by adding the modifier -90 to the usual procedure number.	Fee according to contract
-91	*Repeat Clinical Diagnostic Laboratory Test:* In the course of treatment of the patient, it may be necessary to repeat the same laboratory test on the same day to obtain subsequent (multiple) test results. Under these circumstances, the laboratory test performed can be identified by its usual procedure number and the addition of modifier -91. **NOTE:** This modifier may not be used when tests are rerun to confirm initial results; due to testing problems with specimens or equipment; or for any other reason when a normal, one-time, reportable result is all that is required. This modifier may not be used when other code(s) describe a series of test results (e.g., glucose tolerance tests, evocative/suppression testing). This modifier may only be used for laboratory test(s) performed more than once on the same day on the same patient.	Decrease fee
-92	*Alternative Laboratory Platform Testing:* When laboratory testing is performed using a kit or transportable instrument that wholly or in part consists of a single-use, disposable analytical chamber, the service may be identified by adding modifier -92 to the usual laboratory procedure code (HIV testing 86701-86703). The test does not require permanent dedicated space; hence, by its design, it may be hand carried or transported to the vicinity of the patient for immediate testing at the site, although location of the testing is not in itself determinative of the use of the modifier.	Use standard fee
-99	*Multiple Modifiers:* Under certain circumstances, two or more modifiers may be necessary to completely delineate a service. In such situations, modifier -99 should be added to the basic procedure, and other applicable modifiers may be listed as part of the description of the service.	Variable

Table 3. Mock Fee Schedule					
			Medicare*		
Code Number	Description	Mock Fees	Participating	Nonparticipating	Limiting Charge
EVALUATION AND MANAGEMENT†					
Office					
New Patient					
99201	Level 1 Problem Focused	33.25	30.43	28.91	33.25
99202	Level 2 Expanded Prob Foc	51.91	47.52	45.14	51.91
99203	Level 3 Detailed	70.92	64.92	61.67	70.92
99204	Level 4 Comprehensive	106.11	97.13	92.27	106.11
99205	Level 5 Comprehensive	132.28	121.08	115.03	132.28
Established Patient					
99211	Level 1 Nurse Visit	16.07	14.70	13.97	16.07
99212	Level 2 Problem Focused	28.55	26.14	24.83	28.55
99213	Level 3 Expanded Prob Foc	40.20	36.80	34.96	40.20
99214	Level 4 Comprehensive	61.51	56.31	53.79	61.51
99215	Level 5 Comprehensive	96.97	88.76	84.32	96.97
Hospital					
Observation Services (new or established patient)					
99217	Observation Care Dischg	66.88	61.22	58.16	66.88
99218	Dhx/exam SF/LC MDM	74.22	67.94	64.54	74.22
99219	Chx/exam MC MDM	117.75	107.78	102.39	117.75
99220	Chx/exam HC MDM	147.48	134.99	128.24	147.48
Inpatient Services (new or established patient)					
99221	30 min Dhx, Dpx, SF or low MDM	73.00	66.84	63.48	73.00
99222	50 min Comp/Comp/Moderate	120.80	110.57	105.04	120.80
99223	70 min Comp/Comp/High MDM	152.98	140.03	133.03	152.98
Subsequent Hospital Care					
99231	15 min PF, PF, SF MDM	37.74	34.55	32.82	37.74
99232	25 min EPF, EPF, Moderate	50.85	48.31	55.56	
99233	35 min D, D, HC MDM	76.97	70.45	66.93	76.97
99238	Discharge <30 min	65.26	59.74	56.75	65.26
99239	Discharge >30 min				
Consultations					
Office (new or established patient)					
99241	Level 1 PF, PF, SF	51.93	47.54	45.16	51.93
99242	Level 2 EPF, EPF, SF	80.24	73.44	69.77	80.24
99243	Level 3 D, D, LC MDM	103.51	94.75	90.01	103.51
99244	Level 4 C, C, Moderate MDM	145.05	132.77	126.13	145.05
99245	Level 5 C, C, HC MDM	195.45	178.93	169.98	195.45
Inpatient (new or established patient)					
99251	Level 1 PF, PF, SF	53.29	48.78	46.34	53.29
99252	Level 2 EPF, EPF, SF	80.56	73.74	70.05	80.56
99253	Level 3 D, D, LC MDM	106.10	97.12	92.26	106.10
99254	Level 4 C, C, Moderate MDM	145.26	132.96	126.31	145.26
99255	Level 5 C, C, HC MDM	196.55	179.91	170.91	196.55
Emergency Department (new/established patient)					
99281	PF hx/exam SF MDM	24.32	22.26	21.15	24.32
99282	EPF hx/exam LC MDM	37.02	33.88	32.19	37.02
99283	EPF hx/exam MC MDM	66.23	60.62	57.59	66.23
99284	D hx/exam MC MDM	100.71	92.18	87.57	100.71
99285	C hx/exam HC MDM	158.86	145.41	138.14	158.86

*Some services and procedures may not be considered a benefit under the Medicare program and when listed on a claim form, no reimbursement may be received. However, it is important to include these codes when billing because Medicare policies may change without an individual knowing of a new benefit. For this reason, some of the services shown in this Mock Fee Schedule do not have any amounts listed under the three Medicare columns.

†See Tables 6-3 and 6-4 in the *Handbook* for more descriptions of E/M codes 99201 through 99255.

Table 3. Mock Fee Schedule—cont'd

Code Number	Description	Mock Fees	Medicare* Participating	Medicare* Nonparticipating	Medicare* Limiting Charge
Critical Care Services					
99291	First hour	208.91	191.22	181.66	208.91
99292	Each addl. 30 min	102.02	92.46	87.84	102.02
Neonatal Intensive Care					
99468	Initial	892.74	817.16	776.30	892.74
99469	Subsequent unstable case	418.73	383.27	364.11	418.73
Initial Nursing Facility					
99304	25 min (Low Severity)	64.11	58.68	55.75	64.11
99305	35 min (Moderate Severity)	90.55	82.88	78.74	90.55
99306	45 min (High Severity)	136.76	125.18	118.92	136.76
Subsequent NF Care					
99307	PF hx/exam SF DM	37.95	34.74	33.00	37.95
99308	15 min EPF hx/exam LC DM	55.11	50.44	47.92	55.11
99309	25 min D hx/exam MC DM	69.61	63.72	60.53	69.61
99310	35 min C hx/exam HC DM	84.73	77.00	73.14	84.73
Domiciliary, Rest Home, Custodial Care					
New Patient					
99324	PF hx/exam SF DM	46.10	42.20	40.09	46.10
99325	EPF hx/exam LC DM	65.02	59.53	56.54	65.02
99326	D hx/exam MC DM	86.18	78.88	74.94	86.18
99327	C hx/exam MC DM	107.34	98.23	93.34	107.34
99328	C hx/exam HC DM	128.50	117.58	111.74	128.50
Established Patient					
99334	PF hx/exam SF MDM	37.31	34.15	32.44	37.31
99335	EPF hx/exam LC MDM	49.22	45.05	42.80	49.22
99336	D hx/exam Moderate MDM	60.61	55.47	52.70	60.61
99337	C hx/exam M-H DM	72.00	65.89	62.60	72.00
Home Services					
New Patient					
99341	PF hx/exam SF DM	70.32	64.37	61.15	70.32
99342	EPF hx/exam LC DM	91.85	84.07	79.87	91.85
99343	D hx/exam MC DM	120.24	110.06	104.56	120.24
99344	C hx/exam MC DM	148.63	136.05	129.25	148.63
99345	C hx/exam HC DM	177.02	162.04	153.50	177.02
Established Patient					
99347	PF hx/exam SF DM	54.83	50.19	47.68	54.83
99348	EPF hx/exam LC DM	70.06	64.13	60.92	70.06
99349	D hx/exam MC DM	88.33	80.85	76.81	88.33
99350	C hx/exam M-H DM	106.60	97.57	92.70	106.60
Prolonged Services With Direct (Face-to-Face) Patient Contact (Report in Addition to the Designated E/M Service at Any Level)					
Outpatient					
99354	First hour	96.97	88.76	84.32	96.97
99355	Each addl. 30 min	96.97	88.76	84.32	96.97
Inpatient					
99356	First hour	96.42	88.25	83.84	96.42
99357	Each addl. 30 min	96.42	88.25	83.84	96.42

*Some services and procedures may not be considered a benefit under the Medicare program and when listed on a claim form, no reimbursement may be received. However, it is important to include these codes when billing because Medicare policies may change without an individual knowing of a new benefit. For this reason, some of the services shown in this Mock Fee Schedule do not have any amounts listed under the three Medicare columns.

Continued

Table 3. Mock Fee Schedule—cont'd					
			Medicare*		
Code Number	Description	Mock Fees	Participating	Nonparticipating	Limiting Charge
Prolonged Services Without Direct Contact					
99358	First hour	90.00			
99359	Each addl. 30 min	90.00			
Physician Standby Service					
99360	Each 30 min	95.00			
Case Management Services					
Team Conferences					
99366		85.00			
99367-99368		105.00			
Telephone Calls					
99441	5-10 min	30.00			
99442	11-20 min	40.00			
99443	21-30 min	60.00			
Care Plan Oversight Services					
99375	30 min or more/month	93.40	85.49	81.22	93.40
Preventive Medicine					
New Patient					
99381	Infant younger than 1 year	50.00			
99382	1-4 years	50.00			
99383	5-11 years	45.00			
99384	12-17 years	45.00			
99385	18-39 years	50.00			
99386	40-64 years	50.00			
99387	65 years and older	55.00			
Established Patient					
99391	Infant younger than year	35.00			
99392	1-4 years	35.00			
99393	5-11 years	30.00			
99394	12-17 years	30.00			
99395	18-39 years	35.00			
99396	40-64 years	35.00			
99397	65 years and older	40.00			
Counseling (new/est pt)					
Individual					
99401	15 min	35.00			
99402	30 min	50.00			
99403	45 min	65.00			
99404	60 min	80.00			
Group					
99411	30 min	30.00			
99412	60 min	50.00			
Other Preventive Medicine Services					
99420	Health hazard appraisal	50.00			
99429	Unlisted preventive med service	Variable			
Newborn Care					
99460	Birthing room delivery	102.50	93.50	88.83	102.15
99461	Other than birthing room	110.16	100.83	95.79	110.16
99462	Subsequent hospital care	54.02	49.44	46.97	54.02
99465	Newborn resuscitation	255.98	234.30	222.59	255.98

*Some services and procedures may not be considered a benefit under the Medicare program and when listed on a claim form, no reimbursement may be received. However, it is important to include these codes when billing because Medicare policies may change without an individual knowing of a new benefit. For this reason, some of the services shown in this Mock Fee Schedule do not have any amounts listed under the three Medicare columns.

Table 3. Mock Fee Schedule—cont'd					
			Medicare*		
Code Number	Description	Mock Fees	Participating	Nonparticipating	Limiting Charge
Anesthesiology					
Anesthesiology fees are presented here for CPT codes. However, each case would require a fee for time, e.g., every 15 minutes would be worth $55. This fee is determined according to the relative value system, calculated, and added into the anesthesia (CPT) fee. Some anesthetists may list a surgical code using an anesthesia modifier on a subsequent line for carriers that do not acknowledge anesthesia codes.					
99100	Anes for pt younger than 1 yr or older than 70 years	55.00			
99116	Anes complicated use total hypothermia	275.00			
99135	Anes complicated use hypotension	275.00			
99140	Anes complicated emer cond	110.00			
Physician Status Modifier Codes					
P-1	Normal healthy patient	00.00			
P-2	Patient with mild systemic disease	00.00			
P-3	Patient with severe systemic disease	55.00			
P-4	Patient with severe systemic disease that is a constant threat to life	110.00			
P-5	Moribund pt not expected to survive without operation	165.00			
P-6	Declared brain-dead pt, organs being removed for donor	00.00			
Head					
00160	Anes nose/sinus (NEC)	275.00			
00172	Anes repair cleft palate	165.00			
Thorax					
00400	Anes for proc ant integumentary system of chest, incl SC tissue	165.00			
00402	Anes breast reconstruction	275.00			
00546	Anes pulmonary resection with thoracoplasty	275.00			
00600	Anes cervical spine and cord	550.00			
Lower Abdomen					
00800	Anes for proc lower ant abdominal wall	165.00			
00840	Anes intraperitoneal proc lower abdomen: NOS	330.00			
00842	Amniocentesis	220.00			
00914	Anes TURP	275.00			
00942	Anes colporrhaphy, colpotomy, colpectomy	220.00			
Upper Leg					
01210	Anes open proc hip joint; NOS	330.00			
01214	Total hip replacement	440.00			

*Some services and procedures may not be considered a benefit under the Medicare program and when listed on a claim form, no reimbursement may be received. However, it is important to include these codes when billing because Medicare policies may change without an individual knowing of a new benefit. For this reason, some of the services shown in this Mock Fee Schedule do not have any amounts listed under the three Medicare columns.

Continued

Table 3. Mock Fee Schedule—cont'd

Code Number	Description	Mock Fees	Medicare* Participating	Medicare* Nonparticipating	Medicare* Limiting Charge
Upper Arm and Elbow					
01740	Anes open proc humerus/elbow; NOS	220.00			
01758	Exc cyst/tumor humerus	275.00			
Radiologic Procedures					
01922	Anes CAT scan	385.00			
Miscellaneous Procedure(s)					
01999	Unlisted anes proc	variable			
Neurology					
95812	Electroencephalogram	129.32	118.37	112.45	129.32
95819	Electroencephalogram—awake	126.81	116.07	110.27	126.81
95860	Electromyography, 1 extremity	88.83	81.31	77.24	88.83
95864	Electromyography, 4 extremities	239.99	219.67	208.69	239.99
96101	Psychological testing (per hour)	80.95	74.10	70.39	80.95
Physical Medicine					
97024	Diathermy	14.27	13.06	12.41	14.27
97036	Hubbard tank, each 15 min	24.77	22.67	21.54	24.77
97110	Therapeutic proc, one or more areas, each 15 min	23.89	21.86	20.77	23.89
97140	Manual therapy (manipulation, traction), one or more regions, each 15 min	16.93	15.49	14.72	16.93
Special Services and Reports					
99000	Handling of specimen (transfer from Dr.'s office to lab)	5.00			
99024	Postoperative visit (bundled)	No Charge			
99050	Services provided, in the office at times other than regularly scheduled office hours or days when office is normally closed (e.g., holidays, Saturday, or Sunday) in addition to basic service	25.00			
99053	Services between 10:00 PM and 8:00 AM in addition to basic service (24 hr fac)	35.00			
99056	Services normally provided in office requested by pt in location other than office in addition to basic service	20.00			
99058	Office services provided on an emergency basis, which causes disruption of other sched svcs.				
99070	Supplies and materials (itemize drugs and materials provided)	10.00			
99080	Special reports: insurance forms				
	Review of data to clarify pt's status	20.00			
	WC reports	50.00			
	WC extensive review report	250.00			

*Some services and procedures may not be considered a benefit under the Medicare program and when listed on a claim form, no reimbursement may be received. However, it is important to include these codes when billing because Medicare policies may change without an individual knowing of a new benefit. For this reason, some of the services shown in this Mock Fee Schedule do not have any amounts listed under the three Medicare columns.

Table 3. Mock Fee Schedule—cont'd

Code Number	Description	Mock Fees	Medicare Participating	Medicare Non-participating	Medicare Limiting Charge	Medicare Follow-Up Days*
10060	I & D furuncle, onychia, paronychia; single	75.92	69.49	66.02	75.92	10
11040	Débridement; skin, partial thickness	79.32	75.60	68.97	79.32	10
11044	Débridement; skin, subcu. muscle, bone	269.28	246.48	234.16	269.28	10
11100	Biopsy of skin, SC tissue &/or mucous membrane; 1 lesion	65.43	59.89	56.90	65.43	10
11200	Exc, skin tags; up to 15	55.68	50.97	45.42	55.68	10
11401	Exc, benign lesion, 0.6-1.0 cm trunk, arms, legs	95.62	87.53	83.15	96.62	10
11402	1.1-2.0 cm	121.52	111.23	105.67	121.52	10
11403	2.1-3.0 cm	151.82	138.97	132.02	151.82	10
11420	Exc, benign lesion, 0.5 cm or less scalp, neck, hands, feet, genitalia	75.44	69.05	65.60	75.44	10
11422	Exc, benign lesion scalp, neck, hands, feet, or genitalia; 1.1-2.0 cm	131.35	120.23	114.22	131.35	10
11441	Exc, benign lesion face, ears, eyelids, nose, lips, or mucous membrane	119.08	109.00	103.55	119.08	10
11602	Exc, malignant lesion, trunk, arms, or legs; 1.1-2.0 cm dia	195.06	178.55	169.62	195.06	10
11719	Trimming of nondystrophic nails, any number	30.58	27.82	26.33	30.58	0
11720	Débridement of nails, any method, 1-5	32.58	29.82	28.33	32.58	0
11721	6 or more	32.58	29.82	28.33	32.58	0
11730	Avulsion nail plate, partial or complete, simple repair; single	76.91	70.40	66.88	76.91	0
11750	Exc, nail or nail matrix, partial or complete	193.45	177.07	168.22	193.45	10
11765	Wedge excision of nail fold	57.95	53.04	50.39	57.95	10
12001	Simple repair (scalp, neck, axillae, ext genitalia, trunk, or extremities incl hands & feet); 2.5 cm or less	91.17	83.45	79.28	91.17	10
12011	Simple repair (face, ears, eyelids, nose, lips, or mucous membranes); 2.5 cm or less	101.44	92.85	88.21	101.44	10
12013	2.6-5.0 cm	123.98	113.48	107.81	123.98	10
12032	Repair, scalp, axillae, trunk (intermediate)	169.73	155.36	147.59	169.73	10

*Data for the surgical follow-up days from St. Anthony's *CPT'96 Companion: A Guide to Medicare Billing*.

Continued

Table 3. Mock Fee Schedule—cont'd

			Medicare			
Code Number	Description	Mock Fees	Participating	Non-participating	Limiting Charge	Follow-Up Days*
12034	Repair, intermediate, wounds (scalp, axillae, trunk, or extremities) excl hands or feet; 7.6-12.5 cm	214.20	196.06	186.26	214.20	10
12051	Repair, intermediate, layer closure of wounds (face, ears, eyelids, nose, lips, or mucous membranes); 2.5 cm or less	167.60	153.41	145.74	167.60	10
17000	Cauterization, 1 lesion	52.56	48.11	45.70	52.56	10
17003	Second through 14 lesions, each	15.21	17.77	16.88	5.21	
17004	Destruction (laser surgery), 15 or more lesions					10
19020	Mastotomy, drainage/exploration deep abscess	237.36	217.26	206.40	237.36	90
19100	Biopsy, breast, needle	96.17	88.03	83.63	96.17	0
19101	Biopsy, breast, incisional	281.51	257.67	244.79	281.51	10
20610	Arthrocentesis, aspiration or injection major joint (shoulder, hip, knee, or bursa)	52.33	47.89	45.50	52.33	0
21330	Nasal fracture, open treatment complicated	599.46	548.71	521.27	599.46	90
24066	Biopsy, deep, soft tissue, upper arm, elbow	383.34	350.88	333.34	383.34	90
27455	Osteotomy, proximal tibia	1248.03	1142.36	1085.24	1248.03	90
27500	Treatment closed femoral shaft fracture without manipulation	554.90	507.92	482.52	554.90	90
27530	Treatment closed tibial fracture, proximal, without manipulation	344.24	315.09	299.34	344.24	90
27750	Treatment closed tibial shaft fracture, without manipulation	400.94	366.99	348.64	400.94	90
27752	With manipulation	531.63	486.62	462.29	531.63	90
29280	Strapping of hand or finger	35.13	31.36	29.79	35.13	0
29345	Appl long leg cast (thigh to toes)	123.23	112.80	107.16	123.23	0
29355	Walker or ambulatory type	133.75	122.42	116.30	133.75	0
29425	Appl short leg walking cast	102.10	93.45	88.78	102.10	0
30110	Excision, simple nasal polyp	145.21	132.92	126.27	145.21	10
30520	Septoplasty	660.88	604.93	574.68	660.88	90
30903	Control nasal hemorrhage; unilateral	118.17	108.17	102.76	118.17	0

*Data for the surgical follow-up days from St. Anthony's *CPT'96 Companion: A Guide to Medicare Billing.*

Table 3. Mock Fee Schedule—cont'd

Code Number	Description	Mock Fees	Medicare			
			Participating	Non-participating	Limiting Charge	Follow-Up Days*
30905	Control nasal hemorrhage, posterior with posterior nasal packs and/or cautery; initial	190.57	174.43	165.71	190.57	0
30906	Subsequent	173.01	158.36	150.44	173.01	
31540	Laryngoscopy with excision of tumor and/or stripping of vocal cords	488.95	447.55	425.17	488.95	0
31541	With operating microscope	428.33	392.06	372.46	428.33	0
31575	Laryngoscopy, flexible fiberoptic; diagnostic	138.48	126.76	120.42	138.48	0
31625	Bronchoscopy with biopsy	312.87	286.38	272.06	312.87	0
32310	Pleurectomy	1234.79	1130.24	1073.73	1234.79	90
32440	Pneumonectomy, total	1972.10	1805.13	1714.87	1972.10	90
33020	Pericardiotomy	1289.25	1180.09	1121.09	1289.25	90
33206	Insertion of pacemaker; atrial	728.42	666.75	633.41	728.42	90
33208	Atrial and ventricular	751.57	687.89	653.50	751.57	90
35301	Thromboendarterectomy, with or without patch graft; carotid, vertebral, subclavian, by neck incision	1585.02	1450.82	1378.28	1585.02	90
36005	Intravenous injection forcontrast venography	59.18	54.17	51.46	59.18	0
36248	Catheter placement (selective) arterial system, 2nd, 3rd order and beyond	68.54	62.74	59.60	68.54	0
36415	Routine venipuncture for collection of specimen(s)	10.00				
38101	Splenectomy, partial	994.44	910.24	864.73	994.44	90
38220	Bone marrow; aspiration only	73.52	67.29	63.93	73.52	NA
38221	Biopsy, needle or trocar	90.65	82.98	78.83	90.65	NA
38510	Biopsy/excision deep cervical node/s	327.42	299.69	284.71	327.42	10
39520	Hernia repair	1436.50	1314.87	1249.13	1436.50	90
42820	T & A under age 12 years	341.63	312.71	297.07	341.63	90
42821	T & A over age 12 years	410.73	375.96	357.16	410.73	90
43234	Upper GI endoscopy, simple primary exam	201.86	184.77	175.53	201.86	0
43235	Upper GI endoscopy incl esophagus, stomach, duodenum, or jejunum; complex	238.92	218.69	207.76	238.92	0
43255	With control of bleeding, any method	281.51	257.67	244.79	281.51	0
43456	Dilation esophagus	254.52	232.97	221.32	254.52	0
43820	Gastrojejunostomy	971.86	889.58	845.10	971.86	90
44150	Colectomy, total, abdominal	1757.81	108.98	1528.53	1757.81	90
44320	Colostomy or skin level cecostomy	966.25	884.44	840.22	966.25	90

*Data for the surgical follow-up days from St. Anthony's *CPT'96 Companion: A Guide to Medicare Billing*.

Continued

Table 3. Mock Fee Schedule—cont'd

Code Number	Description	Mock Fees	Medicare Participating	Medicare Non-participating	Medicare Limiting Charge	Medicare Follow-Up Days*
44950	Appendectomy	568.36	520.24	494.23	568.36	90
45308	Proctosigmoidoscopy; removal of polyp	135.34	123.88	117.69	135.34	0
45315	Multiple polyps	185.12	169.44	160.97	185.12	0
45330	Sigmoidoscopy (flexible), diagnostic (with or without biopsy or collection of specimen by brushing or washing)	95.92	87.80	83.41	95.92	0
45333	Sigmoidoscopy (flexible) with removal of polyps	183.99	168.41	159.99	183.99	0
45380	Colonoscopy with biopsy	382.35	349.98	332.48	382.35	0
46255	Hemorrhoidectomy int &ext, simple	503.57	460.94	437.89	503.57	90
46258	Hemorrhoidectomy with fistulectomy	636.02	582.17	553.06	636.02	90
46600	Anoscopy; diagnostic	32.86	30.07	28.57	32.86	0
46614	With control of hemorrhage	182.10	166.68	158.35	182.10	0
46700	Anoplasty, for stricture, adult	657.39	601.73	571.64	657.39	90
47562	Cholecystectomy; laparoscopic	714.99	654.45	621.73	714.99	90
47600	Cholecystectomy; abdominal excision	937.74	858.35	815.43	937.74	90
49505	Inguinal hernia repair, age 5 or over	551.07	504.41	479.19	551.07	90
49520	Repair, inguinal hernia, any age; reducible	671.89	615.00	584.25	671.89	90
50080	Nephrostolithotomy, percutaneous	1323.93	1211.83	1151.24	1323.93	90
50780	Ureteroneocystostomy	1561.23	1429.84	1357.59	1561.23	90
51900	Closure of vesicovaginal fistula, abdominal approach	1196.82	1095.48	1040.71	1196.82	90
52000	Cystourethroscopy	167.05	152.90	145.26	167.05	0
52601	Transurethral resection of prostate	1193.53	1092.47	1037.85	1193.53	90
53040	Drainage of deep periurethral abscess	379.48	347.35	329.98	379.48	90
53060	Drainage of Skene's gland	147.45	134.97	128.22	147.45	10
53230	Excision, female diverticulum (urethral)	859.69	786.91	747.56	859.69	90
53240	Marsupialization of urethral diverticulum, M or F	520.11	476.07	452.27	520.11	90
53270	Excision of Skene's gland(s)	184.39	168.78	160.34	184.39	10
53620	Dilation, urethra, male	100.73	92.20	87.59	100.73	0
53660	Dilation urethra, female	48.32	44.23	42.02	48.32	0
54150	Circumcision	111.78	102.32	97.20	111.78	10
54520	Orchiectomy, simple	523.92	479.56	455.58	523.92	90
55700	Biopsy of prostate, needle or punch	156.22	142.99	135.84	156.22	0

*Data for the surgical follow-up days from St. Anthony's *CPT'96 Companion: A Guide to Medicare Billing*.

Table 3. Mock Fee Schedule—cont'd

Code Number	Description	Mock Fees	Medicare Participating	Medicare Non-participating	Medicare Limiting Charge	Medicare Follow-Up Days*
55801	Prostatectomy, perineal subtotal	1466.56	1342.39	1275.27	1466.56	90
57265	Colporrhaphy AP with enterocele repair	902.24	825.85	784.56	902.24	90
57452	Colposcopy	84.18	77.05	73.20	84.18	0
57510	Cauterization of cervix, electro or thermal	115.15	105.40	100.13	115.15	10
57520	Conization of cervix with or without D & C, with or without repair	387.08	354.30	336.59	387.08	90
58100	Endometrial biopsy	71.88	65.79	62.50	71.88	0
58120	D & C, diagnostic and/or therapeutic (non-OB)	272.83	249.73	237.24	272.83	10
58150	TAH w/without salpingo-oophorectomy	1167.72	1068.85	1015.41	1167.72	90
58200	Total hysterectomy, extended, corpus	1707.24	1562.69	1484.56	1707.24	90
58210	Radical abdominal hysterectomy with bilateral total pelvic lymphadenectomy	2160.78	1977.83	1878.94	2160.78	90
	completed surgically	357.39	327.13	310.77	357.39	90
58300	Insertion of intrauterine device	100.00	93.45	88.78	100.00	0
58340	Hysterosalpingography, inj proc for	73.06	66.87	63.53	73.06	0
58720	Salpingo-oophorectomy, complete or partial, unilateral or bilateral surgical treatment of ectopic pregnancy	732.40	670.39	636.87	732.40	90
59120	Ectopic pregnancy requiring salpingectomy and/or oophorectomy	789.26	722.43	686.31	789.26	90
59121	Without salpingectomy and/or oophorectomy	638.84	584.75	555.51	638.84	90
59130	Abdominal pregnancy	699.12	639.93	607.93	699.12	90
59135	Total hysterectomy, interstitial, uterine pregnancy	1154.16	1056.44	1003.62	1154.16	90
59136	Partial uterine resection, interstitial uterine pregnancy	1154.16	1056.44	1003.62	1154.16	90
59140	Cervical, with evacuation	489.68	448.22	425.81	489.68	90
59160	Curettage postpartum hemorrhage (separate proc)	293.46	268.61	255.18	293.46	10
59400	OB care—routine, incl. antepartum/postpartum care	1864.30	1706.45	1621.13	1864.30	N/A
59510	C-section including antepartum and postpartum care	2102.33	1924.33	1828.11	2102.33	N/A
59515	C-section, postpartum care only	1469.80	1345.36	1278.09	1469.80	N/A

*Data for the surgical follow-up days from St. Anthony's *CPT'96 Companion: A Guide to Medicare Billing*.

Continued

Table 3. Mock Fee Schedule—cont'd

Code Number	Description	Mock Fees	Medicare			
			Participating	Non-participating	Limiting Charge	Follow-Up Days*
59812	Treatment of incompl abortion, any trimester;	357.39	327.13	310.77	357.39	90
61314	Craniotomy infratentorial	2548.09	2332.35	2215.73	2548.09	90
62270	Spinal puncture, lumbar; diagnostic	77.52	70.96	67.41	77.52	0
65091	Evisceration of eye, without implant	708.22	648.25	615.84	708.22	90
65205	Removal of foreign body, ext eye	56.02	51.27	48.71	56.02	0
65222	Removal of foreign body, corneal, with slit lamp	73.81	67.56	64.18	73.81	0
69420	Myringotomy	97.76	89.48	85.01	97.76	10

*Data for the surgical follow-up days from St. Anthony's *CPT'96 Companion: A Guide to Medicare Billing*.

Table 3. Mock Fee Schedule—cont'd					
			Medicare*		
Code Number	Description	Mock Fees	Participating	Nonparticipating	Limiting Charge
RADIOLOGY, NUCLEAR MEDICINE, AND DIAGNOSTIC ULTRASOUND					
70120	X-ray mastoids, less than 3 views per side	38.96	35.66	33.88	38.96
70130	Complete, min., 3 views per side	56.07	51.33	48.76	56.07
71010	Chest x-ray, 1 view	31.95	29.24	27.78	31.95
71020	Chest x-ray, 2 views	40.97	37.50	35.63	40.97
71030	Chest x-ray, compl, 4 views	54.02	49.44	46.97	54.02
71060	Bronchogram, bilateral	143.75	131.58	125.00	143.75
72100	X-ray spine, LS; 2 or 3 views	43.23	39.57	37.59	43.23
72114	Complete, incl. bending views	74.97	68.62	65.19	74.97
73100	X-ray wrist, 2 views	31.61	28.94	27.49	31.61
73500	X-ray hip, 1 view, 1 side	31.56	28.88	27.44	31.56
73540	X-ray pelvis & hips, infant or child, minimum 2 views	37.94	34.73	32.99	37.94
73590	X-ray tibia & fibula, 2 views	33.35	30.53	29.00	33.35
73620	Radiologic exam, foot; 2 views	31.61	28.94	27.49	31.61
73650	X-ray calcaneus, 2 views	30.71	28.11	26.70	30.71
74241	Radiologic exam, upper gastrointestinal tract; with/without delayed films with KUB	108.93	99.71	94.72	108.93
74245	With small bowel, serial films	161.70	148.01	140.61	161.70
74270	Barium enema	118.47	108.44	103.02	118.47
74290	Cholecystography, oral contrast	52.59	48.14	45.73	52.59
74400	Urography (pyelography), intravenous, with or without KUB	104.78	95.90	91.11	104.78
74410	Urography, infusion	116.76	106.87	101.53	116.76
74420	Urography, retrograde	138.89	127.13	120.77	138.89
75982	Percutaneous placement of drainage catheter	359.08	328.67	312.24	359.08
76805	Ultrasound, pregnant uterus, or real time; complete, first gestation	154.18	141.13	134.07	154.18
76810	Ultrasound, pregnant uterus, complete: each additional gestation, after first trimester	306.54	280.59	266.56	306.54
76946	Ultrasonic guidance for amniocentesis	91.22	83.49	79.32	91.22
77055	Mammography, unilateral	62.57	57.27	54.41	62.57
77056	Mammography, bilateral	82.83	75.82	72.03	82.83
77300	Radiation dosimetry	97.58	89.32	84.85	97.58
77315	Teletherapy, isodose plan, complex	213.59	195.51	185.73	213.59
78104	Bone marrow imaging, whole body	230.56	211.04	200.49	230.56
78215	Liver and spleen imaging	160.44	146.85	139.51	160.44
78800	Tumor localization, limited area	191.53	175.32	166.55	191.53

*Some services and procedures may not be considered a benefit under the Medicare program and when listed on a claim form, no reimbursement may be received. However, it is important to include these codes when billing because Medicare policies may change without an individual knowing of a new benefit. For this reason, some of the services shown in this Mock Fee Schedule do not have any amounts listed under the three Medicare columns.

PATHOLOGY AND LABORATORY[1]

Laboratory tests done as groups or combination "profiles" performed on multichannel equipment should be billed using the appropriate code number (80048 through 80076). Following is a list of the tests. The subsequent listing illustrates how to find the correct code.

Alanine aminotransferase (ALT, SGPT)
Albumin
Aspartate aminotransferase (AST, SGOT)
Bilirubin, direct
Bilirubin, total
Calcium
Carbon dioxide content
Chloride
Cholesterol
Creatinine
Glucose (sugar)
Lactate dehydrogenase (LD)
Phosphatase, alkaline
Phosphorus (inorganic phosphate)
Potassium
Protein, total
Sodium
Urea nitrogen (BUN)
Uric acid

[1]Mock fees for laboratory tests presented in this schedule may not be representative of fees in your region due to the variety of capitation and managed care contracts, as well as discount policies made by laboratories. At the time of this edition, Medicare guidelines may or may not pay for automatic multichannel tests where a large number of tests are performed per panel. Some cases require documentation and a related diagnostic code for each test performed. Provider must have the CLIA level of licensure to bill for tests, and test results must be documented.

Continued

Table 3. Mock Fee Schedule—cont'd

Code Number	Description	Mock Fees	Medicare* Participating	Medicare* Nonparticipating	Medicare* Limiting Charge
ORGAN OR DISEASE-ORIENTED PANELS					
80048	Basic metabolic panel	15.00	14.60	13.87	16.64
80050	General health panel	20.00	19.20	15.99	21.87
80051	Electrolyte panel	20.00	19.20	15.99	21.87
80053	Comprehensive metabolic panel	25.00	20.99	19.94	23.93
80055	Obstetric panel	25.00	20.99	19.94	23.93
80061	Lipid panel	30.00	28.60	25.97	32.16
80074	Acute hepatitis panel	27.00	25.00	20.88	24.88
80076	Hepatic function panel	27.00	25.00	20.88	24.98
81000	Urinalysis, non-automated, with microscopy	8.00	7.44	5.98	8.84
81001	Urinalysis, automated, with microscopy	8.00	7.44	5.98	8.84
81002	Urinalysis, non-automated without microscopy	8.00	7.44	5.98	8.84
81015	Urinalysis, microscopy only	8.00	7.44	5.98	8.84
82270	Blood, occult; feces screening 1-3	4.05	3.56	3.31	4.05
82565	Creatinine; blood	10.00	9.80	8.88	12.03
82947	Glucose; quantitative	15.00			
82951	Glucose tol test, 3 spec	40.00	41.00	36.80	45.16
82952	Each add spec beyond 3	30.00	28.60	25.97	32.16
83020	Hemoglobin, electrophoresis	25.00	20.00	19.94	23.93
83700	Lipoprotein, blood; electrophoretic separation	25.00	20.00	19.94	23.93
84478	Triglycerides, blood	20.00	19.20	15.999	21.87
84480	Triiodothyronine (T-3)	20.00	19.20	15.99	21.87
84520	Urea nitrogen, blood (BUN); quantitative	25.00	20.99	19.94	23.93
84550	Uric acid, blood chemical	20.00	19.20	15.99	21.87
84702	Gonadotropin, chorionic; quantitative	20.00	19.20	15.99	21.87
84703	Gonadotropin, chorionic; qualitative	20.00	19.20	15.99	21.87
85013	Microhematocrit (spun)	20.00	19.20	15.99	21.87
85025	Complete blood count (hemogram), platelet count, automated, differential WBC count	25.00	20.00	19.94	23.93
85032	Manual cell count (erythrocyte, leukocyte, or platelet) each	20.00	19.20	15.99	21.87
85345	Coagulation time; Lee & White	20.00	19.20	15.99	21.87
86038	Antinuclear antibodies	25.00	20.00	19.94	23.93
86580	Skin test; TB, intradermal	11.34	10.38	9.86	11.34
87081	Culture, bacterial, screening for single organisms	25.00	20.00	19.94	23.93
87181	Sensitivity studies, antibiotic; per antibiotic	20.00	19.20	15.99	21.87
87184	Disk method, per plate (12 disks or less)	20.00	19.20	15.99	21.87
87210	Smear, primary source, wet mount with simple stain, for bacteria, fungi, ova, and/or parasites	35.00	48.35	45.93	55.12
88150	Papanicolaou, cytopath	35.00	48.35	45.93	55.12
88302	Surgical pathology, gross & micro exam (skin, fingers, nerve, testis)	24.14	22.09	20.99	24.14
88305	Bone marrow, interpret	77.69	71.12	67.56	77.69

*Some services and procedures may not be considered a benefit under the Medicare program and when listed on a claim form, no reimbursement may be received. However, it is important to include these codes when billing because Medicare policies may change without an individual knowing of a new benefit. For this reason, some of the services shown in this Mock Fee Schedule do not have any amounts listed under the three Medicare columns.

Table 3. Mock Fee Schedule—cont'd					
			Medicare*		
Code Number	**Description**	**Mock Fees**	**Participating**	**Nonparticipating**	**Limiting Charge**
MEDICINE PROCEDURES					
Immunization Injections					
90701	Diphtheria, tetanus, pertussis	34.00			
90703	Tetanus toxoid	28.00			
90712	Poliovirus vaccine, oral	28.00			
Therapeutic Injections					
96372	Therapeutic prophylactic or Dx injection; IM or SC	5.22	4.37	4.15	5.22
96374	Intravenous push, single or initial substance/drug	21.33	19.53	18.55	21.33
96379	Intravenous therapeutic prophylactic, or diagnostic	21.33	19.53	18.55	21.33
Psychiatry					
90816	Individual psychotherapy 20-30 min	60.25	55.15	52.39	60.25
90853	Group therapy	29.22	26.75	25.41	29.22
Hemodialysis					
90935	Single phys evaluation	117.23	107.31	101.94	117.23
90937	Repeat evaluation	206.24	188.78	179.34	206.24
Gastroenterology					
91000	Esophageal incubation	69.82	63.91	60.71	69.82
91055	Gastric incubation	87.41	80.01	76.01	87.41
Ophthalmologic Services					
92004	Comprehensive eye exam	90.86	83.17	79.01	90.86
92100	Tonometry	47.31	43.31	41.14	47.31
92230	Fluorescein angioscopy	55.49	50.79	48.25	55.49
92275	Electroretinography	81.17	74.29	70.58	81.17
92531	Spontaneous nystagmus	26.00			
Audiologic Function Tests					
92557	Comprehensive audiometry	54.33	49.73	47.24	54.33
92596	Ear measurements	26.81	24.54	23.31	26.81
Cardiovascular Therapeutic Services					
93000	Electrocardiogram (ECG)	34.26	31.36	29.79	34.26
93015	Treadmill ECG	140.71	128.80	122.36	140.71
93040	Rhythm ECG, 1-3 leads	18.47	16.90	16.06	18.47
93306	Doppler echocardiography	250.73	229.50	218.03	250.73
93307	Echocardiography without Doppler	114.60	104.90	99.65	114.60
Pulmonary					
94010	Spirometry	38.57	35.31	33.54	38.57
94060	Spirometry before and after bronchodilator	71.67	65.60	62.32	71.67
94150	Vital capacity, total	13.82	12.65	12.02	13.82

*Some services and procedures may not be considered a benefit under the Medicare program and when listed on a claim form, no reimbursement may be received. However, it is important to include these codes when billing because Medicare policies may change without an individual knowing of a new benefit. For this reason, some of the services shown in this Mock Fee Schedule do not have any amounts listed under the three Medicare columns.

Continued

Table 3. Mock Fee Schedule—cont'd

Code Number	Description	Mock Fees	Medicare* Participating	Medicare* Nonparticipating	Medicare* Limiting Charge
Allergy and Clinical Immunology					
95024	Intradermal tests; immediate reaction	6.58	6.02	5.72	6.85
95028	Intradermal tests; delayed reaction	9.32	8.85	10.18	9.32
95044	Patch tests	8.83	8.08	7.68	8.83
95115	Treatment for allergy, single inj.	17.20	15.75	14.96	17.20
95117	2 or more inj.	22.17	20.29	19.28	22.17
95165	Allergen immunotherapy, single or multiple antigens, multiple-dose vials (professional svcs for preparation supervision)		6.50	6.18	7.11
Neurology					
95812	Electroencephalogram, 41-60 min	129.32	118.37	112.45	129.32
95819	Electroencephalogram—awake and	126.81	116.07	110.27	126.81
95860	Electromyography, 1 extremity	88.83	81.31	77.24	88.83
95864					
96101	Psychological testing (per hour)	80.95	74.10	70.39	80.95
Physical Medicine					
97024	Diathermy	14.27	13.06	12.41	14.27
97036	Hubbard tank, each 15 min	24.77	22.67	21.54	24.77
97110	Physical therapy, initial 30 min	23.89	21.86	20.77	23.89
97140	Manual therapy (manipulation, traction), one or more regions, each 15 min	16.93	15.49	14.72	16.93
Chiropractic Manipulative Treatment					
98940	Chiropractic manipulative treatment; spinal 1-2 regions	75.00			
Special Services and Reports					
99000	Handling of specimen (transfer from Dr.'s office to lab)	5.00			
99050	Services provided after office hours, or on Sundays and holidays in addition to basic service in the office	25.00			
99053	Services between 10 PM and 8 AM in addition to basic service	35.00			
99056	Services normally provided in office requested by pt in location other than office	20.00			
99058	Office services provided on an emergency basis	65.00			
99070	Supplies and materials (itemize drugs and materials provided)	25.00			
99080	Special reports:				
	Insurance forms	10.00			
	Review of data to clarify pt's status	20.00			
	WC reports	50.00			
	WC extensive review report	250.00			

*Some services and procedures may not be considered a benefit under the Medicare program and when listed on a claim form, no reimbursement may be received. However, it is important to include these codes when billing because Medicare policies may change without an individual knowing of a new benefit. For this reason, some of the services shown in this Mock Fee Schedule do not have any amounts listed under the three Medicare columns.

INDEX

A

B

C

Colectomy	44140-44160
Colonoscopy, fiberoptic	45355-45385
Colostomy, separate procedure	44320
Colporrhaphy	57240-57265, 57289
Colposcopy	57452-57460
Complete blood count	85022-85031
Conization, cervix	57520-57522
Consultation	
during surgery (pathology)	88329-88332
initial	99251-99255
office	99241-99245
telephone calls	99371-99373
with examination and evaluation	99241-99255
Counseling—Preventive Medicine	
group	99411, 99412
individual	99401-99404
Craniotomy	61314
Creatinine	82540, 82565-82570
Critical care	
first 30-74 minutes	99291
each additional 30 minutes	99292
neonatal	99295-99297
Culture, bacterial	87040-87088
Custodial care medical services	
established patient	99334-99337
new patient	99324-99328
Cystourethroscopy	52000-52340

D

Débridement	
nails	11720-11721
skin	11040-11044
Destruction benign lesion, any method	
face	17000-17010
other than face	17100-17105
Dentition, prolonged physician attendance	99354-99360
Dilation	
dilatation and curettage	57820, 58120, 59160, 59840, 59851
esophagus	43450-43460
urethra, female	53660-53661
urethra, male	53620-53621
Diathermy	97024
Domiciliary visits	
established patient	99334-99337
new patient	99324-99328
Dosimetry	77300, 77331

E

Ear	
excision, benign lesion, external	11440-11446
layer closure, wounds	12051-12057
simple repair, wounds	12011-12018
Echocardiography	93307
Echography, pregnant uterus	76805-76816
Electrocardiogram	93000-93042
Electroencephalogram	95819-95827
Electromyography	95858, 95860-95869
Electroretinography	92275

Emergency department services	99281-99288
Endoscopy, gastrointestinal, upper	43234-43264
Esophageal intubation	91000
Excision—see organ, region, or structure involved	
Eye	
excision	65091
removal foreign body	65205-65222
Eyelid	
excision, benign lesion	11440-11446
layer closure, wounds	12051-12057
repair, simple	12011-12018

F

Face	
excision, benign lesion	11440-11446
layer closure, wounds (intermediate)	12051-12057
simple repair, wounds	12011-12018
Feces screening; blood occult	82270
Feet—see foot	
Fluorescein angioscopy, ophthalmoscopy	92230
Foot	
excision, benign lesion, skin	11420-11426
radiologic exam	73620-73630
simple repair, wounds	12001-12007
Fracture	
femur shaft	27500-27508
nasal	21300-21339
tibia proximal, plateau	27530-27537
tibia shaft	27750-27758

G

Gastric intubation	91055
Gastrointestinal tract, radiologic examination	74210-74340
Gastrojejunostomy	43632, 43820-43825, 43860-43865
Genitalia	
excision, benign lesion	11420-11426
repair, simple	12001-12007
Glucose, quantitative	82947
Glucose tolerance test	82951, 82952
Gonadotropin, chorionic	84702, 84703

H

Handling of specimen	99000
Hands	
excision, benign lesion	11420-11426
simple repair, wounds	12001-12007
Hemodialysis	90935-90937
insertion of cannula	36800-36815
placement, venous catheter	36245-36248
Hemoglobin electrophoresis	83020
Hemorrhage, nasal	30901-30906
Hemorrhoidectomy	46221-46262
Hernia, inguinal	49495-49525
Hip, radiologic examination	73500-73540
Home visits	
established patient	99347-99350
new patient	99341-99345

Physical medicine services	97010-97150
Platelet count	85590
Pleurectomy	32310
Pneumonectomy	32440-32450
Preventive medicine	
established patient	99391-99397
health hazard appraisal	99420
new patient	99381-99387
unlisted	99429
Proctosigmoidoscopy	45300-45321
Prolonged services	
inpatient or outpatient setting	99354-99359
Prostatectomy, perineal, subtotal	55801
Psychiatric evaluation of records, reports, and/or tests	90825
Psychological testing	96101
Psychotherapy	
pharmacologic management	90862
family (conjoint)	90847
group medical	90853
individual	90816
multiple-family	90849
Puncture, lumbar spine	62270, 62272

Q

Quadriceps repair	27430

R

Radiology	
dosimetry	77300, 77331
teletherapy	77305-77315, 77321
therapeutic	77261-77799
treatment delivery	77401-77417
Repair—see procedure, organ, structure, or region involved	
Reports, special	99080
Resection, prostate, transurethral	52601-54640

S

Salpingectomy and/or oophorectomy	59120-59140
excision, benign lesion	11420-11422
layer closure, wounds	12031-12037
simple repair, wounds	12001-12007
Salpingo-oophorectomy	58720
Sensitivity studies, antibiotic	87181-87192
Septum, nasal septoplasty	30520
Sigmoidoscopy	45330-45333
Skene's gland	53060-53270
Skin excision, skin tags	11200, 11201
Splenectomy	38100-38115
Smear, primary source	87205-87211
Spine, radiologic exam	72010-72120
Spirometry	94010-94070
Standby services	99360
Supplies and materials	99070, 99071

T

TB skin test	86580
Teletherapy	77305-77321

Telephone calls	99441-99443
Thromboendarterectomy	35301-35381
Tibia, radiologic exam	73590
Tonometry	92100
Tonsillectomy	42820-42826
TURP	52601-52648
Treadmill exercise	93015-93018
Triglycerides	84478
Triiodothyronine	84479-84482
Trunk	
excision, malignant lesion	11600-11606
layer closure—intermediate	12031-12037
simple repair	12001-12007
Tumor localization	78800-78803

U

Ureteroneocystostomy	50780-50800
Urethral diverticulum, excision	53230-53235
Uric acid	84550-84560
Urinalysis	81000-81099
Urography	74400-74425

V

Venipuncture	36400-36425
Vesicovaginal fistula, closure	51900, 57320, 57330
Vital capacity (pulmonary function)	94010, 94150, 94160

W

Wrist, radiologic examination	73100, 73110

X

Xenograft	15400

Y

Y-plasty, bladder	51800

Z

Z-plasty	14000, 26121, 41520

B Medicare Level II HCPCS Codes

The following pages provide a partial alphanumeric list of the Centers for Medicare and Medicaid Services (CMS), referred to as Healthcare Common Procedure Coding System (HCPCS) (pronounced "hick-picks"). These Level II codes and modifiers were adopted by the Medicare program in 1984; additional codes and modifiers are added and deleted every year. This system was developed to code procedures not listed in the American Medical Association's *Current Procedural Terminology* (CPT) code book. This second level is a national standard used by all regional Medicare carriers.

Partial List of the Medicare Healthcare Common Procedure Coding System (HCPCS)

In certain circumstances, a code may need a modifier to show that the procedure has been changed by a specific situation. Remember that CPT and national modifiers apply to both CPT and HCPCS code systems. When applicable, indicate the appropriate modifier on the insurance claim form (Tables 1 and 2). Sometimes a special report may be needed to clarify the use of the modifier to the insurance company.

Table 1. Medicare HCPCS Modifiers

Modifier	Short Description
A1	Dressing for one wound
A2	Dressing for two wounds
A3	Dressing for three wounds
A4	Dressing for four wounds
A5	Dressing for five wounds
A6	Dressing for six wounds
A7	Dressing for seven wounds
A8	Dressing for eight wounds
A9	Dressing for nine or more wounds
AA	Anesthesia performed personally by anesthesiologist
AD	Physician supervision; more than four concurrent anesthesia procedures
AE	Registered dietitian
AF	Specialty physician
AG	Primary physician
AH	Clinical psychologist
AJ	Clinical social worker
AK	Nonparticipating physician
AM	Physician, team member service
AP	No determination of refractive state
AR	Physician scarcity area
AS	Non-NPP assistant-at-surgery service
AT	Acute treatment
AU	Uro, ostomy, or trach item
AV	Item with prosthetic/orthotic
AW	Item with a surgical dressing
AX	Item with dialysis services
AY	Item or service furnished to an end-stage renal disease patient that is not for the treatment of ESRD
AZ	Physician providing service in dental health professional–shortage area for electronic health record incentive pmt
BA	Item with pen services
BO	Nutrition oral admin no tube
BP	Beneficiary elected to purchase item
BR	Beneficiary elected to rent item
BU	Beneficiary undecided on purch/rent
CA	Procedure payable inpatient
CB	ESRD beneficiary Part A SNF-sep pay
CC	Procedure code change
CD	AMCC test for ESRD or MCP physician
CE	Med necessity AMCC test sep reimbursement
CF	AMCC test not composite rate
DA	Oral health assessment by licensed health professional other than dentist
E1	Upper left eyelid
E2	Lower left eyelid
E3	Upper right eyelid
E4	Lower right eyelid
EJ	Subsequent claim
EM	Emergency reserve supply (ESRD)
EP	Medicaid EPSDT program SVC
ET	Emergency treatment
EY	No physician/health care provider order for item/service
FA	Left hand, thumb
FP	Service provided as part of family planning program
F1	Left hand, second digit
F2	Left hand, third digit

Continued

Table 1. Medicare HCPCS Modifiers—cont'd

Modifier	Short Description
F3	Left hand, fourth digit
F4	Left hand, fifth digit
F5	Right hand, thumb
F6	Right hand, second digit
F7	Right hand, third digit
F8	Right hand, fourth digit
F9	Right hand, fifth digit
G1	URR reading of less than 60
G2	URR reading of 60 to 64.9
G3	URR reading of 65 to 69.9
G4	URR reading of 70 to 74.9
G5	URR reading of 75 or greater
G6	ERSD patient less than 6 dialysis/mth
G7	Pregnancy as result of rape or incest or pregnancy certified by physician as life threatening
G8	Monitored anesthesia care
G9	MAC for at-risk patient
GA	Waiver of liability statement issued, as required by payer policy (for covered charges)
GB	Claim resubmitted
GC	Resident/teaching phys serv
GE	Resident primary care exception
GF	Nonphysician serv in critical access hosp
GG	Payment screen mam diag mam, same pt, same day
GH	Diag mammo to screening mammo
GJ	Opt out physician or practitioner of ER serv
GK	Reasonable and necessary service associated with modifier GA or GZ
GL	Upgraded item, no charge
GM	Multiple transports per ambulance
GN	OP speech language service
GO	OP occupational therapy serv
GP	OP PT services
GQ	Telehealth store and forward
GT	Interactive telecommunication
GU	Waiver of liability statement issued as required by payer policy, routine notice
GV	Attending phys not hospice
GW	Service unrelated to terminal condition of hospice pt
GX	Notice of liability issued, voluntary under payer policy (services excluded from coverage) for noncovered charges
GY	Statutorily excluded
GZ	Not reasonable and necessary
H9	Court ordered
HA	Child/adolescent program
HB	Adult program nongeriatric
HC	Adult program geriatric
HD	Pregnant/parenting women's program
HE	Mental health program
HF	Substance abuse program
HG	Opioid addiction tx program
HH	Mental hlth/substance abs pr
HI	M health/m retrdtn/dev dis pro
HJ	Employee assistance program
HK	Spec high-risk mntl hlth pop p
HL	Intern
HM	Less than bachelor's degree level
HN	Bachelor's degree level
HO	Master's degree level
HP	Doctoral level
HQ	Group setting
HR	Family/couple with client present
HS	Family/couple without client present
HT	Multidisciplinary team
HU	Child welfare agency funded
HV	Funded state addiction agency
HW	State mntl hlth agency funded
HX	County/local agency funded
HY	Funded by juvenile justice agency
HZ	Criminal justice agency fund
JW	Discarded drug not administered
K0	LWR EXT PROST FUNCTNL LVL 0
K1	LWR EXT PROST FUNCTNL LVL 1
K2	LWR EXT PROST FUNCTNL LVL 2
K3	LWR EXT PROST FUNCTNL LVL 3
K4	LWR EXT PROST FUNCTNL LVL 4
KA	Wheelchair add-on option/acc
KB	More than four modifiers on claim, based on beneficiary request for ABN upgrade
KC	Replace special power wheelchair interface
KD	Drug/biological dme infused
KF	FDA class III device
KH	DME POS INI CLM, PUR/1 MO RNT
KI	DME POS 2nd or 3rd mo rental
KJ	DME POS PEN PMP or 4-15 mo rent
KM	RPLC facial prosth new imp
KN	RPLC facial prosth old mod
KO	Single drug unit dose form
KP	First drug of multidrug UD
KQ	2nd/subsqnt drg multi DRG UD
KR	Rental item partial month
KS	Glucose monitor supply
KX	Documentation on file
KZ	New cov not implement by MC
LC	Left circumflex coronary artery
LD	Left anterior descending coronary artery
LL	Lease/rental (Applied to purchase price)
LR	Laboratory round trip
LS	FDA-monitored intraocular lens implant
LT	Left side
MS	6 mo maint/svc fee parts/lbr if services not covered under warranty
NB	Nebulizer system, any type, FDA cleared for use with specific drug

Table 1. Medicare HCPCS Modifiers—cont'd

Modifier	Short Description
NR	New when rented
NU	New equipment
PL	Progressive addition lenses
PT	Colorectal cancer screening test; converted to diagnostic test or other procedure
Q0	Investigational clinical service provided in a clinical research study that is in an approved clinical research study
Q1	Routine clinical service provided in a clinical research study that is in an approved clinical research study
Q2	HCFA/ord demo procedure/svc
Q3	Live donor surgery/services
Q4	Service exempt ordering/referring physician
Q5	Substitute physician service, recip bill arrangement
Q6	Locum tenens physician service
Q7	One Class A finding
Q8	Two Class B findings
Q9	One Class B and two Class C findings
QB	Physician providing SVC in rural HPSA
QC	Single-channel monitoring
QD	Recording/storage in solid-state memory
QE	Prescribed oxygen <1 LPM
QF	Prescribed oxygen >4 LPM & port
QG	Prescribed oxygen >4 LPM
QH	Oxygen-conserving device with delivery system
QJ	Patient in state/local custody
QK	Med dir 2-4 concurrent anes proc
QL	Patient died after Amb call
QM	Ambulance arrangement by hospital
QN	Ambulance furnished by provider
QP	Individually ordered lab test
QQ	SOI submitted with claim
QS	Monitored anesthesia care
QT	Recording/storage tape analog recorder
QU	Physician providing service urban HPSA
QW	CLIA waived test
QX	CRNA service with physician med direction
QY	Medically directed CRNA
QZ	CRNA service: without medical direction by physician
RC	Right coronary artery
RD	Drug admin not incident-to
RR	Rental (DME)
RT	Right side
SA	Nurse practitioner with physician
SB	Nurse midwife
SC	Medically necessary serv/sup
SD	Service by home infusion RN
SE	State/Fed funded program/serv
SF	Second opinion ordered by PRO
SG	Ambulatory surgical center facility service
SH	Second concurrent infusion therapy
SJ	Third concurrent infusion therapy
SK	High-risk population
SL	State supplied vaccine
SM	Second opinion
SN	Third opinion
SQ	Item ordered by home health
ST	Related to trauma or injury
SU	Performed in phys office
SV	Drugs delivered not used
SW	Serv by cert diab educator
SY	Contact w/high-risk pop
T1	Left foot, second digit
T2	Left foot, third digit
T3	Left foot, fourth digit
T4	Left foot, fifth digit
T5	Right foot, great toe
T6	Right foot, second digit
T7	Right foot, third digit
T8	Right foot, fourth digit
T9	Right foot, fifth digit
TA	Left foot, great toe
TC	Technical component
TD	RN
TE	LPN/LVN
TF	Intermediate level of care
TG	Complex/high tech level care
TH	OB tx/servcs prenatl/postpart
TJ	Child/adolescent program GP
TK	Extra patient or passenger
TL	Early intervention IFSP
TM	Individualized ED prrm (EP)
TN	Rural/out of service area
TP	Med transprt unloaded vehicle
TQ	Bls by volunteer amb provider
TR	School-based IEP out of district
TS	Follow-up service
TT	Additional patient
TU	Overtime payment rate
TV	Holiday/weekend payment rate
TW	Back-up equipment
U1	Medicaid care Level 1 state def
U2	Medicaid care Level 2 state def
U3	Medicaid care Level 3 state def
U4	Medicaid care Level 4 state def
U5	Medicaid care Level 5 state def
U6	Medicaid care Level 6 state def
U7	Medicaid care Level 7 state def
U8	Medicaid care Level 8 state def
U9	Medicaid care Level 9 state def
UA	Medicaid care Level 10 state def
UB	Medicaid care Level 11 state def

Continued

Table 1. Medicare HCPCS Modifiers—cont'd

Modifier	Short Description	Modifier	Short Description
UC	Medicaid care Level 12 state def	UK	Service on behalf client-collateral
UD	Medicaid care Level 13 state def	UN	Two patients served
UE	Used durable medical equipment	UP	Three patients served
UF	Services provided, morning	UQ	Four patients served
UG	Services provided, afternoon	UR	Five patients served
UH	Services provided, evening	US	Six or more patients served
UJ	Services provided, night	VP	Aphakic patient

Table 2. HCPCS Alphanumeric Index

Description	Code
A	
above-elbow endoskeletal prostheses	L6500
above-elbow prostheses	L6250
acetazolamide sodium (Diamox), injection	J1120
actinomycin D, injection	J9120
adjustable arms, wheelchair	E0973
adjustable chair, dialysis	E1570
adrenaline, injection	J0170
ambulance oxygen and oxygen supplies	A0422
air bubble detector, dialysis	E1530
air travel and nonemergency transport	A0140
alarm, pressure dialysis	E1540
alcohol	A4244
alcohol wipes	A4245
alternating pressure pad, powered pressure	E0181
aminophylline, injection	J0280
amitriptyline HCl (Elavil), injection	J1320
ammonia test paper	A4774
amobarbital sodium (Amytal sodium), injection	J0300
ampicillin, injection	J0290
ampicillin sodium (Omnipen-N), injection	J2430
amputee adapter, wheelchair	E0959
amputee wheelchair, detachable elevating leg rests	E1170
amputee wheelchair, detachable foot rests	E1200
amygdalin, injection	J3570
anesthetics, topical, for dialysis	A4736
ankle prostheses, Syme's, metal frame	L5060
ankle prostheses, Syme's, molded socket	L5050
antineoplastic drugs, not otherwise classified (NOC)	J9999
antitipping device, wheelchair	E0971
appliance, pneumatic	E0655
arm rest, wheelchair	E0994
arms, adjustable, wheelchair	E0973
asparaginase (Elspar), injection	J9020
atropine sulfate, injection	J0460
aurothioglucose (Solganal), injection	J2910
axillary crutch extension	L0978

Table 2. HCPCS Alphanumeric Index—cont'd

Description	Code
B	
bath conductivity meter, dialysis	E1550
BCNU (carmustine, bis-chloroethyl-nitrosourea), injection	J9050
bed accessories: boards, tables	E0315
bed pan	E0276
below-elbow endoskeletal prostheses	L6400
belt, extremity	E0945
belt, ostomy	A4367
belt, pelvic	E0944
bench, bathtub	E0245
benztropine, injection	J0515
bethanechol chloride, injection	J0520
bethanechol chloride (Myotonachol), injection	J0520
bethanechol chloride (Urecholine), injection	J0520
bicarbonate concentrate for hemodialysis per gallon	A4706
bilirubin (phototherapy) light	E0202
biperiden HCl (Akineton), injection	J0190
bis-chloroethyl-nitrosourea, injection	J9050
bleomycin sulfate, injection	J9040
blood, mucoprotein	P2038
blood (split unit), specify amount	P9011
blood (whole), for transfusion, per unit	P9010
blood leak detector, dialysis	El560
blood pressure monitor	A4670
blood pump, dialysis	El620
blood strips	A4253
blood testing supplies	A4770
bond or cement, ostomy skin	A4364
brompheniramine maleate (Dehist), injection	J0945
C	
calcitonin (salmon) (Calcimar), injection	J0630
calcium disodium edetate (Versenate), injection	J0600
calcium gluconate, injection	J0610
calcium glycerophosphate and calcium lactate (Calphosan), injection	J0620
calcium leucovorin, injection	J0640
calf rest, wheelchair	E0995
calibrator solution	A4256
canes	E0100
carbon filters	A4680
carmustine, injection	J9050
cast supplies	
long leg, adult (11 years), cylinder, fiberglass	Q4034
long leg, adult (11 years), cylinder, plaster	Q4033
long leg, adult (11 years), fiberglass	Q4030
catheter caps, disposable (dialysis)	A4860
catheter insertion tray	A4354
catheter irrigation set	A4355
cefazolin sodium, injection	J0690
ceftriaxone sodium (Rocephin), 250-mg injection	J0696
cellular therapy	M0075
cement, ostomy	A4364
centrifuge	A4650

Continued

Table 2. HCPCS Alphanumeric Index—cont'd

Description	Code
cephalin flocculation, blood	P2028
cephalothin sodium (Keflin), injection	J1890
cephapirin sodium, injection	J0710
cervical head harness/halter	E0942
chair, adjustable, dialysis	E1570
chelation therapy, intravenous (chemical endarterectomy)	M0300
chin cup, cervical	L0150
chloramphenicol (Chloromycetin Sodium Succinate), injection	J0720
chlordiazepoxide HCl (Librium), injection	J1990
chloroprocaine HCl (Nesacaine), injection	J2400
chloroquine HCl (Aralen HCl), injection	J0390
chlorothiazide sodium (Diuril), injection	J1205
chlorpromazine (Thorazine), injection	J3230
chorionic gonadotropin, injection	J0725
clamps, dialysis, venous pressure	A4918
clotting time tube	A4771
codeine phosphate, injection	J0745
Colchicine injection	J0760
colistimethate sodium (Coly-Mycin M), injection	J0770
commode seat, wheelchair	E0968
compressor	E0565
compressor, pneumatic	E0650
conductive paste or gel	A4558
Congo red blood	P2029
contracts, repair and maintenance, ESRD	A4890
corticotropin, injection	J0800
crutches	E0110
cryoprecipitate, each unit	P9012
culture sensitivity study	P7001
Cycler, hemodialysis	E1590
Cycler dialysis machine	E1594
cyclophosphamide, injection	J9070
D	
dactinomycin (Cosmegen) or actinomycin, injection	J9120
daunorubicin HCl, injection	J9150
decubitus care pad	E0185
deionizer, water purification system	El615
detector, blood leak, dialysis	El560
dexamethasone sodium phosphate, injection	J1100
dextrose/normal saline, solution	J7042
Dextrostix	A4772
dialysate concentrate additives	A4765
dialysate testing solution	A4760
dialysis, bath conductivity, meter	E1550
dialysis supplies, miscellaneous	A4913
dialyzers	A4690
diazepam (Valium), injection	J3360
diazoxide (Hyperstat), injection	J1730
dicyclomine HCl (Bentyl), injection	J0500
digoxin, injection	J1160
dihydroergotamine mesylate (D.H.E. 45), injection	J1110
dimenhydrinate (Dramamine), injection	J1240

Table 2. HCPCS Alphanumeric Index—cont'd

Description	Code
dimercaprol in peanut oil (BAL in Oil), injection	J0470
dimethyl imidazole carboxamide (DIC) (dacarbazine, DTIC-DOME), 100-mg vial	J9130
dimethyl sulfoxide (DMSO) (Rimso-50), injection	J1212
diphenhydramine HCl (Benadryl), injection	J1200
disarticulation, elbow, prostheses	L6200
doxorubicin (Adriamycin), injection	J9000
drainage bag	A4358
drainage board	E0606
droperidol (Inapsine), injection	J1790
droperidol and fentanyl citrate (Innovar), injection	J1810
drugs, nonprescription	A9150
dyphylline (Dilor), injection	J1180
E	
elbow protector	E0191
electrical work or plumbing, home, dialysis equipment	A4870
electrocardiogram, routine ECG with 12 leads, with interpret and report	G0403
electrocardiogram, routine ECG with 12 leads, without interpret and report	G0404
electrocardiogram, routine ECG with 12 leads, interpret and report only	G0405
electrodes	A4556
elevating leg rest, wheelchair	E0990
endarterectomy, chemical	M0300
epinephrine, injection	J0170
ergonovine maleate (Ergotrate Maleate), injection	J1330
estradiol cypionate (Depo-Estradiol Cypionate), injection	J1000
estradiol valerate (Delestrogen), injection	J0970
estradiol valerate, up to 20 mg (Estraval-2X), injection	J1390
estradiol valerate, up to 10 mg (Estraval P.A.), injection	J1380
estrone, injection	J1435
etoposide, 50 mg, injection	J9181
examination, initial preventive physical	G0402
external ambulatory infusion pump with administration equipment	E0781
extremity belt-harness	E0945
F	
faceplate, ostomy	A4361
fentanyl citrate (Sublimaze), injection	J3010
fistula cannulation set	A4730
flotation mattress	E0184
flotation pad gel pressure	E0185
floxuridine, 500 mg, injection	J9200
fluid barriers, dialysis	El575
fluorouracil, injection	J9190
fluphenazine decanoate (Prolixin Decanoate), injection	J2680
foot rest, for use with commode chair	E0175
footplates, wheelchair	E0970
forearm crutches	E0110
furosemide (Lasix), injection	J1940
G	
gamma globulin, 1 ml, injection	J1460
gel, conductive	A4558
gel flotation pad	E0185
gentamicin, injection	J1580

Continued

Table 2. HCPCS Alphanumeric Index—cont'd

Description	Code
gentamicin sulfate (Garamycin), injection	J1580
gloves, nonsterile, per 100	A4927
glucose test strips	A4772
gold sodium thiosulfate, injection	J1600
Grade-Aid, wheelchair	E0974
gravity traction device	E0941
Gravlee Jet Washer	A4470
H	
hair analysis	P2031
hallux-valgus dynamic splint	L3100
haloperidol (Haldol), injection	J1630
halter, cervical head	E0942
hand rims, wheelchair	E0967
harness, extremity	E0945
harness, pelvic	E0944
harness/halter, cervical head	E0942
head rest extension, wheelchair	E0966
heater for nebulizer	E1372
heel or elbow protector	E0191
heel stabilizer	L3170
Hemastix	A4773
hemipelvectomy prostheses	L5280
hemodialysis, monthly capitation	E0945
hemodialysis unit	E1590
heparin infusion pump, dialysis	E1520
hexachlorophene (pHisoHex) solution	A4246
Hexcelite, cast material—see Q codes under "cast supplies" for specific casts	A4590
HN2 (nitrogen mustard)	J9230
hot water bottle	E0220
hyaluronidase (Wydase), injection	J3470
hydralazine HCl (Apresoline), injection	J0360
hydrocortisone, injection	J1720
hydrocortisone acetate, up to 25 mg, injection	J1700
hydrocortisone phosphate, injection	J1710
hydrocortisone sodium succinate (Solu-Cortef), injection	J1720
hydromorphone (Dilaudid), injection	J1170
hydroxyzine HCl (Vistaril), injection	J3410
hyoscyamine sulfate (Levsin), injection	J1980
hypertonic saline solution	J7130
I	
ice cap or collar	E0230
incontinence clamp	A4356
infusion pump, external ambulatory with administration equipment	E0781
infusion pump, heparin, dialysis	E1520
infusion pump, implantable	E0782
installation and/or delivery charges for ESRD equipment	E1600
insulin, injection	J1815
intercapsular thoracic endoskeletal prostheses	L6570
interferon, injection	J9213
intermittent peritoneal dialysis (IPD) system, automatic	E1592
intermittent positive-pressure breathing (IPPB) machine	E0500

Table 2. HCPCS Alphanumeric Index—cont'd

Description	Code
intraocular lenses, anterior chamber	V2630
intraocular lenses, iris supported	V2631
intraocular lenses, posterior chamber	V2632
iodine I-123 sod. iodide capsule(s) diag.	A9516
iodine swabs/wipes	A4247
irrigation kits, ostomy	A4400
irrigation set, catheter	A4355
IV pole	E0776
K	
kanamycin sulfate, injection	J1840
kanamycin sulfate (Kantrex), up to 75 mg, pediatric, injection	J1850
Kartop patient lift, toilet or bathroom	E0625
L	
laetrile, amygdalin (vitamin B17), injection	J3570
lancets	A4259
lead wires	A4557
leg rest, wheelchair, elevating	E0990
leukocyte-poor blood, each unit	P9016
levorphanol tartrate (Levo-Dromoran), injection	J1960
lidocaine (Xylocaine) injection	J2001
lightweight wheelchair	E1087
lincomycin, injection	J2010
liquid barrier, ostomy	A4363
lubricant, ostomy	A4402
M	
mannitol, injection	J2150
mechlorethamine HCl (Mustargen), injection	J9230
meperidine, injection	J2175
meperidine HCl and promethazine HCl (Mepergan), injection	J2180
metaraminol bitartrate (Aramine), injection	J0380
meter, bath conductivity, dialysis	E1550
methadone HCl, injection	J1230
methocarbamol (Robaxin), injection	J2800
methyldopate HCl (Aldomet Ester HCl)	J0210
methylergonovine maleate (Methergine), injection	J2210
methylprednisolone acetate (Depo-Medrol), injection	J1020
methylprednisolone sodium succinate (Solu Medrol), injection	
up to 40 mg	J2920
up to 125 mg	J2930
metoclopramide HCl (Reglan)	J2765
microbiology tests	P7001
mini-bus, nonemergency transportation	A0120
miscellaneous dialysis supplies	A4913
mithramycin, injection	J9270
mitomycin (Mutamycin), injection	J9280
monitor, blood pressure	A4670
morphine, injection	J2270
mucoprotein, blood	P2038
N	
nandrolone decanoate, up to 50 mg, injection	J2320
nandrolone decanoate, up to 200 mg, injection	J2322

Continued

Table 2. HCPCS Alphanumeric Index—cont'd

Description	Code
narrowing device, wheelchair	E0969
nasal vaccine inhalation	J3530
nebulizer, with compressor	E0570
nebulizer heater	E1372
needle with syringe	A4206
needles	A4215
neonatal transport, ambulance, base rate	A0225
neostigmine methylsulfate (Prostigmin), injection	J2710
neuromuscular stimulator	E0745
nikethamide (Coramine), injection	J3490
nitrogen mustard, injection	J9230
noncovered procedure	A9270
nonprescription drugs	A9150
nonprofit transport, nonemergency	A0120
O	
occipital/mandibular support, cervical	L0160
orphenadrine citrate (Norflex), injection	L2360
orthoses, thoracic-lumbar-sacral (scoliosis)	L1200
orthotic, knee	L1830
ostomy supplies	A4421
oxacillin sodium (Bactocill), injection	J2410
oxymorphone HCl (Numorphan), injection	J2700
oxytetracycline, injection	J2460
oxytocin (Pitocin), injection	J2590
P	
pacemaker monitor, includes audible/visible check systems	E0610
pacemaker monitor, includes digital/visible check systems	E0615
pad for water circulating heat unit	E0249
pail or pan for use with commode chair	E0167
papaverine HCl, injection	J2440
paraffin	A4265
paraffin bath unit	E0235
paste, conductive	A4558
pelvic belt/harness/boot	E0944
penicillin G benzathine (Bicillin L-A), injection	J0560
penicillin G potassium (Pfizerpen), injection	J2540
penicillin procaine, aqueous, injection	J2510
pentazocine HCl (Talwin), injection	J3070
percussor	E0480
peritoneal straps	L0980
peroxide	A4244
perphenazine (Trilafon), injection	J3310
phenobarbital, injection	J2560
phenobarbital sodium, injection	J2515
phentolamine mesylate (Regitine), injection	J2760
phenylephrine HCl (Neo-Synephrine), injection	J2370
phenytoin sodium (Dilantin), injection	J1165
phototherapy, light	E0202
plasma, single donor, fresh frozen, each unit	P9017
platelet concentrate, each unit	P9019
platelet-rich plasma, each unit	P9020

Table 2. HCPCS Alphanumeric Index—cont'd

Description	Code
portable hemodialyzer system	E1635
postural drainage board	E0606
pralidoxime chloride (Protopam Chloride), injection	J2730
prednisolone acetate, injection	J2650
pressure alarm, dialysis	E1540
procainamide HCl (Pronestyl), injection	J2690
prochlorperazine (Compazine), injection	J0780
progesterone, injection	J2675
prolotherapy	M0076
promazine HCl (Sparine), injection	J2950
promethazine HCl (Phenergan), injection	J2550
propiomazine (Largon), injection	J1930
propranolol HCl (Inderal), injection	J1800
prostheses, above elbow, endoskeletal	L6500
prostheses, below elbow, endoskeletal	L6400
prostheses, hemipelvectomy	L5280
prostheses, intercapsular thoracic, endoskeletal	L6570
prostheses, lower extremity, NOC	L5999
prosthetic services, NOC	L8499
protamine sulfate, injection	J2720
protector, heel or elbow	E0191
Q	
Quad cane	E0105
R	
rack/stand, oxygen	E1355
reciprocating peritoneal dialysis system	E1630
red blood cells, each unit	P9021
regulator, oxygen	E1353
reserpine (Sandril), injection	J2820
restraints, any type	E0710
reverse osmosis water purification, ESRD	E1610
Rh_O(D) immune globulin, injection	J2790
rims, hand (wheelchair)	E0967
Ringer's injection	J7120
rings, ostomy	A4404
S	
safety equipment	E0700
safety visit, wheelchair	E0980
seat attachment, walker	E0156
seat insert, wheelchair	E0992
sensitivity study	P7001
serum clotting time tube	A4771
shunt accessories, for dialysis	A4740
sitz bath, portable	E0160
skin bond or cement, ostomy	A4364
sling, patient lift	E0621
slings	A4565
social worker, nonemergency transport	A0160
sodium succinate, injection	J1720
sorbent cartridges, ESRD	E1636
spectinomycin dihydrochloride (Trobicin), injection	J3320

Continued

Table 2. HCPCS Alphanumeric Index—cont'd

Description	Code
sphygmomanometer with cuff and stethoscope	A4660
spinal orthosis, NOC	L1499
splint	A4570
splint, hallux-valgus, night, dynamic	L3100
stand/rack, oxygen	E1355
streptokinase-streptodornase, injection	J2995
streptomycin, injection	J3000
streptozocin, injection	J9320
succinylcholine chloride (Anectine), injection	J0330
suction pump, portable	E0600
supplies for self-administered injections	A4211
surgical stockings, above-knee length	A4490
surgical supplies, miscellaneous	A4649
surgical trays	A4550
swabs, povidone-iodine (Betadine) or iodine	A4247
syringe	A4213
T	
taxi, nonemergency transportation	A0100
terbutaline sulfate, 0.5 mg, injection	J3105
testosterone cypionate (Depo-Testosterone), injection	J1070
testosterone cypionate and estradiol cypionate (Depo-Testadiol), injection	J1060
testosterone propionate, injection	J3150
testosterone suspension, injection	J3140
tetanus immune human globulin (Homo-Tet), injection	J1670
tetracycline, injection	J0120
tetracycline HCl (Achromycin), injection	J0120
theophylline and mersalyl (Salyrgan), injection	J2810
thiethylperazine maleate (Torecan), injection	J3280
thiotepa (triethylenethiophosphoramide), injection	J9340
thymol turbidity, blood	P2033
thyrotropin (TSH), exogenous, up to 10 IU, injection	J3240
tobramycin sulfate (Nebcin), injection	J3260
toilet rail	E0243
toilet seat, raised	E0244
tolazoline HCl (Priscoline), injection	J2670
tolls, nonemergency transport	A0170
traction device, gravity-assisted	E0941
traction equipment, overdoor	E0860
travel hemodialyzer system	E1635
trays, surgical	A4550
triflupromazine HCl (Vesprin), injection	J3400
trimethaphan camsylate (Arfonad)	J0400
trimethobenzamide HCl (Tigan), injection	J3250
U	
unclassified drugs (contraceptives)	J3490
underarm crutches, wood	E0112
unipuncture control system, dialysis	E1580
urea (Ureaphil), injection	J3350
urinary drainage bag	A4357
urinary leg bag	A4358
urine control strips or tablets	A4250
urine sensitivity study	P7001

Table 2. HCPCS Alphanumeric Index—cont'd

Description	Code
V	
vancomycin HCl (Vancocin), injection	J3370
vaporizer	E0605
vascular catheters	A4300
venous pressure clamps, dialysis	A4918
ventilator, volume	E0450
vest, safety, wheelchair	E0980
vinblastine sulfate, injection	J9360
vinblastine sulfate (Velban), injection	J9360
vitamin B12, injection	J3420
vitamin K, injection	J3430
volume ventilator, stationary or portable	E0450
W	
walker, wheeled, without seat	E0141
walker attachments, platform	E0154
warfarin sodium (Coumadin), injection—unclassified	J3490
washed red blood cells, each unit	P9022
water softening system, ESRD	E1625
wearable artificial kidney (WAK), each	E1632
wheelchair, Heavy duty with detachable arms	E1280
Y	
youth wheelchair	E1091

C ICD-10-PCS Section 0 Medical and Surgical, Character 3, Operation Definitions*

Alteration
Definition: Modifying the anatomic structure of a body part without affecting the function of the body part
Explanation: Principal purpose is to improve appearance
Includes/Examples: Face lift, breast augmentation

Bypass
Definition: Altering the route of passage of the contents of a tubular body part
Explanation: Rerouting contents of a body part to a downstream area of the normal route, to a similar route and body part, or to an abnormal route and dissimilar body part. Includes one or more anastomoses, with or without the use of a device.
Includes/Examples: Coronary artery bypass, colostomy formation

Change
Definition: Taking out or off a device from a body part and putting back an identical or similar device in or on the same body part without cutting or puncturing the skin or a mucous membrane
Explanation: All CHANGE procedures are coded using the approach EXTERNAL.
Includes/Examples: Urinary catheter change, gastrostomy tube change

Control
Definition: Stopping, or attempting to stop, postprocedural bleeding
Explanation: The site of the bleeding is coded as an anatomic region and not to a specific body part.
Includes/Examples: Control of post-prostatectomy hemorrhage, control of post-tonsillectomy hemorrhage

Creation
Definition: Making a new genital structure that does not take over the function of a body part
Explanation: Used only for sex change operations
Includes/Examples: Creation of vagina in a male, creation of penis in a female

Destruction
Definition: Physical eradication of all or a portion of a body part by the direct use of energy, force, or a destructive agent
Explanation: None of the body part is physically taken out.
Includes/Examples: Fulguration of rectal polyp, cautery of skin lesion

Detachment
Definition: Cutting off all or a portion of the upper or lower extremities
Explanation: The body part value is the site of the detachment, with a qualifier if applicable to further specify the level where the extremity was detached.
Includes/Examples: Below-the-knee amputation, disarticulation of shoulder

Dilation
Definition: Expanding an orifice or the lumen of a tubular body part
Explanation: The orifice can be a natural orifice or an artificially created orifice. Accomplished by stretching a tubular body part using intraluminal pressure or by cutting part of the orifice or wall of the tubular body part.
Includes/Examples: Percutaneous transluminal angioplasty, pyloromyotomy

Division
Definition: Cutting into a body part, without draining fluids and/or gases from the body part, in order to separate or transect a body part
Explanation: All or a portion of the body part is separated into two or more portions.
Includes/Examples: Spinal cordotomy, osteotomy

Drainage
Definition: Taking or letting out fluids and/or gases from a body part
Explanation: The qualifier DIAGNOSTIC is used to identify drainage procedures that are biopsies.
Includes/Examples: Thoracentesis, incision and drainage

Excision
Definition: Cutting out or off, without replacement, a portion of a body part
Explanation: The qualifier DIAGNOSTIC is used to identify excision procedures that are biopsies.
Includes/Examples: Partial nephrectomy, liver biopsy

Extirpation
Definition: Taking or cutting out solid matter from a body part
Explanation: The solid matter may be an abnormal by-product of a biologic function or a foreign body; it may be embedded in a body part or in the lumen of a tubular body part. The solid matter may or may not have been previously broken into pieces.
Includes/Examples: Thrombectomy, choledocholithotomy

*Centers for Medicare and Medicaid Services. *ICD-10 Procedure Coding System (ICD-10-PCS) 2013 Tables and Index*. Washington DC, 2013.

Extraction — **Definition:** Pulling or stripping out or off all or a portion of a body part by the use of force
Explanation: The qualifier DIAGNOSTIC is used to identify extraction procedures that are biopsies.
Includes/Examples: Dilation and curettage, vein stripping

Fragmentation — **Definition:** Breaking solid matter in a body part into pieces
Explanation: Physical force (e.g., manual, ultrasonic) applied directly or indirectly is used to break the solid matter into pieces. The solid matter may be an abnormal by-product of a biologic function or a foreign body. The pieces of solid matter are not taken out.
Includes/Examples: Extracorporeal shockwave lithotripsy, transurethral lithotripsy

Fusion — **Definition:** Joining together portions of an articular body part rendering the articular body part immobile
Explanation: The body part is joined together by fixation device, bone graft, or other means.
Includes/Examples: Spinal fusion, ankle arthrodesis

Insertion — **Definition:** Putting in a nonbiologic appliance that monitors, assists, performs, or prevents a physiologic function but does not physically take the place of a body part
Explanation: A device is put into a body part.
Includes/Examples: Insertion of radioactive implant, insertion of central venous catheter

Inspection — **Definition:** Visually and/or manually exploring a body part
Explanation: Visual exploration may be performed with or without optical instrumentation. Manual exploration may be performed directly or through intervening body layers.
Includes/Examples: Diagnostic arthroscopy, exploratory laparotomy

Map — **Definition:** Locating the route of passage of electrical impulses and/or locating functional areas in a body part
Explanation: Applicable only to the cardiac conduction mechanism and the central nervous system
Includes/Examples: Cardiac mapping, cortical mapping

Occlusion — **Definition:** Completely closing an orifice or the lumen of a tubular body part
Explanation: The orifice can be a natural orifice or an artificially created orifice.
Includes/Examples: Fallopian tube ligation, ligation of inferior vena cava

Reattachment — **Definition:** Putting back in or on all or a portion of a separated body part to its normal location or other suitable location
Explanation: Vascular circulation and nervous pathways may or may not be reestablished.
Includes/Examples: Reattachment of hand, reattachment of avulsed kidney

Release — **Definition:** Freeing a body part from an abnormal physical constraint by cutting or by the use of force
Explanation: Some of the restraining tissue may be taken out but none of the body part is taken out.
Includes/Examples: Adhesiolysis, carpal tunnel release

Removal — **Definition:** Taking out or off a device from a body part
Explanation: If a device is taken out and a similar device put in without cutting or puncturing the skin or mucous membrane, the procedure is coded to the root operation CHANGE. Otherwise, the procedure for taking out a device is coded to the root operation REMOVAL.
Includes/Examples: Drainage tube removal, cardiac pacemaker removal

Repair — **Definition:** Restoring, to the extent possible, a body part to its normal anatomic structure and function
Explanation: Used only when the method to accomplish the repair is not one of the other root operations
Includes/Examples: Colostomy takedown, suture of laceration

Replacement — **Definition:** Putting in or on biologic or synthetic material that physically takes the place and/or function of all or a portion of a body part
Explanation: The body part may have been taken out or replaced, or it may be taken out, physically eradicated, or rendered nonfunctional during the Replacement procedure. A Removal procedure is coded for taking out the device used in a previous replacement procedure.
Includes/Examples: Total hip replacement, bone graft, free skin graft

Reposition — **Definition:** Moving to its normal location, or other suitable location, all or a portion of a body part
Explanation: The body part is moved to a new location from an abnormal location, or from a normal location where it is not functioning correctly. The body part may or may not be cut out or off to be moved to the new location.
Includes/Examples: Reposition of undescended testicle, fracture reduction

Resection — **Definition:** Cutting out or off, without replacement, all of a body part
Explanation: To remove part or all of an organ or tissue.
Includes/Examples: Total nephrectomy, total lobectomy of lung

Restriction — **Definition:** Partially closing an orifice or the lumen of a tubular body part
Explanation: The orifice can be a natural orifice or an artificially created orifice.
Includes/Examples: Esophagogastric fundoplication, cervical cerclage

Revision **Definition:** Correcting, to the extent possible, a portion of a malfunctioning device or the position of a displaced device

Explanation: Revision can include correcting a malfunctioning or displaced device by taking out or putting in components of the device such as a screw or pin.

Includes/Examples: Adjustment of position of pacemaker lead, recementing of hip prosthesis

Supplement **Definition:** Putting in or on biologic or synthetic material that physically reinforces and/or augments the function of a portion of a body part

Explanation: The biologic material is nonliving, or is living and from the same individual. The body part may have been previously replaced, and the Supplement procedure is performed to physically reinforce and/or augment the function of the replaced body part.

Includes/Examples: Herniorrhaphy using mesh, free nerve graft, mitral valve ring annuloplasty, put a new acetabular liner in a previous hip replacement

Transfer **Definition:** Moving, without taking out, all or a portion of a body part to another location to take over the function of all or a portion of a body part

Explanation: The body part transferred remains connected to its vascular and nervous supply.

Includes/Examples: Tendon transfer, skin pedicle flap transfer

Transplantation **Definition:** Putting in or on all or a portion of a living body part taken from another individual or animal to physically take the place and/or function of all or a portion of a similar body part

Explanation: The native body part may or may not be taken out, and the transplanted body part may take over all or a portion of its function.

Includes/Examples: Kidney transplant, heart transplant

D ICD-10-PCS Section 0 Medical and Surgical, Character 5, Approach Definitions*

External	**Definition:** Procedures performed directly on the skin or mucous membrane and procedures performed indirectly by the application of external force through the skin or mucous membrane
Open	**Definition:** Cutting through the skin or mucous membrane and any other body layers necessary to expose the site of the procedure
Percutaneous	**Definition:** Entry, by puncture or minor incision, of instrumentation through the skin or mucous membrane and any other body layers necessary to reach the site of the procedure
Percutaneous Endoscopic	**Definition:** Entry, by puncture or minor incision, of instrumentation through the skin or mucous membrane and any other body layers necessary to reach and visualize the site of the procedure
Via Natural or Artificial Opening	**Definition:** Entry of instrumentation through a natural or artificial external opening to reach the site of the procedure
Via Natural or Artificial Opening Endoscopic	**Definition:** Entry of instrumentation through a natural or artificial external opening to reach and visualize the site of the procedure
Via Natural or Artificial Opening With Percutaneous Endoscopic Assistance	**Definition:** Entry of instrument through a natural or artificial external opening and entry, by puncture or minor incision, of instrumentation through the skin or mucous membrane and any other body layers necessary to aid in the performance of the procedure

*Centers for Medicare and Medicaid Services. *ICD-10 Procedure Coding System (ICD-10-PCS) 2013 Tables and Index*. Washington DC, 2013.